THE ROUTLEDGE HANDBOOK OF DISABILITY IN SOUTHERN AFRICA

This comprehensive ground-breaking southern African-centred collection spans the breadth of disability research and practice. Reputable and emerging scholars, together with disability advocates, adopt a critical and interdisciplinary stance to prove, challenge and shift commonly held social understanding of disability in traditional discourses, frontiers and practices in prominent areas such as inter/national development, disability studies, education, culture, health, religion, gender, sports, tourism, ICT, theatre, media, housing and legislation.

This handbook provides a body of interdisciplinary analyses suitable for the development of disability studies in southern Africa. Through drawing upon and introducing resources from several disciplines, theoretical perspectives and personal narratives from disability activists, it reflects on disability and sustainable development in southern Africa. It also addresses a clear need to bring together interdisciplinary perspectives and narratives on disability and sustainable development in ways that do not undermine disability politics advanced by disabled people across the world. The handbook further acknowledges and builds upon the huge body of literature that understands the social, cultural, educational, psychological, economic, historical and political facets of the exclusion of disabled people.

The handbook covers the following broad themes:

- Disability inclusion, ICT and sustainable development
- Access to education, from early childhood development up to higher education
- Disability, employment, entrepreneurship and community-based rehabilitation
- Religion, gender and parenthood
- Tourism, sports and accessibility
- Compelling narratives from disability activists on societal attitudes toward disability, media advocacy, accessible housing and social exclusion.

Thus, this much-awaited handbook provides students, academics, practitioners, development partners, policy makers and activists with an authoritative framework for critical thinking and debates that inform policy and practice in incomparable ways, with the view to promoting inclusive and sustainable development.

Tsitsi Chataika is the editor of this handbook and also a senior lecturer in inclusive education in the Department of Educational Foundations, University of Zimbabwe. She is an ardent supporter of disability rights. Chataika's research interests allow her to understand how disability intersects with education, gender, religion, childhood studies, poverty, policy, development and postcolonial theory. Her goal is to promote inclusive sustainable development, hence influencing policy and practice. She conducts disability awareness and mainstreaming workshops in various African countries. Chataika has presented at various national and international platforms and she has also published widely in her areas of research interests.

THE ROUTLEDGE
HANDBOOK OF DISABILITY
IN SOUTHERN AFRICA

Edited by Tsitsi Chataika

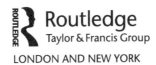

LONDON AND NEW YORK

First published 2019
by Routledge
2 Park Square, Milton Park, Abingdon, Oxon OX14 4RN

and by Routledge
52 Vanderbilt Avenue, New York, NY 10017

First issued in paperback 2020

Routledge is an imprint of the Taylor & Francis Group, an informa business

British Library Cataloguing in Publication Data
A catalogue record for this book is available from the British Library

Library of Congress Cataloging in Publication Data
A catalog record for this book has been requested

ISBN 13: 978-0-367-58059-9 (pbk)
ISBN 13: 978-1-138-24233-3 (hbk)

Typeset in Bembo
by Swales & Willis Ltd, Exeter, Devon, UK

This book is dedicated to all the efforts of the disability activists and their allies, who ensured that the African Disability Protocol was endorsed by 30 African leaders in Addis Ababa in January 2018 and all the disabled people and their allies across southern Africa.

CONTENTS

FIGURES

TABLES

CONTRIBUTORS

Gloria Azalde is a researcher at SINTEF Technology and Society, Norway. She has a background in public health and experience in research projects concerning global health, as well as expertise in coordinating EU-funded research projects. Azalde's research interests include poverty, disability, policy and participation from a public health perspective. She has broad international experience from several African countries, including Malawi and Zambia, as well as countries in South America and Europe.

Sarah Banda is a Senior Social Welfare Officer working for the Zambian Government in the Ministry of Community Development and Social Services. She is a Social Worker and Child and Adolescent Psychologist by profession. She has worked for the government for over ten years with a focus on child-related, disability, and ageing issues. She has participated in a number of researches, key ones being on child development and disability and was one of the coordinators for the 2015 Zambia National Disability Survey.

Diane Bell is the Director of the Carel du Toit Trust. Previously, she worked as a member of the Global Cooperation on Assistive Technologies (GATE) team at the World Health Organization, aiming to make high-quality assistive products accessible and affordable, especially in low-income countries. She is the mother of a daughter born with a profound hearing impairment. Her PhD thesis focused on students with hearing impairment in higher education and she has authored several journal articles and a book chapter on disability and higher education. She also serves as a member of the South African Presidential Working Group on Disability.

John Charema is the Director of Mophato Education Centre in Botswana. He has authored two books and contributed ten chapters in edited books. He has presented papers at international conferences in different countries both in Europe and in Africa. Charema has authored many publications in special needs education, counselling, inclusive education, health and wellness and medicinal plants, which are his research interests. He is a consulting editor for different journals and has edited a number of articles. He is a member of the Board of Worldwide Disabilities, a PhD supervisor and a University External Examiner.

Tsitsi Chataika is the editor of this handbook and also a senior lecturer in inclusive education in the Department of Educational Foundations, University of Zimbabwe. She is an ardent supporter of disability rights. Chataika's research interests allow her to understand how disability intersects with education, gender, religion, childhood studies, poverty, policy, development and postcolonial theory. Her goal is to promote inclusive sustainable development, hence influencing policy and practice. She conducts disability awareness and mainstreaming workshops in various African countries. Chataika has presented at various national and international platforms and she has also published widely in her areas of research interests.

Lovemore Chidemo is the founder and Executive Director of Zimbabwe Deaf Media Trust. He teaches Sign Language at Great Zimbabwe University. He is also the producer of *Action Power*, the television show for the deaf on Zimbabwe Broadcasting Corporation Television. His research interests include disability and the media, disability arts, disability and entrepreneurship, and Sign Language.

Oliver Chikuta is the Dean of the School of Hospitality and Tourism at Chinhoyi University of Technology, Zimbabwe. He holds a PhD in Tourism Management (NWU-SA). His research areas include universal accessibility in the tourism sector, sustainable tourism and domestic tourism. He has published several articles in the above areas.

Agness Chindimba works with Deaf Women Included, a grassroots deaf women's organisation that she founded. She worked with deaf children as a teacher for more than ten years. She also teaches Sign Language at Great Zimbabwe University. Her research interests include disability and feminism, inclusive education, and deaf education.

Nehemiah Chivandikwa is a full-time senior lecturer at the University of Zimbabwe. He teaches theatre and development communication and playmaking. His research interests are in performance and body politics, gender, disability, applied theatre performances and media. He has published several articles in both regional and international journals in these areas. Chivandikwa has been involved in several projects in applied theatre on gender, political violence, disability and rural and urban development.

Helen Dunbar-Krige is a senior lecturer in the Department of Educational Psychology at the University of Johannesburg on the Soweto Campus. She is involved in the postgraduate professional training of Masters students in Educational Psychology and Honours students as counsellors working in schools. Her main research interests are service learning, professional ethics and social justice for inclusion.

Arne H. Eide is the Chief Scientist at SINTEF Technology and Society, Norway, Professor at the Norwegian University for Science and Technology and Guest Professor at Stellenbosch University, South Africa. He has 20 years of experience in research on disability and poverty, community-based rehabilitation and studies on living conditions in low-income countries. Eide has been engaged by the World Health Organization and the United Nations as an expert on disability statistics, disability and development and on the provision of assistive technology. He has published widely and has contributed to the *World Report on Disability* (WHO and World Bank 2011) as well as the *2012 Education for All Global Monitoring Report* (UNESCO).

Anthony G. Giannoumis is currently an associate professor of universal design at the Department of Computer Science at Oslo and Akershus University College. He is also an international research fellow at the Burton Blatt Institute at Syracuse University. Anthony's research focuses on technology law and policy. Giannoumis is currently researching the implementation of policies aimed at ensuring equal access to technology. His research interests include universal design, international governance, sustainable development, social regulation, and standardisation, and he has also conducted research on assistive technology and intellectual property.

Megan Giljam is Clinical Strategic Lead at Shonaquip Social Enterprise. Her role is to guide and support the team of occupational and physiotherapists as they provide holistic and sustainable seating services, support and training across southern Africa. Informed by her experience working in rural Eastern Cape and now her work at Shonaquip, her interests are in the impact of the appropriate wheelchair as well as holistic, community-based support services on the inclusion and participation for persons with disabilities.

Sitshengisiwe Gweme is a specialist teacher for children with intellectual impairment at Nechibondo Primary School in Hwange, Zimbabwe. She is an emerging writer who has interest in researching on intellectual impairment, inclusive education and the special class model. She believes that the special class model appears complex to most mainstream teachers in Zimbabwe, and needs further research in order to ensure that learners benefit from this model.

Tanya Healey is currently employed by the University of the Witwatersrand in the Academic Planning Office. She managed the disability programme of the Foundation of Tertiary Institutions of the Northern Metropolis from 2007 to 2011. Projects included a national investigation into the status of disability in higher education and an exploration of librarians' support to students with disabilities. Healey's research interest is on higher education students with learning difficulties and she is passionate about disability issues.

Johan van Heerden is a Professor in Human Movement/Sport Scientist. He has been an academic for over 23 years and has authored/co-authored 43 scientific publications and presented at 16 international conferences. Since joining the University of KwaZulu-Natal, he has served as the Head of the School for Physiotherapy, Sport Science and Optometry and is currently the Academic Leader for Research and Chair of the Research Ethics in the Higher Degrees Committee in the School of Health Science. He is a member of the Education Committee for the Board for Physiotherapy, Biokinetics and Podiatry on the Health Professions Council of South Africa.

Rebecca Irvine is a research fellow and coordinator of the Conflict, Terrorism, and Development Collaboratory at Michigan State University. She also maintains strong links with Queen's University Belfast, where she was a founding member of the Disability Research Network. She holds a BA in International Relations (Michigan State University), an MA in Comparative Ethnic Conflict and a PhD in Social Policy (both from Queen's University Belfast). Irvine regularly works on issues related to public policy and the participation of people with disabilities in political and public life. You can find her on Twitter @rshea_irvine.

Forbes Kabote is a research assistant at the Chinhoyi University of Technology, Zimbabwe in the School of Hospitality and Tourism. Forbes has more than 14 years experience in the hospitality and tourism industry holding various posts, including hotel manager, tourism and hospitality degree coordinator, lecturer, teaching assistant and research assistant. His research interests are in domestic tourism, sustainable tourism development and tourism economics where he has published a number of journal articles.

Rachel K. Kachaje has over 25 years of experience in advocating for disability rights in Malawi and globally. She has a strong track record of performance with success as a turn-around expert with a talent for leading teams and regional bodies. Rachel is a creative visionary with exceptional ability to communicate and motivate. She has proven ability in advancing the agendas of disabled people, identifying needs for change and resolving problems. She is the former Malawian Minister for Persons with Disability and Elderly Affairs, Chairperson for Disabled Peoples International and Founder/Executive Director for Disabled Women in Africa.

Bhekuzulu Khumalo recently graduated with a PhD in Sports Science at the University of KwaZulu-Natal in Durban, South Africa; studying Wheelchair Basketball. He is a Sports Science and Coaching lecturer at the National University of Science and Technology in Bulawayo, Zimbabwe. Khumalo's main areas of teaching and researching are theory and methodology of coaching, sports administration and track and field athletics. He has been engaged in sports education for the International Association of Athletics Federations, Sports Recreation Commission (Zimbabwe), and Zimbabwe's National Paralympic Committee since the late 1990s.

Mari Koistinen has worked in the field of Disability and Development in various roles for more than 20 years in several countries. Currently, she works at the Disability Partnership Finland as a Programme Advisor. In this position, she has worked on disability mainstreaming in countries such as Burundi, Kenya, Ivory Coast, Malawi and Mozambique. She also recently edited a book called *Development for All: Experiences on disability mainstreaming in the development sector* (Disability Partnership Finland 2017), in which several non-governmental organisations reflect on their experiences with disability mainstreaming. Her research interests include social exclusion, inclusion in education and participatory research methods.

Elina Lehtomäki holds the chair of global education at the University of Oulu, Finland. She has worked in several African countries and continues collaborating with colleagues, researchers and disability rights activists. Her research focuses on social meaning of education, equity and inclusion in and through education, cross-cultural collaboration and internationalisation in higher education. Lehtomäki has been the principal investigator of the research project 'Educated Girls and Women: Socio-cultural meaning of education in Tanzania' funded by the Academy of Finland. Other projects include 'Global Responsibility' and 'Equity in International Student Mobility in Nordic Higher Education'.

Margaret Linegar has, for the past ten years, applied her experience as both clinical occupational therapist and educator to support the monitoring and evaluation, research and training activities of Shonaquip Social Enterprise in South Africa. Shonaquip strives to reduce the medical and community barriers that prevent children with mobility challenges from achieving full participation in all spheres of life. Linegar shares the organisation's vision to build an inclusive society using a rights-based and networked approach. In alignment with this vision, she helps to build the capabilities and resources of our outreach teams, and to provide inputs into policy affecting children with mobility limitations and other impairments.

Francis Machingura is an Associate Professor in Biblical Studies at the University of Zimbabwe, Faculty of Education, Curriculum and Arts Education Department, which he is currently chairing. His areas of special interest are on interaction of the Bible and gender, politics, health, inclusivity, sexuality, music and Pentecostal Christianity in Africa.

Messiah R. Makuane has 20 years' experience working in the disability and rehabilitation field. She holds a Masters of Rehabilitation Counselling and Bachelor of Health Science (University of Sydney, Australia) and Diploma in Social Youth Work (Mindolo Ecumenical Foundation, Zambia). Makuane's major research interest is community oriented, focusing on inclusion and participation in livelihoods for people with disabilities. She is also interested in identification/interventions for people with disabilities, school and job placement, return to work programmes, counselling and community work. She has extensively dealt with public awareness strategies development, empowerment, advocacy, wellness programmes for people with disabilities and their care givers.

Jacob R. S. Malungo is the first Zambian Professor of Demography with the University of Zambia. He is the Deputy Vice-Chancellor at Rusangu University. Malungo has conducted 60 baseline, midline, process, endline evaluative and policy and programme-oriented studies, censuses and Millennium Development Goals with the United Nations, World Bank, USAID, Zambian Government, ChildFund and Care International and other agencies. He has presented 220 scientific papers in more than 30 publications. Malungo has also been departmental head, dean, director, executive secretary, president (board chair), board member of the National Institute of Allergy and Infectious Diseases in the United States of America.

Jorge Manhique is the Programme Officer for Africa for the Disability Rights Fund and the Disability Rights Advocacy Fund. He is responsible for grant making, grants oversight and technical support to disabled persons' organisations in Malawi and Rwanda. Jorge has over six years of experience working with persons with disabilities in Mozambique. He served as the project manager at the Forum of Mozambican Association of Disabled People (FAMOD). Manhique established the first monitoring unit within FAMOD, with the mandate to advocate for law reform in critical areas, such as education, health, accessibility and mental health.

France Maphosa is an Associate Professor of Sociology and Anthropology at the University of Botswana. His research interests include the sociology of organisations, participation, disability, rural livelihoods, labour studies and alternative dispute resolution. He has been awarded several research grants including the ORREA Senior Scholars Research Grant, CODESRIA Advanced Research Fellowship Grant and the CODESRIA National Working Group Research Grant. He has more than 15 years' experience of university teaching. He has taught at both undergraduate and graduate levels and successfully supervised many PhD theses and several Masters' dissertations.

Edmore Masendeke holds an Honours degree in Business Studies from the University of Zimbabwe, a Master of Arts degree in Leadership and Management from the Africa Leadership and a Master of Law degree in International and European Human Rights Law at the University of Leeds in the UK. In 2010, Masendeke founded Endless Possibilities, an organisation that empowers disabled people and advocates for their rights. In 2015, he participated in an Open Society Foundation-sponsored research internship at the University of Pretoria in South Africa. He researched on the implementation of Article 19 of the Convention on the Rights of Persons with Disabilities in South Africa.

Abraham Mateta is a lawyer by training and a disability rights activist by calling. He holds, among other qualifications, a Bachelor of Law from the University of Zimbabwe and a Masters in International and European Human Rights from the University of Leeds. Mateta has worked in government and the civic society and currently he is in private practice. He works with various organisations engaging in disability. Mateta is currently the Secretary for the Lawyers with Disabilities Association Zimbabwe Trust, which seeks to advance the rights of disabled lawyers and the rights of all disabled people to get access to justice.

Lincoln Matongo is the Programmes Director at Zimbabwe Deaf Media Trust. Previously, Matongo taught deaf children for more than ten years. He is a Sign Language trainer with Zimbabwe Open University. He was one of the coordinators in the development of the Zimbabwe Sign Language dictionary and is the Director on *Action Power*. His research interests include deafness and Sign Language, including its variations.

Magreth Matonya is employed as a lecturer at the University of Dar es Salaam. She completed her Master's degree in Education at the University of Dar es Salaam in 2008. In 2017, she was awarded a PhD in Education from the University of Jyväskylä, Finland. Her research was on disability, gender and inclusive higher education. She was involved in the research project 'Educated Girls and Women in Tanzania: Social Cultural Interpretations of the Meaning of Education', funded by the Academy of Finland.

Knowledge R. Matshedisho is a senior lecturer in the Department of Sociology at the University of the Witwatersrand in South Africa. He researches on disability in higher education, diversity in public urban spaces and, lately, scholarships of learning and teaching. He has published in several journals.

Shona McDonald is the founder and chief executive officer of Uhambo-Shonaquip, a social enterprise inspired by her daughter, Shelly, who was born with cerebral palsy. Her family experienced first-hand how difficult it was to find information, accessible affordable support services and appropriate assistive devices and understood that the right wheelchair was far more than just a means of transport, but an assistive device which, if correctly assessed, prescribed, fitted and reviewed, would ensure that the users does not develop life threatening secondary complications. She strives to ensure that wheelchairs are appropriately provided for each individual and the environment in which they are used while ensuring excellent support services and training that improve the user's function, opportunities for inclusion, independence, health and dignity.

Elias Mpofu is a Professor of Rehabilitation and Health Services Research at the University of North Texas. He also is Affiliate Professor of Rehabilitation and Health Sciences at the University of Sydney and the University of Wisconsin-Madison. Mpofu is a distinguished Visiting Professor of Educational Psychology and Inclusive Education at the University of Johannesburg in South Africa. His major area of research focus is on community-oriented health care, applying the World Health Organization's International Classification of Functioning, Disability and Health.

Chibesa Musamba is a senior statistician in the Department of Population and Demography, Central Statistical Office. He is also one of the co-Principal Investigators on the Zambia National Disability Survey and a number of other surveys conducted by the CSO such as the Zambia Demographic and Health Survey and the Zambia Population based HIV Impact Assessment.

His areas of interest include the demographics associated with disability and how to measure disability more accurately by using the W-6 questions and Child module.

Martin Musengi is an Associate Professor of Special Needs Education at Great Zimbabwe University, where he is the chairperson of the Jairos Jiri Centre for Special Needs Education. He taught in a special school for the deaf for 15 years before becoming a specialist teacher-educator initially in a teachers' college. Musengi has been teaching at the Great Zimbabwe University for the past 13 years. He has published numerous empirical studies and book chapters on deaf education.

Phillipa C. Mutswanga is a senior lecturer at the Zimbabwe Open University. Previously, she worked as Education Officer, school head and special needs teacher. Her research interest is in deaf education. She is also interested in art, developing new courses responding to contemporary issues, talking to youths and the aged. Mutswanga has authored and co-authored 38 publications, 18 modules and she was a consultant in three projects.

Joanne Neille is employed in the Speech Therapy Department at the University of Witwatersrand, Johannesburg in South Africa. She completed her PhD in 2013 for which she explored the lived experiences of adults with disabilities in rural areas. Joanne is passionate about disability studies, with a focus on promoting equitable and accessible services for all. Joanne has published a number of articles and book chapters in the field of disability studies.

Nchimunya Nkombo is a Principal Statistician in the Central Statistical Office of Zambia. A demographer by profession, Nkombo also holds a Master's degree in Population and Development. She is in charge of the Population and Demography branch. Having worked for about 22 years in the statistical office, she has been a manager of several national data generation initiatives including the 2010 Census of Population and Housing and the Demographic and Health surveys. She coordinated the 2015 National Disability Survey for Zambia funded by UNICEF with technical assistance from SINTEF Technology of Science.

Kayi Ntinda is a Senior Lecturer of Educational Counselling and Mixed-methods Inquiry Approaches at the University of Swaziland. Her research interests are in assessment, learner support services, inclusive education and social justice research among vulnerable populations. She is a former International Union of Psychological Science Advanced Research Training Seminars awardee (2012), International Society for the Study of Behaviourial Development conference scholar (2010) and the Australian Leadership Fellowship Awardee (2011). Ntinda has authored and co-authored several research articles and book chapters addressing assessment, inclusive education and counselling practices in diverse contexts.

Barbra Nyangairi is the Executive Director of Deaf Zimbabwe Trust, a research and advocacy think tank on deaf issues in Zimbabwe. She is interested in disability education with a focus on deaf people, elections, gender, women and politics among others. She has researched on deaf issues and access to information, Sign Language variations and deaf education. Her research interests are education, democracy, election, disability and political participation.

Mari-Anne Okkolin works as a senior lecturer at the Department of Education, University of Jyväskylä, Finland, and post-doctoral fellow at the Institute for Reconciliation and Social Justice, University of the Free State, South Africa. She is a sociologist and educationalist whose research interests focus on sociology of education, gender and development, teacher education and the teaching profession, human capabilities, and qualitative research methodology. Her recent publications include the book *Education, Gender and Development: A Capabilities Perspective* (Routledge 2016) and the book chapter 'Well-being and agency freedoms to construct and decide upon one's educational career: Narratives from Tanzania and South-Africa' (with B. Ramamoorthi).

Ravi Paul is the Head of the Department of Psychiatry at the University of Zambia. He pioneered the MMed Psychiatry programme in Zambia. He is also a consultant psychiatrist at the University Teaching Hospital in Lusaka, Zambia. Paul started the Child and Adolescent Psychiatry Unit, Cognitive Behaviour and ART Therapy units and the Addictions Unit at the University Teaching Hospital. His areas of interest include child and adolescent psychiatry with special interest in learning disabilities, HIV and neurocognitive functioning, HIV and psychiatric co-morbidities, HIV and secondary mania, epilepsy and paroxysmal non-epileptic seizures, alcohol dependence and brief relapse prevention, HIV and postnatal depression.

Christine Peta is a public healthcare practitioner who holds a PhD in Disability Studies. Her research interests are in the intersections of disability with sexuality, maternal and child health, mental health, human rights, livelihoods and education. Christine Peta has authored a number of publications in scientific journals and has written a book entitled *Disability and Sexuality: Voices from the Periphery* (Routledge 2017). She is currently based at Ukwanda Rural Clinical School in South Africa, under the Centre for Rehabilitation Studies, Division of Global Health, Faculty of Medicine and Health Sciences, Stellenbosch University.

Anlia Pretorius is a registered counselling psychologist and is currently the Head of the University of the Witwatersrand Disability Rights Unit in South Africa. Pretorius previously worked at the University of Johannesburg as a psychologist where she started the Office for People with Disabilities, and is also one of the founding members of Higher Education Disability Services Association. She serves on advisory bodies advising on policy formulation, including as Chair of the Ministerial Committee to Develop a Disability Policy Framework for the Post School Environment in South Africa. Pretorius is the author and co-author of research papers in the field of disability and student support, which is her research interest.

Tafadzwa Rugoho is a part-time lecturer at Great Zimbabwe University and a doctoral candidate with University of KwaZulu-Natal where he is specialising in participation of persons with disabilities in empowerment initiatives in Zimbabwe. He holds an MSc in Development Studies and MSc Strategic Management. He has vast experience in disability issues, having worked in the field for more than ten years. He has authored a number of scientific journal papers and two book chapters. Rugoho is a disability activist.

Nkhasi Sefuthi is an Advocate of the Courts of Lesotho and is currently working as the Executive Director of the Lesotho National Federation of Organisations of the Disabled. The mandate of his organisation is to advocate for the inclusive laws and policies through domestication of the United Nations Convention on the Rights of Persons with Disabilities. His research interests include access to justice for persons with disabilities and universal design, with the intention of breaking down barriers faced by people with disabilities. Sefuthi is a football fan and he is also fond of reading historical books.

Masekara Sekoankoetla is an advocacy and human rights officer at Lesotho National Federation of Organisations of the Disabled. She holds an LLM in Human Rights and Democratization in Africa from the Centre for Human Rights, University of Pretoria and an LLB from the National University of Lesotho. She is also an advocate of the High Court of Lesotho. Her research interests include human rights of marginalised groups and development. Sekoankoetla is also interested in international, regional and national conflict resolution and humanitarian laws.

Irene Sithole is an independent consultant and researcher. She is a qualified lawyer and gender specialist with extensive experience in capacity development, advocacy work and gender programming in the development sector. She is also a founding member and former chairperson of Zimbabwe Blind Women Trust, an organisation established to advance the rights of visually impaired women. Her greatest passion is to use her qualifications, personal and professional experiences in contributing meaningfully in the uplifting of lives of vulnerable groups in Zimbabwe, Africa and globally.

Thomas Skalko is a Professor Emeritus of Recreational Therapy at the East Carolina University and Honorary Professor at the College of Health Sciences, University of KwaZulu-Natal. Skalko has been engaged in Recreational Therapy service delivery, teaching and research since 1974, with roles in healthcare and human service delivery including: Advisor for Wheelchair Basketball, Director of Recreational Therapy and Director of Child Life Services, Walter Reed Army Medical Center. Skalko is a founding member and past president of the American Therapeutic Recreation Association (ATRA). He has also chaired the ATRA World Health Organization – International Classification of Functioning, Disability and Health Committee.

Veronica I. Umeasiegbu is an assistant professor at the University of Texas Rio Grande Valley, USA. She has an MSc in Physiotherapy from the University of Nigeria and an MSc in Rehabilitation Counselling from the University of Pittsburgh, USA. She obtained her PhD in Rehabilitation Counselling Education, Research and Policy in 2013 from the University of Kentucky, USA. In 2008, she served as an intern with the World Health Organization. Her research interests include health disparities and disability, social determinants of health and disability, community participation in disability and chronic illness, self-advocacy and spinal cord injury, and health outcomes research.

Ronique Walters is a physiotherapist working in the field of wheelchair and assistive device service provision at Shonaquip. Since Shonaquip and the Uhambo Foundation, together, are a social enterprise working toward building an inclusive society for persons with disabilities in South Africa, her work extends to train parents, caregivers, social workers and other therapists. Training programmes form part of sustainable community development projects that are delivered at community level. The mobile outreach seating clinics provide parent training – on the importance of appropriate wheelchair prescription; and positioning. In this capacity, she provides improved wheelchair service delivery to persons with disabilities and their families.

ACKNOWLEDGEMENTS

The writing of a handbook of this magnitude is never an individual effort. Its final production represents months (and years) of sharing and collaborations. This handbook is a collective effort that emerged out of several critical moments and dialogue held by fellow academics, disability activists, family and friends.

I am indebted to various communities who are presented in this volume (especially emerging writers), who allowed me to be with them, travel with them, learn with them, listen to them and write with them; and at times 'cry with them'. Sincere thanks are conveyed to all the contributors, who were generous enough to endure deadlines and push the boundaries of their own practice. I am also very much indebted to all the blind reviewers of all the chapters who executed a sterling job and they are too many to mention. They made this handbook what it is today.

To the publishers, I am especially thankful for the guidance and support along the way and I will be forever grateful for giving me the opportunity to publish this edited collection. I specifically extend my gratitude to Georgia Priestley (editorial assistant) for guiding and supporting me throughout in keeping the entire project together. She endured with me personal and family challenges that I went through during the production of this handbook.

While writing and editing this book, my family and friends have been supportive. They were my cheer leaders and prayer warriors. Their encouragement along the journey has been more than expected, especially Fortune Chataika (sonny!), who endured long periods of house chores during the period of putting this handbook together. For this, I extend my heartfelt and special thanks to you all. Above all, I thank God for giving me the strength when illnesses and deaths in the family tested my resilience. Despite all that, God directed me up to the end of this project.

PART I

Disability inclusion and sustainable development

Part I, with the introductory chapter, provides the overview of the handbook and what each chapter focuses on. It also maps out key conceptual, theoretical and disciplinary domains or spaces within the disability and development agenda. Thus, Part I focuses on issues of disability inclusion with implications for policy and practice and promoting inclusive sustainable development.

1

INTRODUCTION

Critical connections and gaps in disability and development

Tsitsi Chataika

Introduction

To produce this edited volume took several months of hard work. Although the process of drawing together the relevant authors working with different perspectives and approaches was strenuous, the worthwhile learning experience was profound to me. This edited book draws from a body of interdisciplinary analyses for development of disability studies using the southern African regional context. Thus, the handbook sets the southern Africa research agenda by redefining existing areas within the context of international multidisciplinary research, highlighting emerging areas and providing readers with guidance (and ideas) for policy and practice, and signposting areas for further research. This introductory chapter sets the scene and provides the structure of the handbook. Specifically, it emphasises the importance of inclusive sustainable development and how various authors bring together a wide range of diverse research evidence and personal southern African experiences.

Note on terminology

I am aware that definitions are powerful and words/statements we choose to use when making reference to disability issues play an essential part in the way we view people with various forms of impairments (Oliver & Barnes, 1998). Hence, the language used to describe impairments and the people who experience them is constantly evolving. It is almost impossible to always 'get it right' and avoid offence completely. Al Ju'beh (2015) argues that the language used to describe people with disabilities is important as it is about fundamental respect for their integrity and dignity. The use of 'people/persons with disabilities', is known as 'people first' language. It is based on the need 'to affirm and define the person first, before the impairment or disability' (Al Ju'beh, 2015, p. 25). This term is preferred in many low-income countries (including the southern African region) and the language used in the United Nations Convention on the Rights of Persons with Disabilities (CRPD) (Al Ju'beh, 2015; United Nations, 2006). Disability activists in the United Kingdom and in other parts of Africa prefer the term 'disabled people'. Their argument is that 'people do not have disabilities, but rather have impairments that interact with society that does not take into account the diverse needs of all people as a result of attitudinal, environmental and institutional barriers' (WHO & World Bank, 2011). Hence, persons with disabilities become

3

disabled due to society that is not comprehensively accessible and inclusive (Al Ju'beh, 2015). Therefore, in this handbook, the terms people/persons with disabilities and disabled people are used interchangeably. My understanding of disabled people or persons/people with disabilities is informed by the CRPD definition:

> Persons with disabilities include those who have long-term physical, mental, intellectual or sensory impairments which in interaction with various barriers may hinder their full and effective participation in society on an equal basis with others.
>
> *(United Nations, 2006, p. 4)*

Setting the scene

Disability is both a cause and consequence of poverty, and poverty and disability reinforce each other, contributing to increased vulnerability and exclusion (Trani & Loeb, 2012). Nonetheless, the presence of impairment does not necessarily imply limited well-being and poverty. There is a growing body of evidence indicating that disabled people also face various forms of barriers and intersecting inequalities, which can result in multi-dimensional poverty, exclusion and marginalisation. Exclusion in one area of life can have negative repercussions in other areas (Groce, Kett, Lang & Trani, 2011; Mitra, Posarac & Vick, 2013).

In this book, I acknowledge that disability manifests itself through the interaction of individuals' impairments with attitudinal, environmental (physical and communication) and institutional (policy and practice) barriers imposed by society (Bruijn et al., 2012; Wapling & Downie, 2012; WHO & World Bank, 2011). Institutional barriers include many laws, policies, strategies or practices that discriminate against disabled people. Hence, the evidence makes it clear that these inequalities are a result of barriers, rather than any inherent limitations of people with disabilities (Groce & Kett, 2014; Bruijn et al., 2012; WHO & World Bank, 2011). This unfortunately has an adverse effect on nearly one billion disabled people in the world, with the majority of them, particularly in the global South, who struggle to access education, employment and health services (WHO & World Bank, 2011). They also constitute the largest population of the world's minority groups, yet discrimination, stigmatising and exclusion are common (*ibid.*). Over the past decade, some fundamental changes have begun to take place and, currently, disability is arguably the hottest, fastest-rising issue in international development. When the CRPD came into being (United Nations, 2006), State Parties that had ratified this legal instrument had the prerogative of realigning their national legislation and policies. Thus, most work on disability inclusion is framed around the CRPD.

People with disabilities are mentioned under five of the United Nations' 17 Sustainable Development Goals (SDGs): education (SDG4); growth and employment (8); inequality (10); accessibility of human settlements (11); and data collection and monitoring (17). Thus, as disability has moved up the development agenda, this edited text brings to light disability issues from southern Africa. It provides a body of interdisciplinary analyses suitable for the development of disability studies within the southern African region. Southern Africa encompasses countries in the Southern African Development Cooperation (SADC) region. The SADC region is comprised of 15 member countries, namely: Angola, Botswana, Democratic Republic of Congo (DRC), Lesotho, Madagascar, Malawi, Mauritius, Mozambique, Namibia, Seychelles, South Africa, Swaziland, United Republic of Tanzania, Zambia and Zimbabwe. It is in sub-Saharan Africa where 60% of the countries fall within the low human development support index on key dimensions of health and education (WHO & World Bank, 2011). This handbook, however, is informed by research evidence from eight SADC countries, although the contributors are from this region and beyond.

Through drawing upon and introducing resources from a number of disciplines, theoretical perspectives and personal narratives of disability activists, this handbook reflects on disability and sustainable development within the SADC region. It addresses a clear need to bring together interdisciplinary perspectives and narratives on disability and sustainable development in ways that do not undermine the disability politics advanced by disabled people. It also acknowledges and builds upon the huge body of literature that understands the social, cultural, educational, psychological, economic, historical and political facets of the exclusion of people with various forms of impairments.

There seems to be a dominance of disability studies texts from the global North when compared with those emerging from the global South. Hence, the deliberate effort of bringing the voices of emerging African disability activists such as Mateta (Chapter 26), Sefuthi and Sekoankoetla (Chapter 3), Masendeke (Chapter 25), Chidemo, Chindimba and Matongo (Chapter 24) into this volume. Such voices are hardly heard as disability studies literature is usually dominated by the usual 'suspects', who in most cases reside in the global North. While I acknowledge that there are various forms of physical, sensory, intellectual and neurological impairments, some of which are covered in this text, it is not the impairment, but the barriers in society, that limit people from reaching their full potential (Goodley, 2011; WHO & World Bank, 2011). The compelling contributions from emerging disabled activists in this text are clear testimony that, if they are given the opportunity, they can reach their full potential. Therefore, by creating this space for emerging disabled writers,

> the struggle is about challenging oppression, voicelessness, stereotyping, undermining, neo-colonisation, postcolonisation, 'them and us', and bridging the gap between the global North and global South spaces in the disability and development research agenda.
>
> *(Chataika, 2012, p. 252)*

At the same time, I am mindful of the contribution of seasoned disability studies writers, hence their inclusion. Also, the world has now turned into a global village, hence the presence of contributors from the global North working alongside those from African countries. Key to bridging this gap is to deliberately promote 'productive exchange and cross-fertilization' (Barker & Murray, 2010, p. 219) between the two spaces while, at the same time, addressing the inequalities and silent voices of emerging African disability activists that have not been traditionally contributing to the disability studies discourse.

The book is broadly split into seven parts, traversing conceptual, practice, personal experiences and cross-cutting research terrains. Introductions to these parts explain the importance and relevance of the chapters in the disability studies field. Thus, these snapshots are extraordinary opportunities to make general observations about the field and to stress, rank, order, or otherwise analyse various perspectives that are most important to understanding the subject matter at hand. While Chapter 1 provides the overview of the handbook, Chapters 2 to 27 are distinctive chapters, highlighting the cross-cutting themes, which when read together inform the importance of inclusive sustainable development. Finally, Chapter 28 brings the handbook to a conclusion by drawing lessons, best practices, challenges and opportunities tabled by various authors. It also reflects on how each chapter feeds into the sustainable development agenda and how the conclusions can inform policy and practice. The handbook is divided into the following parts.

Part I: Disability inclusion and sustainable development

Part I maps out key conceptual, theoretical and disciplinary domains or spaces within the disability and development agenda. It focuses on issues of disability inclusion with implications for policy and practice and promoting inclusive sustainable development. Chapter 1 is the scene-setting chapter and it provides the overview of the handbook and what each chapter focuses on.

Chapter 2, by Koistinen, reflects upon the experiences and practices based on the work of the Disability Partnership Finland (DPF) on disability mainstreaming since 2013, using case studies drawn mainly from Malawi and Mozambique. DPF is a non-governmental organisation with nine member disability organisations that has been working in the two countries. She argues that disabled people have been largely invisible in poverty-reduction programmes and in the development agenda. Consequently, continued neglect of disabled people by national governments and international development agencies remains one of the great gaps of national and international poverty-reduction efforts (Groce, 2011). She argues that disability is a development issue, despite being ignored in the international development agenda for a long period. It is from this context that she highlights some of the main issues that DPF have been found to be important in the process of disability mainstreaming. Finally, lessons learned for disability mainstreaming are discussed from the development practitioner's point of view so that no one is left behind in development processes.

In Chapter 3, Sefuthi and Sekoankoetla reflect on the development of the National Disability Mainstreaming Plan in Lesotho. They start by providing the country's situational analysis of disabled people before discussing the process of the development of the disability mainstreaming plan. The two disability activists outline how the Lesotho National Federation of Organisations of the Disabled (LNFOD) was involved in the development of the country's National Disability Mainstreaming Plan, which was adopted in 2015. They articulate what prompted the development of the plan, the level of participation of disabled people, challenges encountered and how the plan was adopted. They also discuss the challenges being currently faced as the country attempts to implement this plan in government policies, programmes and services, as well as how some of these challenges could be overcome. Sefuthi and Sekoankoetla conclude by sharing lessons learned during the development of the National Disability Mainstreaming Plan, a process that can also inform others who are contemplating developing such a plan.

In Chapter 4, Chivandikwa acknowledges and analyses the unrecognised (and private) resistive powers or 'hidden transcripts' (Scott, 1985, 1990) of young disabled people and how this power and agency can be nurtured and appropriated for transition into the public domain (resistive public transcript) in Theatre for Development (TfD) discourses. The 'hidden transcripts' are in sharp contrast to the feigned respect, obedience and docility of oppressed people (public transcripts), when they are in the presence of their dominators (Scott, 1990). He argues that the 'hidden transcripts' as resistance are necessary for the liberation and self-construction of disabled young people in publicly challenging their oppression and marginalisation.

Deploying the concepts of 'hidden transcripts' and 'public transcripts' as theoretical frameworks, and drawing from a TfD project that he facilitated at the University of Zimbabwe between 2008 and 2013, he further argues that preliminaries and informal engagements with disabled people before the actual theatre performances, are sites in which we may access and nurture the private forms of resistance from disabled young people. These methods of engagement with the private forms of resistance help researchers and development activists to access and appreciate the multiplex and sophisticated resistive powers of disabled young people which are usually overlooked by both popular opinion and disability scholarship. The chapter further shows how these forms of resistance might be strengthened to challenge disability oppression in a public theatrical production.

Drawing from the experiences of South Africa, Mozambique, Zimbabwe and Angola, Chapter 5 by Irvine focuses on the development and implementation of policies aimed at increasing the social inclusion of disabled people during conflict transformation. It highlights the benefits of including disabled people in the transition process and provides recommendations for improving the implementation of the policies introduced. Thus, Irvine explores the relationship between the inclusion of disabled people and sustainable communities by focusing on the experiences of societies that have undergone conflict transformation in southern Africa. Countries emerging from conflict have been selected to represent circumstances in which the potential for change is heightened, as new policies are developed at unprecedented rates in order to address historic inequalities and create a new post-conflict identity (Irvine, 2015).

In Chapter 6, Manhique and Giannoumis consider accessibility as a precondition for enjoying all other substantive rights as prescribed by the CRPD (United Nations, 2006). This chapter examines the experience of Mozambique in implementing both the CRPD and SDGs in promoting Information and Communication Technology accessibility. Thus, they investigated the experiences of Disabled People's Organisations (DPOs) in influencing Information and Communication Technology accessibility legislation in Mozambique, while informing the above international frameworks. The analysis is supported by qualitative data from 14 semi-structured interviews with key stakeholders in the Information and Communication Technology sector including government agencies, regulators, private businesses, standard organisations, civil society organisations and DPOs.

Part II: Access to education

In Part II, authors discuss issues of access to education of disabled people from early childhood to secondary education, with a leaning toward deaf learners, an aspect that has not received much attention in southern Africa. Peta's Chapter 7 emerges from an ongoing study, which is exploring the outcome of access to early childhood education of disabled people in Zimbabwe. Using a case study approach, she explores the extent to which 15 disabled women aged between 18 and 30 accessed early childhood education during their early years. The study indicates that children with disabilities confront difficulties in accessing early childhood education programmes due to some traditional belief systems. For families that value such education, identifying an appropriate early childhood learning centre, which caters for the specific needs of children with disabilities, is not easy. There is evidence that the violation of the rights of children with disabilities, in relation to education, perpetuates into later years, with life-time consequences such as increased poverty and vulnerability to sexual and emotional abuse.

In Chapter 8, Musengi and Nyangairi analyse the inclusion of deaf children in mainstream and special secondary schools in Zimbabwe. The chapter discusses the evolution of the concept of the least restrictive environment with particular focus on deaf learners. Eighteen deaf school leavers shared their experiences on the extent to which schools are either inclusive or exclusionary. The study established that both special and mainstream schools do not meet the criteria of 'schools for all'. This is because there is inadequate training of teachers in Sign Language and there are no teaching materials for this language in the schools. These inadequacies have created environments that are unsuitable for the effective participation of children who are deaf. The chapter argues that inclusive education should not mainly be about placement but successful participation in learning. The chapter concludes that the practice of inclusive education for deaf children should enable not just their physical access to schools, but also their epistemological access, regardless of whether this occurs in mainstream or special schools.

In Chapter 9, through analysis of survey and qualitative data of the Zambia National Disability Study conducted in 2015, Azalde *et al.* use the International Classification of Functioning, Disability and Health (ICF) model in changing the discourse of disability to promote inclusive education in Zambia, in a context with few resources. They argue that by viewing functioning as continuous, and in interaction with its surroundings, the ICF model can help create opportunities and enabling environments in schools to ensure that all children learn to their potential regardless of vulnerability.

In Chapter 10, Gweme and Chataika explore the effectiveness of the special class model on three randomly selected primary schools that are also implementing the special class model in Hwange urban, which is in Zimbabwe. This model targets children with specific learning difficulties (SpLDs). They focus on dyslexia and dyscalculia as these are the SpLDs that are considered for placement in Zimbabwe's special class model. Gweme and Chataika established that there is a lack of understanding on the special class model among teachers, parents and learners. Also negative attitudes and lack of understanding on the selection criteria of learners have adversely affected the implementation of this model. Hence, the good intention of this model is being compromised. Therefore, there is a need to raise awareness and capacitate teachers, parents and learners so that such a class is not labelled; an aspect that works against improving learning outcomes. They recommend further research at a larger scale in order to evaluate the effectiveness of this model. This would allow policy makers and implementers to come up with more effective ways of supporting learners with SpLDs.

Part III: Inclusion in higher education

Part III brings out the challenges, opportunities and threats faced by disabled students in accessing higher education in southern Africa. Having impairments appears to be used as exclusionary criteria, yet disabled people make up approximately 15% of the world's population. Chapter 11 by Matshedisho focuses on disability and higher education in southern Africa. He indicates that some researchers across Africa argue that the right to education for disabled people is important. However, it is fraught with difficulties and exclusions (Kochung, 2011; Emong & Eron, 2016), aspects that he interrogates. This chapter makes references to Angola, Botswana, Lesotho, Malawi, Mozambique, Namibia, South Africa, Swaziland, Zambia and Zimbabwe. It begins by explaining the international and national disability rights templates that exist to situate southern African advocacy on disability and higher education. It then problematises disability rights, illustrating how they can lie in tension to one another. Matshedisho further explains how neoliberal values become correlated to disability rights. He concludes with some reflective questions and the way forward for disability inclusion in higher education in southern Africa.

In Chapter 12, Pretorius, Bell and Healey present the current state of inclusion within higher and further education institutions of South Africa. Their focus is on equity and inclusion, including access and reasonable accommodation. They allow disabled students to share their lived experiences in higher education. While some progress has been made in mainstreaming disability, this chapter argues that a consolidated framework needs to be implemented in the sector in order to ensure and regulate access, equality and full inclusion for all students with disabilities in South Africa. The authors note that although the transition of students with disabilities to the labour market after graduation is not addressed in this chapter, it forms an interesting area for further research.

Part IV: Disability, employment, entrepreneurship and CBR

Part IV presents employment and entrepreneurship issues affecting disabled people and the relevance of community-based rehabilitation (CBR) in promoting sustainable development. In Chapter 13, Ntinda, Mpofu, Dunbar-Krige, Makuane and Umeasiegbu draw lessons from several southern African countries to argue for CBR as a preferred development strategy in promoting disability-inclusive social development. They believe that a socially inclusive CBR implements development strategies that promote full participation of people with disabilities. Such disability-inclusive community development strategies seek to create and sustain structures that optimise the participation of people with disabilities in their diversity, rather than expecting them to fit in within existing sub-optimal arrangements. Also, the authors argue that full collaboration of governmental and civic community in the design and delivery of community development initiatives in which persons with disabilities actively contribute, are crucial elements of a successful CBR programme.

Chapter 14 explores options of self-employment, entrepreneurship and sustainable development among disabled people, drawing examples from southern African countries. Charema examines the roles of the governments, educational institutions, vocational and industrial institutions. Environmental, socio-economic, personal and family factors that impact disabled people's welfare and social lives are taken into consideration. The chapter further discusses various challenges that disabled people face, thereby exposing them to employment and social discrimination. Charema argues that with proper planning and government support, the process of consumer empowerment and the impact of the entrepreneurship programmes on the lives of disabled people can benefit the country and individuals involved.

In Chapter 15, Mutswanga, explores the impetus of guidance and counselling in empowering deaf people to have realistic hopes and aspirations for socio-economic sustainable development. She employed a mixed approach where Becker's reading-free vocational interest inventory quantitatively analysed the consistency in vocational choices of the 50 purposively selected deaf students. Deaf students' responses reflect a high mismatch between pursued subjects and desired vocational interests. The findings further revealed that district career guidance days were of less help in informing deaf students in pursuing realistic hopes and aspirations. Mutswanga established that teachers' voices proposed the need for robust and fully funded policies, which mandate positions of career guidance counsellors.

Part V: Religion, gender and parenthood

In Part V, parenthood, gender and religion are discussed to illustrate how they intersect with disability. This results in the exclusion of disabled people, thus highlighting the importance of promoting inclusive sustainable development.

Chapter 16 explores how the interpretation of Judaeo-Christian and African Traditional religio-cultural traditions impact on the well-being of disabled people in Zimbabwe. Machingura advocates for a liberative approach to indigenous traditions, biblical traditions, biblical texts, beliefs and practices on disability. He also engages and interrogates cultural beliefs that fuel the negative beliefs and practices toward disabled people. Machingura's main argument is that all human rights initiatives come to note if men and women of God or religious practitioners in their 'holy talks, spaces, places, platforms and scriptures', do not interrogate certain cultural, religious beliefs, practices and teachings where disability is taken as a sign of: sin, curses, disobedience, evil spirits, demons and witchcraft.

In Chapter 17, Lehtomäki, Okkolin and Matonya examine the global approaches, processes and (policy) frameworks on disability and gender, focusing on similarities and differences over decades, their extent and how they intersect. They focus on what can be learned by looking at the intersection, instead of each dimension separately, to improve and better implement various inclusive development initiatives. The chapter focuses on Tanzania, but the authors claim that the intersection of gender and disability requires more attention also elsewhere. Their argument is that by analysing disability and gender together, as intersecting issues in education, research can better inform policy and practice about critical factors in development toward equality and equity in the southern African region.

Rugoho and Maphosa's Chapter 18 discusses the factors that have caused women with disabilities to remain at the periphery of society in Zimbabwe. It highlights institutionalised discrimination and the weakness of the disability movement as the major factors responsible for the marginalisation of women with disabilities. Rugoho and Maphosa interrogate legal instruments on gender and disability and how their implementation (or non-implementation) has contributed to the perpetuation of the marginalisation of women with disabilities. The chapter ends by proffering some recommendations on how women with disabilities achieve self-representation in development processes.

In Chapter 19, Neille explores the experiences of disabled people in the establishment and maintenance of long-term intimate relationships and their experiences of pregnancy and child-rearing with 30 disabled adults with various impairments in rural South Africa. She established that contextual and stereotypical beliefs regarding sexuality among disabled people, together with a high incidence of violence, negatively impact on identity development. These results highlight the need for contextually relevant information, which supports freedom of choice, while at the same time, protecting disabled people from becoming victims of violence. Neille argues for a need to evaluate ways in which human rights policies are put into practice and the extent to which they relate to contextual beliefs pertaining to disability, intimacy and parenthood.

Part VI: Tourism, sports and accessibility

In Part VI, authors challenge discrimination of disabled people in tourism and sports and suggest ways of increasing accessibility for them to participate in recreational activities. In Chapter 20, Chikuta and Kabote interrogate disability policy issues as applied in southern African countries' tourism industry. The two concepts, disability and tourism are discussed in unison with the aim of identifying legal frameworks that provide disabled people with opportunities to participate in tourism. By analysing government documents of Botswana, Zambia, Zimbabwe and South Africa, Chikuta and Kabote address questions such as: what legal frameworks exist in these countries to promote tourism access by disabled people? How inclusive are these policies especially looking at the diversity of disabilities? The main findings from these countries are lack of implementation and enforcement of frameworks. As such, southern African countries must take disability issues seriously if the desires of disabled people are to be met. It is evident in the countries that they have disjointed legal instruments to deal with disability and tourism, with only South Africa having what looks like a more tourism-specific document. Of concern in this chapter is that in all the tourism policies discussed, there is little or no mention of disability issues. However, legal documents developed in these countries since the 1960s, have helped shape organisational mandates to serve disabled people by offering tailor-made services.

Chapter 21 by Khumalo, Heerden and Skalko is informed by a survey conducted on wheelchair basketball facilities in selected Zimbabwean cities. It investigates the levels of adaptation of facilities toward standards for use by people with mobility impairments. A facility inspection tool derived from the United Nations manual for a barrier-free environment, designed to guide and set standards for built environment accessibility by disabled people, was used. Physical measurements or those derived from construction plans were used to check if the facilities met the recommended specifications. Facilities used by 11 wheelchair clubs registered with the Zimbabwe Paralympic Committee in 2015, were inspected. The variables of interest were obstruction and signage, street furniture and pathways, public phones, mail boxes and water fountains, curb ramps and parking, pedestrian crossing (traffic lights) and ramps, elevators and platform lifts, stairs, railing and hand rails, entrances, vestibules and doors, corridors and rest rooms. The results show that the majority of the expected features fall short of the specifications or are non-existent. The authors' main recommendation is the need for educating those responsible for designing and constructing buildings and sports facilities, on the needs of disabled people and the fundamentals of universal design.

In Chapter 22, Linegar, Giljam, McDonald and Walters illustrate how mobile outreach seating clinics, run by trained seating practitioners, can increase the access of children with posture support needs to assistive equipment and holistic services close to where they live. They share internal reflections of Shonaquip's holistic model of service delivery which has evolved over 25 years' experience in diverse contexts and communities across South Africa. In this chapter, an appropriate wheelchair is widely recognised to be a fundamental right and an important pre-requisite for participation, health and well-being of a person with mobility impairment. When accompanied by sustainable seating services, and supported by empowered parents, skilled carers and a disability-aware community, the authors argue that each child is better placed to develop, learn and flourish as a valued member of their community.

Part VII: Narratives from disability activists

In Part VII, disability activists share their vivid personal stories on how they face and deal with exclusionary practices in their everyday lives and the coping mechanisms they use to overcome such practices. In Chapter 23, Sithole discusses the journey of her life as a disabled person, which has given her both positive and negative experiences in society. Being partially sighted has allowed her to look at the world through the lens of both sighted and blind people. She has experienced the stigma and discrimination faced by blind people. Sithole has also experienced the frustration that sighted people face in trying to understand blind people. This story is about her personal experiences in both worlds of sightedness and blindness. It is an expression of her hope and desire that the misunderstandings and lack of trust between the two worlds can be cleared when each group makes a deliberate effort to understand the other. Sithole concludes by challenging the two worlds to work together for the development of humanity.

Chidemo, Chindimba and Matongo's Chapter 24 is based on their journey of starting up a disability advocacy television programme in Zimbabwe entitled *Action Power*. They talk about the birth of the Zimbabwe Disability Media Trust and how *Action Power* came into being. Thus, they share their successes, lessons learned, challenges and what lies ahead in their quest to ensure that the rights of disabled people in general, and deaf people in particular, are upheld in Zimbabwe.

In Chapter 25, Masendeke explains the steps that he took toward the building of an accessible house in Zimbabwe that meets his impairment-specific requirements, which is a first of its kind since many disabled people face several challenges within the housing sector. This chapter is informed by Article 19 of the CRPD (United Nations, 2006), which states that disabled people have the right to live independently and be included in the community. He argues that disabled people should have the opportunity to choose their own place of residence, including where and with whom they should live with, on an equal basis with others. However, due to the scarcity of disability-friendly or accessible houses in Zimbabwe, Masendeke argues that securing appropriate accommodation is a major challenge for disabled people and their families. They face many barriers in the housing sector, including lack of physical accessibility; ongoing discrimination and stigmatisation; institutional hurdles; lack of access to the labour market; low income; and lack of social housing or community support. Hence, part of his advocacy work involves promoting the building of accessible houses in Zimbabwe.

Chapter 26 is a reflection of a legal practitioner by training and a disability rights activist by calling, who believes that his experiences have made him speak out against social exclusion, hence becoming a disability activist. Mateta believes that no one is born an activist. However, life gives us various challenges and how we respond to those challenges often creates what kind of people we end up becoming. He shares a story that was his turning point as a Zimbabwean blind person and how it defined the kind of activism that he has undertaken for the past ten years, as well as some of the work that he is currently doing as an activist.

Chapter 27 is the author's personal story, which starts with a Scripture from Jeremiah 29 verse 11, because she believes that this verse directed her destiny. Kachaje argues that addressing attitudes that people have is an ongoing process and it starts in the family and goes to the clan and then the community. Kachaje narrates how as the beauty icon of her family, she became disabled as a result of poliomyelitis. She takes us on a journey through her personal experiences as a disabled woman in Malawi; her challenges, achievements and how she has managed to live a purpose-driven life.

Chapter 28 brings the handbook to a conclusion by drawing lessons, best practices, challenges and opportunities tabled by various authors. Chataika reflects on how each chapter feeds into the sustainable development agenda and how the conclusions can inform future directions (i.e. policy and practice), with possible implications for improved livelihoods of disabled people in the southern African region and beyond.

Conclusion

It is my hope that readers find this handbook engaging and challenging. I also hope it opens up spaces for critical thought, research and practice in southern Africa and beyond. This handbook is neither complete nor comprehensive, but I feel that a complex and diverse thematic area such as disability can perhaps never be, particularly in southern Africa. Having said this, I hope that this project is one step toward an ongoing quest of amplifying the traditionally silent voices of upcoming disabled African authors. It is also a step toward challenging exclusion and marginalisation, with the view of promoting inclusive development in southern Africa, where diversity is embraced through critical praxis and transformative decolonising revolution.

A visible gap in this volume is limited work on early childhood education, which is crucial in preparing children with disabilities into meaningful adulthood, where they can have more access to inclusive and equitable education and, eventually, employment opportunities. Also, the absence of research on people with intellectual impairment, albinism and dyslexia is of great concern as these categories are among the most marginalised in southern Africa. Thus, these areas and others that might not have been covered in the handbook are recommended for research in order to create critical connections, close gaps and promote inclusive sustainable development in southern Africa. I have deliberately not included a subheading on reflective questions as this chapter is an introductory chapter to the handbook.

References

Al Ju'beh, K. (2015). *Disability Inclusive Development Toolkit*. Bensheim: CBM.

Barker, C. & Murray, S. (2010). Disabled people at the heart of research: a retrospective appreciation of the disability knowledge and research programme. *Disability Dialogue* **6**, 9–10.

Bruijn, P., Regeer, B., Cornielje, H., Wolting, R., van Veen, S., & Maharaj, N. (2012). *Count Me In: Include People with Disabilities in Development Projects – A Practical Guide for Organisations in North and South*. Veenendaal: Light for the World.

Chataika, T. (2012). Postcolonialism, disability and development. In D. Goodley & B. Hughes (eds) *Social Theories of Disability: New Developments and Directions* (pp. 252–269). London: Routledge.

Emong, P. & Eron, L. (2016). Disability inclusion in higher education in Uganda: status and strategies. *African Journal of Disability* **5**(1). Retrieved from www.ajod.org, DOI: 10.4102/ajod.v5i1.193 on 29 August 2017.

Goodley, D. (2011). *Disability Studies: An Interdisciplinary Introduction*. London: Sage Publications Ltd.

Groce, N. E. (2011). *Disability and the Millennium Development Goals: A Review of the MDG Process and Strategies for Inclusion of Disability Issues in Millennium Development Goal Efforts*. New York: UN.

Groce, N. & Kett, M. (2014). *Youth with disabilities* (Working Paper Series: No. 23). London: Leonard Cheshire Disability and Inclusive Development Centre.

Groce, N., Kett, M., Lang, R., & Trani, J.-F. (2011). Disability and poverty: the need for a more nuanced understanding of implications for development policy and practice. *Third World Quarterly* **32**(8), 1493–1513.

Irvine, R. (2015). Prioritising the inclusion of children and young people with disabilities in post-conflict education reform. *Child Care in Practice* **21**(1), 22–32.

Kochung, E. J. (2011). Role of higher education in promoting inclusive education: Kenyan perspective. *Journal of Emerging Trends in Educational Research and Policy Studies (JETERAPS)* **2**(3), 144–149.

Mitra, S., Posarac, A., & Vick, B. (2013). Disability and poverty in developing countries: a multidimensional study. *World Development* **41**, 1–18.

Oliver, M. & Barnes, C. (1998). *From Exclusion to Inclusion: Social Policy and Disabled People*. London: Longman.

Scott, J. C. (1985). *Weapons of the Weak: Everyday Forms of Peasant Resistance*. New Haven, CT: Yale University Press.

Scott, J. C. (1990). *Domination and the Arts of Resistance: Hidden Transcripts*. New Haven, CT: Yale University Press.

Trani, J. F. & Loeb, M. (2012). Poverty and disability: a vicious circle? Evidence from Afghanistan and Zambia. *Journal of International Development* **24**(S1), S19–S52.

United Nations (2006). *Convention on the Rights of Persons with Disabilities*. Retrieved from http://www.un.org/development/desa/disabilities/convention-on-the-rights-of-persons-with-disabilities.html on 18 March 2017.

Wapling, L. & Downie, B. (2012). *Beyond Charity: A Donor's Guide to Inclusion – Disability Funding in the Era of the UN Convention on the Rights of Persons with Disabilities*. Boston: Disability Rights Fund.

World Health Organization [WHO] & the World Bank (2011). *World Report on Disability*. Geneva: WHO.

2

LEAVE NO ONE BEHIND

Disability mainstreaming in action

Mari Koistinen

Introduction

For a long time, the development sector has overlooked the needs of disabled people, who represent a large but highly invisible group (World Health Organization [WHO] & World Bank, 2011). Disabled people were not referenced in the UN's Millennium Development Goals (MDGs), hence they were globally excluded from many important development initiatives and funding opportunities. Disabled people often face discrimination and exclusion in their everyday lives. There is a close relationship between poverty and disability (Groce *et al.*, 2011). Also, disabled persons are more likely to experience poverty due to multiple barriers result-ing in limited opportunities, for instance, in accessing education, health care and employment services (WHO & World Bank, 2011). People living in poverty are at greater risk of having impairments due to the higher risk of malnutrition, disease, lack of access to water supplies and sanitation. This chapter reflects upon experiences and practices collected based on the work of non-governmental organisations on disability mainstreaming. Practical experiences are drawn from Malawi and Mozambique. Lessons learned for disability mainstreaming are discussed from the development project practitioners' point of view.

Disabled people as invisible and excluded

For a long time, disabled people have been largely invisible in poverty-reduction programmes and in the development agenda (Groce, 2011; Yeo, 2001). Consequently, poverty-reduction goals have partly failed because this large group of people has not been included in the develop-ment processes. Accordingly, Groce (2011) noted that continued neglect of disabled people by national governments and international development agencies remains one of the great gaps of national and international poverty-reduction efforts.

The reasons for this exclusion are manifold. Many disabled persons have not had a voice, choice or control over their lives. Consequently, they often cannot easily engage with govern-ments and decision-makers; hence, their voices have remained unheard. Decisions are being made in inaccessible places or in inaccessible forms for many disabled people. In addition, lack of data on disability and weak data-collection systems, which often under-estimate the preva-lence of impairments, continue to create challenges (Department for International Development

[DFID], 2014). This, in turn, makes it easier for decision-makers to overlook the rights of disabled persons. Frequently, organisations are simply not aware of disabled people due to their invisibility. Disability is also attached to aspects that include ignorance, misconceptions and stigma. Exclusion can occur due to the view that including disabled people requires special skills that the organisations do not possess. Disability might not be considered a priority by development agencies in communities where people are struggling for survival. Such perceptions have also contributed to the false impression that disabled people are a very small group, reserved only for specialist attention of health, education or rehabilitation professionals (Mitra *et al.*, 2013). Groce (2011, p. viii) argues that 'this invisibility is of great concern' because a growing consensus of disability advocates, experts and researchers find that the most pressing issue faced by disabled people is not their impairment. Rather, their lack of equitable access to resources such as education, employment and the social support systems excludes them in development processes.

Disability is something everyone is likely to experience, either permanently or temporarily, at some point in their life (WHO & World Bank, 2011). We are not talking about a small group; as disabled people comprise an estimated 15%, or one billion, of the world's population, of whom 80% live in the global South as highlighted in Chapter 1. The number of people affected is even greater if the family members affected by discrimination are also considered (WHO & World Bank, 2011). Based on the research done by the African Child Policy Forum (ACPF, 2014), Africa has one of the largest populations of children with disabilities in the world. The research highlights that like in many other parts of the world, Africa's prevalence of various forms of impairments is difficult to assess accurately due to incomplete data collection and inaccurate statistical information (ACPF, 2014). It highlights that impairments on the continent have been caused by widespread armed conflicts, poverty and lack of adequate healthcare services (ACPF, 2014), among other reasons. Many African governments have not taken adequate and appropriate legislative, administrative, budgetary and governance steps to secure the rights of disabled people (ACPF, 2014, p. xiii). Hence, urgent action is needed to ensure that disabled people can benefit from and access services on an equal basis with others.

Gaining more visibility in the development agenda

Disability is a development issue, despite being ignored in the international development agenda for a long period. The International Disability Rights Movement, however, has called for disability inclusion since its formation in the early 1980s (Miller & Albert, 2005; Albert, 2006). The 1981 International Year of Disabled Persons was a milestone in the long history of the struggle of disabled people against the discrimination that violates their human rights. The consequent proclamation of the United Nations Decade of Disabled Persons (1983–1992), for instance, prompted activities designed to improve the situation and status of disabled people. There were other scattered developments taking place in different parts of the world as well. For instance, some actors in the development sector from Finland joined the mission of promoting the inclusion of disabled persons globally in the late 1980s. Consequently, the government of Finland supported the United Nations Unit for disabled people to produce guidelines on integrating the disability dimension into development cooperation projects (Wiman, 2003). The Finnish National Research and Development Centre for Welfare and Health (STAKES) was seconded by the United Nations office in Vienna to work on disability inclusion in 1990. One of the outputs of this work was the publication *The Disability Dimension in Development Action: Manual on Inclusive Planning* (Wiman, 2003) originally published in 1996 by STAKES for and on behalf of the United Nations. This was one of the first publications strongly supporting the disability mainstreaming dimension in development.

Despite these developments, disability was excluded from the eight MDGs (1990–2015), which guided the development agenda for 15 years; thus, raising a critical concern. This perhaps highlighted the fact that disability was not even considered a development issue. The realisation by some actors, especially disabled people's organisations and their allies, that MDGs had excluded disabled people gradually called for greater attention for disability mainstreaming in development practices (van Veen, 2014).

In 2000, the United Kingdom Department for International Development (DFID) linked poverty and disability in an issue paper called *Disability, Poverty and Development*, which recognised the problem of the exclusion of persons with disabilities (DFID, 2000). One of the measures it called for was to bring disability into the mainstream. Also, a growing number of disability activists and organisations of disabled people started to stress the importance of inclusion of disabled people in the global development agenda. In 2003, at an international conference, delegates of disabled people from more than 20 countries made a strong call for disability mainstreaming in the development agenda (Miller & Albert, 2005). However, it was only when disability started to be seen as a fundamental human rights issue that governments and international development agencies started paying more attention to it. Despite this attention, disability mainstreaming had a slow start among development agencies.

A research carried out on mapping disability within DFID four years after the paper *Disability, Poverty and Development* was released, found that although there were a substantial number of disability-specific projects, 'there is little practical evidence that mainstreaming has taken place and disability has hardly registered at all in the development process' (Thomas, 2004, p. 70).

The International Development Committee found in their report on Disability and Development that in 2012–13, just over 5% of DFID's bilateral programmes were designed to benefit disabled people (DFID, 2014). Hence, there are still many barriers ahead for disability inclusion to become a reality. Disability mainstreaming remains scattered, and most international development agencies do not recognise disability as a legitimate focus of mainstreaming (Bruijn *et al.*, 2012). There is a common assumption that development programmes targeting extreme poverty will automatically include disabled people and other excluded groups. However, it is increasingly recognised that this is not the case and disabled people can remain hidden or excluded unless their active inclusion is planned from the start. In addition, the balance is still mostly 'tipped towards disability-specific services in international development, rather than disability mainstreaming in projects and programmes' (Al Ju'beh, 2015, pp. 55–56).

New paradigms supporting disability-inclusive development

The way societies think about disabled people or define disability is also determined by several cultural variables, including the nature and type of impairment. Consequent models of explaining disability have been developed over the years. Groce (2011, p. ix) argues that one reason for disabled people having been overlooked in the international development agenda is because they are 'people whose lives are defined by medical and rehabilitative needs (the medical model) or as individuals who were considered to be appropriate recipients of social and economic support (the charity model)'.

The medical model of disability considers disability as an individual 'problem' within the health and welfare framework. It is not seen as an issue of concern to anyone other than the persons affected. The social model of disability emphasises the fact that the constraints faced by disabled people reflect attitudinal, environmental and institutional barriers and are not inherently part of living with impairments. This social model has broadened in recent years to include a human rights component, which includes the right to health care, education and social participation (Groce, 2011). The social model of disability has been adopted by the United Nations Convention on the Rights of Persons with Disabilities (CRPD), which came into force in 2008 (United Nations, 2006).

The CRPD was a significant step in reaffirming and highlighting the rights of disabled people worldwide. The fact that disabled people from different parts of the world and their organisations actively took part in the drafting of the Convention was also highly remarkable (Kanter, 2015). This was different from the more usual approach, where disability agendas are set in the global North by non-disabled people only. Thus, the drafting process of this Convention offered a good opportunity to raise the visibility of disability issues (Schulze, 2009). The CRPD also made a push toward disability mainstreaming, as Article 32 recognises the responsibility of countries that have ratified the Convention to include disabled people in the international development agendas. In mid-2017, 174 countries internationally had ratified the CRPD, demonstrating strong global support and increasing regional support for the rights of disabled people (United Nations' Department for Economic and Social Affairs [DESA], 2017).

According to the ACPF (2014), on 30 March 2007, the first day that the CRPD was opened for signature, 16 African countries signed the treaty. By mid-2014, 38 had ratified the treaty, and eight were signatory states. Hence, through their ratification, most African states have committed to take all necessary legislative, administrative and budgetary steps to protect, promote and realise the rights of disabled people (ACPF, 2014). The goal of full participation, equality and inclusion and empowerment of disabled people in Africa is also highlighted in the goals of the Extended African Decade of Persons with Disabilities (2010–19), which followed the first African Decade of Persons with Disabilities (1999–2009). The aim of the Decade is to 'promote awareness and commitment to full participation, equality and empowerment of disabled persons in the region' (ACPF, 2014, p. 24). In 2016, the African Commission on Human and Peoples' Rights (ACHPR) adopted a draft protocol on the rights of persons with disabilities. The purpose of this protocol is to complement the African Charter on Human and Peoples' Rights. According to the ACHPR (2016), the protocol is the culmination of the African Union's focus on the rights of persons with disabilities, which began in 1999 with the declaration of the African Decade of Persons with Disabilities. The protocol guarantees equal protection and political rights to individuals with 'physical, mental, intellectual, developmental or sensory impairments' and will require states parties to implement affirmative actions to advance their equality (ACHPR, 2016). All these frameworks are laying down strong policy-level support for disability inclusion and mainstreaming in the African continent.

The Agenda 2030 for Sustainable Development Goals (SDGs) has, for the first time in history, included disabled people in its universal plan to end poverty and hunger by 2030 (United Nations, 2015). The SDGs have the potential to transform the lives of disabled people. Agenda 2030 includes 11 mentions of the inclusion of disabled people within the wider commitment to *leave no one behind*. Disability inclusion means that all development planning and interventions are inclusive of and accessible to disabled people. By uncovering the mechanisms that exclude disabled people, exclusionary mechanisms will come to light (Coe & Wapling, 2010a). Hence, the argument for disability inclusion is finally getting stronger.

Disability-inclusive development

Disability-inclusive development in the 21st century is framed within a rights-based approach (Bruijn *et al.*, 2012). Disabled people are not only beneficiaries but, more importantly, agents of development as well. An inclusive approach seeks to identify and address barriers that prevent disabled people from participating in and benefiting from development. Disability-inclusive development respects the diversity that disability can bring and appreciates that it is an everyday part of the human experience (Bruijn *et al.*, 2012). The twin-track approach combines disability mainstreaming with disability-specific objectives needed to achieve the full inclusion of disabled people (DFID, 2000). This approach is the most commonly referenced approach by United Nations agencies, bilateral development agencies and non-governmental organisations (NGOs) for including disabled people. Nowadays, a triple-track approach is mentioned, which underlines the importance of addressing the political will and mobilisation as a prerequisite for all effective societal action, especially by the public sector (Wiman, 2012). Disability mainstreaming is a way of promoting inclusion and addressing the barriers that exclude disabled people from the equal enjoyment of their human rights (The United Nations Relief and Works Agency for Palestine Refugees in the Near East [UNRWA], 2013). According to DESA (2011, p. 5), mainstreaming is:

> Simultaneously a method, a policy and a tool for achieving social inclusion, which involves the practical pursuit of non-discrimination and equality of opportunity. Mainstreaming disability is about 'recognizing disabled people as rights-holding, equal members of society who must be actively engaged in the development process irrespective of their impairment or other status, such as race; colour; sex . . .'.

Thus, disability mainstreaming is a process of assessing and addressing the possible impact of any planned action on disabled people. It is a strategy for making the concerns and experiences of disabled people an integral dimension of the design, implementation, monitoring and evaluation of policies, projects and programmes. Nowadays, we have guidelines for disability inclusion and mainstreaming, giving ideas of how to implement projects and programmes in an inclusive manner (see, for example, Coe and Wapling, 2010b; Department of Economic and Social Affairs (DESA), 2011; Bruijn *et al.*, 2012; Christian Blind Mission, 2012; Deutsche Gesellschaft für Internationale Zusammenarbeit (GIZ) & Christian Blind Mission (CBM), 2012; Chataika, 2013; Rohwerder, 2015). However, we would need more evidence-based research and information on the experiences of disability mainstreaming by different actors. This is something that this chapter partly addresses.

Disability mainstreaming in action

Disability Partnership Finland (DPF) is an NGO, with eight member disability organisations. Traditionally, the focus of DPF's work has been disability-specific projects mainly to strengthen the capacity of local disabled people's organisations (DPOs). Its work is based on the core principles of the CRPD. Since 2013, the focus of DPF's work has also increasingly been on disability mainstreaming. This has meant forming new partnerships and cooperation with diverse mainstream actors and organisations in the field of rural development, education, HIV/AIDS, water and sanitation, to mention a few. Thus, DPF offers consultative services to mainstream organisations, including capacity-building of personnel and other relevant actors in the global North and South. Training can include topics such as the rights of disabled people, inclusion in education, HIV and AIDS and employment. Also, regular distant support is available upon request. DPF always works in close partnership with local organisations of disabled people in the global South. Training services are initially provided in partnership between DPF and the local DPO, with the aim of the local partner gradually taking over this responsibility. In the next section, two case studies from Mozambique and Malawi are presented, in which I will explain

18

the way that DPF has worked and also highlight some of the main issues that have been found to be important in the process of disability mainstreaming.

Inclusive teacher training college in Mozambique

The government of Mozambique has prioritised the creation and expansion of opportunities to ensure that all children have access to and complete a basic education of seven years, while at the same time, creating conditions for a sustainable expansion of quality post-primary education. The main objectives of the education sector for 2012–16 included ensuring access, inclusion, equity and retention in schools (Ministry of Education, 2012). Similarly, the government has taken some steps that indicate commitment to advancing the rights of disabled people such as signing and ratifying the CPRD and its Optional Protocol in 2012. The National Plan of Action for the Area of Disability – PNAD II 2012–2019 – guides planning, budgeting, monitoring and evaluation activities, which different social actors develop in favour of disabled people. Despite the above-mentioned provisions there is not yet a comprehensive disability law in Mozambique. Disabled people continue to have limited access to education, livelihood opportunities and skills training, participation in public and political life and health care services (Swedish International Development Agency [SIDA], 2014, p. 3).

The following case study comes from the field of education in 2016. In Mozambique, DPF worked on a project in partnership with a mainstream NGO. The focus was on providing training and technical support to the teaching staff and other relevant partners at a private teacher training college. The college follows the national curriculum for teacher education and also trains teachers for government primary schools. The national curriculum for teacher training includes modules on teaching children with diverse educational needs such as children with disabilities. However, viewing disability from a rights perspective (right to education) was rather new at the college. Consequently, the first activity was to provide sensitisation and training on inclusive education to the whole personnel in line with Article 24 of the CRPD (United Nations, 2006).

To increase the level of participation of disabled people, local DPOs were identified and introduced at the college. Identification of the main barriers for children with disabilities in accessing education was done in cooperation with diverse allies. Two disabled people, acting as focal points for disability inclusion, were hired to coordinate the disability inclusion work and to provide sensitisation and training on disability issues for relevant actors. After the initial awareness-raising sessions, teachers were provided with more specific training on inclusive education. Teachers then forwarded this information to their teacher-training students. Training materials were adapted to better suit children with diverse impairments. Communication with children with hearing impairment was found particularly challenging; hence, the college took the initiative to start providing Sign Language instruction.

Regular disability meetings were organised every month at the teacher training college with 55 participants, including representatives from DPOs, social services, city council, primary school teachers, the provincial hospital and other relevant associations. The aim of these gatherings was primarily to discuss and share ideas on disability mainstreaming and to plan disability awareness events in the area. This approach also contributed toward the aim of including localised knowledge for inclusive education, which was then used in planning inclusive interventions. Hence, at the teacher training college and in the surrounding villages, regular awareness-raising of the rights of disabled people in education was conducted. In addition to the groups mentioned above, this has also been done by disabled people and their organisations together with the college personnel and students. A group of 25 mainstream students has also been formed to perform sensitisation in the community. They go door-to-door, visiting families of children with disabilities in order to provide advice. The families are also given information and referrals to other services in the area such as physiotherapy, social and health services, other disability associations and Sign Language teaching and hospitals.

Another important part of the project was the creation of the Graduated Teachers' Network. The meetings were held twice per year and focused on sensitising the teachers to disability and allowing them to exchange information related to teaching methods, teaching material, classroom interaction and other relevant issues. Also, with the help of local DPOs, the school was made more accessible, bearing in mind environmental and communication-related barriers. For instance, some ramps were built and changes were made in two of the dormitories and toilets. As a result of these developments, the college became more disability-inclusive and, during the first year, it accepted five new disabled students. The greatest challenges encountered were the lack of assistive devices and inclusion of students with visual impairment. The government does not organise entrance examinations for persons with visual impairment. Hence, this needed to be done by the college itself. Alternative routes were looked for and, as a result, one applicant took the entrance examination. This was made possible by someone reading the questions to the applicant, who would then write the answers in braille. The answers were sent to the capital city for grading. The applicant was allowed to have some extra time during the examination. Eventually, this applicant with visual impairment was enrolled as a student.

The Mozambique government has regulated that only people ranging between 18 and 25 years old can apply to teacher training colleges. This poses a problem to many disabled people, as they at times require more time to finish secondary education. The implication is that they are not ready to apply to teacher training colleges until they are already too old. In the future, one idea would be to design a new project for providing support to secondary education courses for disabled people, in order for them to apply to teacher training colleges on time. This could further increase the number of students with disabilities at the college. In the next section, the case study from Malawi is presented.

Inclusive women's farmers clubs in Malawi

Malawi ratified the CRPD in September 2009 and domesticated it through the Disability Act of 2012, which adopted the social model approach to disability. The Disability Act highlights the importance of disability mainstreaming (Malawi Government, 2012). Despite the generally good legal environment, government funding for the disability sector is still minimal (United Nations Children's Fund [UNICEF], 2012).

The Malawi case study comes from the sector of agriculture. Agriculture is one of the fields in which disabled persons face some of the greatest prejudice and exclusion, as they are believed to be less active and less capable of farming. DPF cooperated with a mainstream organisation that was working with women farmers in Malawi from 2014–17. The overall objective of the project is to reduce poverty and promote gender equality in the area. Women farmers form clubs and receive training and support for sustainable agricultural measures. The number of farmers included in the project is more than 4,000. The project organises a number of trainings such as agriculture, conservation farming, group dynamics, cooperative management and agri-business, livestock management and nutrition. Before cooperation with the DPF, women with disabilities were excluded from the project. Disability mainstreaming activities started at the beginning of the second phase of the project in 2015, when 750 new clubs were created.

The first step in disability inclusion activities in this project included training and motivation of project personnel both in Finland and Malawi, where the training was provided in cooperation with local DPOs. Based on our experiences, continuous training and support facilities guarantee a boost in confidence for the personnel and ensure interest and motivation for disability inclusion. It is also important that core local actors on disability issues, such as social services and local organisations for disabled people, participate in the training. This provides a good opportunity for participants to make acquaintances and to initiate cooperation.

A focal person, a disabled woman residing in Malawi, was hired to promote disability mainstreaming. She was in charge of initial identification of disabled people in the project area. There are 4,250 women farmers, 166 of which are women with disabilities (4%). In addition, there are 288 women whose spouses or children have various forms of impairments benefiting from the project. In total, the number is 454 (11%). Most women have physical impairment or epilepsy. However, there are also women with visual, hearing and learning disabilities. Thereafter, by-laws were drafted that promote the inclusion of disabled people in the project activities; thus, ensuring that they are given equal opportunities in community activities. For example, when sharing farming inputs and leadership positions, disabled people have to be considered as well. Sensitisation work started in the communities, with close cooperation with village chiefs and other local decision-makers. With their needed support, sensitisation continued regularly in the communities. It was seen as important for chiefs to lead as examples in ensuring that disabled people are not discriminated against.

After the first year, results looked promising, and women with disabilities were more accepted in the communities and have become members of women farmers' clubs. Many disabled women are now in various leadership positions. These include chairpersons and village water committee leaders' positions. Thirty percent of disabled women now have access and control over their household resources. One disabled woman commented that she could not have imagined being a part of farm clubs, but now she has become an active member and her life has changed positively. Information of the status of disabled people being well-documented at the beginning of the project was crucial to this case study. Hence, indicators were set, so that each target had disaggregated goals for disability inclusion. Monitoring and evaluation were done with disability inclusion goals in mind.

When coming up with village committees to oversee a development such as rural road maintenance, the village chiefs now ensure that a committee member or leader should be someone with some form of impairment. Women with disabilities have also been assisted by assistive technology and referrals to healthcare with the help of local social services. Modifications have been made with regard to water pumps and other equipment for easier accessibility. Assistive technology enables active participation in both social and economic activities. It was established that communities are now more aware of the rights of disabled people, and there is less bullying and exclusion taking place. We have experienced many positive developments taking place in Malawi and Mozambique, and several of the lessons learned are discussed in the next section.

Lessons learned for disability mainstreaming

The first lesson learned is that while the inclusion of disability in the SDGs, CRPD and the African Decade of Persons with Disabilities is a great improvement, they remain powerless if they are not implemented with budgetary allocations. In both case countries (Malawi and Mozambique), the governments have ratified the CRPD but there is still a need to increase their commitment toward disability-inclusive development. While NGOs and DPOs can do their part, only government support to disability inclusion can have a wider and more sustainable impact. Without implementation, disabled people might continue to be excluded. Another issue that remains to be seen in the future is whether these supranational agendas will be effective in responding to the needs of disabled people at grassroots level. The question that has been raised is whether there is a need to create Southern theories and models to critique the CRPD (Chataika *et al.*, 2015; Chataika & McKenzie, 2016).

Second, many development and disability concepts have their origin in the global North. When we talk about disability in the global South, we also talk about survival, social change and structures that keep people in poverty (Stone, 2001). It is important to look at how disability is understood in the local cultures to plan effective and relevant intervention processes of disability mainstreaming into general development activities. This should be the starting point of any action. Thus, there might be a need for considering an African disability agenda that informs development partners and other global North stakeholders when dealing with disability rights and mainstreaming. Also, Chataika and McKenzie (2016) challenge the global South to reclaim and increase its visibility within the global arena when fighting for disability mainstreaming and the eradication of poverty among its habitants in general and disabled people in particular. It is from the above lessons and insights that specific action points are suggested in the next sections, if disability mainstreaming is to be achieved in Malawi and Mozambique specifically, and the southern African region in general. These include meaningful inclusion of disabled people, powerful partnerships, continuous support to the personnel, accessibility for all, inclusion in the full project cycle and investments in inclusion.

Meaningful inclusion of disabled people

Planning together with local disabled people and their allies, such as DPOs, gives the best starting point for any intervention (Koistinen, 2017). It is essential that disabled people and their organisations play an active and meaningful role from the beginning up to the end of the project. One research on mainstreaming found that the most relevant and effective interventions were those 'supporting building advocacy and capacity of DPOs' (Nordic Consulting Group, 2012, p. 76). Hence, when relevant, it is also important to provide capacity development to local DPOs on disability mainstreaming activities. Cooperation with disabled people and their organisation is important, as they are the experts in their cause and in identifying barriers for inclusion. It is important to also remember that disabled people are not a homogeneous group. This diversity should be respected when making choices. For example, there is a need to include both men and women representing diverse impairment-specific groups in any activity. It is also important that someone is in charge of disability inclusion; ideally, a disabled person in a key decision-making position.

Many disabled people have been excluded for a long time, and patience should be exercised in the inclusion process. Once identified, disabled people should be empowered to participate in the whole project cycle. An important step of the process is the removal of attitudinal, environmental and institutional barriers that prevent participation. Consequently, to ensure successful participation, disabled people also need access to medical or rehabilitation care or assistive technology such as wheelchairs (Bruijn *et al.*, 2012).

Powerful partnerships

Disability mainstreaming becomes much easier and more powerful through diverse partnerships with, for instance, private and public sectors, NGOs, DPOs as well as people from the communities and government offices. Government offices can be reminded of their responsibility to deliver on the commitments stated in the CRPD through policy dialogue. Thus, adequate budget allocations for disability mainstreaming should be considered. It is also important to provide training to various stakeholders such as policy makers and community leaders on disability mainstreaming. Also, DPOs might need further information on the SDGs and the CRPD. Partnerships are also vital, if there is any hope of recording real impact of the SDGs by 2030. Furthermore, there is a need to maintain pressure on the governments to include disabled people in the development agenda and any national development plans targeting poverty reduction.

Continuous support to the personnel

A crucial step forward is the identification/mapping of training needs of the project personnel. Challenging staff and community attitudes are key first steps to 'achieving positive progress towards the inclusion of disabled people in development work' (Coe & Wapling, 2010a, p. 881). They should be made aware of the rights, needs and capabilities of disabled people. This should be done as soon as possible and could be done by or with local organisations of disabled people who can also act as role models. Awareness encourages identification of incidence, type and impact of impairments of individuals and how communities can positively respond to their needs. It is very typical that in areas where disabled people are invisible, many are identified after raising awareness and building capacity in the identification process. It is important to remember that in many societies, disability is a taboo topic or is seen from a purely medical and/or traditional model. Most importantly, attitudes also usually take a while to change, hence the need to use any available avenues of raising awareness such as community gatherings and various forms of media.

Accessibility for all

A comprehensive accessibility audit is one of the most important practical preconditions for inclusion. Without being able to access the facilities and services in the community, disabled people will never be fully included (United Nations, 2017). In most communities, however, there are several obstacles that hinder disabled people from participation and inclusion. These barriers include, for instance, inaccessible school and community buildings and public transportation and a lack of information in accessible formats. What is key to Article 9 of the CRPD is that everyone should have the right to access public places such as schools, hospitals and government offices. Accessibility should be taken into account at the beginning of any intervention, and disabled people should be consulted in the process (United Nations, 2006).

Inclusion in the full project cycle

It is important that efforts toward mainstream disability begin with the analysis of barriers and careful planning. There should be a plan for inclusion. Disability inclusion should be included from the beginning and continue until the end of the project. It is important to include disabled people in the monitoring system and evaluation of the project. The United Nations Expert Group on Disability Data and Statistics, Monitoring and Evaluation noted that data disaggregated by impairment in all areas is essential to ensuring progress is measured and disabled people are not left behind in future mainstream development programmes (United Nations, 2014, p. 9). Hence, setting both quantitative and qualitative targets is important. Disabled people should be involved at every stage of the process – from collecting data to analysing the results. This approach will not only build their capacity, but is also likely to deliver more reliable and sustainable results and address barriers more effectively (DFID, 2015).

Investments in inclusion

Mainstreaming has so far been recognised as the most cost-effective and efficient way to achieve equality for disabled people (DESA, 2011; Coe & Wapling, 2010a). Experience suggests that an estimated 80% of disabled people can be included without any specific additional intervention, or with low-cost interventions that do not require specific expertise (Bruijn *et al.*, 2012). Hence, a high level of participation can be achieved with some additional resources. In some cases, though, more impact can be achieved by including some additional costs. For instance, modifications to buildings, accessible markets, cost of Sign Language interpreters, assistive technology and physiotherapy. Most importantly, inclusive approaches are more cost-effective than piecemeal disability interventions, where the needs of disabled people are met as an afterthought (Walton, 2012; Bruijn *et al.*, 2012). Research indicates that extra costs that are incurred as a result of meeting access needs of disabled people range from 0% to 3% (WHO & World Bank, 2011). Thus, any additional costs associated with including disabled people are far outweighed by the long-term financial benefits to individuals, families and society (Christian Blind Mission, 2012).

Conclusion

The development agenda has started embracing disability inclusion in line with the global vision, which aspires that by 2030 we will have a world where no one is left behind. This would mean a world where disabled people can participate equally in everyday life. Disability mainstreaming is still rather new as an approach for many organisations as they are taking their first steps toward disability inclusion. Monitoring and evaluation of this progress is critical. Collecting and sharing good practices on disability mainstreaming is equally important. This chapter reviewed some experiences and discussed some good practices that have worked in Malawi and Mozambique. Other authors have documented what has worked best in other contexts (see, for instance, Coe & Wapling, 2010a; Bruijn, 2013; van Veen, 2014). Documenting such success stories might assist development partners in coming up with development programmes and tools that can benefit disabled people and their diverse needs in the global South. What is certain is that no sustainable development initiative can afford to leave disabled people at the periphery of its agenda, if the SDGs are to be achieved in southern Africa and beyond.

Reflective questions

1   Why are disabled people being excluded from the inter/national development agenda?
2   What are the greatest opportunities and challenges the SDGs can offer for disable people?
3   Why is culture an important concept when discussing disability mainstreaming?
4   What are the main lessons learned from disability mainstreaming based on the experiences highlighted in this chapter?

References

African Charter on Human and Peoples' Rights (2016). *Draft Protocol to the African Charter on Human and Peoples' Rights on the Rights of Persons with Disabilities in Africa*. Retrieved from www.achpr.org/files/news/2016/04/d216/disability_protocol.pdf on 25 June 2017.

African Child Policy Forum (2014). *The African Report on Children with Disabilities: Promising Starts and Persisting Challenges*. Retrieved from www.asksource.info/resources/african-report-children-disabilities-promising-starts-and-persisting-challenges on 20 November 2016.

Albert, B. (ed.) (2006). *In or Out of the Mainstream? Lessons from Research on Disability and Development Cooperation*. Leeds: The Disability Press.

Al Ju'beh, K. (2015). *Disability Inclusive Development Toolkit*. Bensheim, Germany: CBM. Retrieved from www.cbm.org/article/downloads/54741/CBM-DID-TOOLKIT-accessible.pdf on 18 September 2016.

Bruijn, P. (2013). *Inclusion works! Lessons learned on the inclusion of people with disabilities in a food security project for ultra-poor women in Bangladesh*. Retrieved from www.licht-fuer-die-welt.at/sites/default/files/inclusionworks.pdf on 15 September 2016.

Bruijn, P., Regeer, B., Cornielje, H., Wolting, R., van Veen, S. & Maharaj, N. (2012). *Count Me In: Include People with Disabilities in Development Projects – A Practical Guide for Organisations in North and South*. Veenendaal: Light for the World. Retrieved from www.light-for-the-world.org/sites/lfdw_org/files/download_files/count-me-in-include-people-with-disabilities-in-development-projects.pdf on 10 April 2018.

Chataika, T. (2013). *Gender and Disability Mainstreaming Training Manual: Prepared for Disabled Women in Africa*. Germany: GMZ and GIZ.

Chataika, T., Berghs, M., Mateta, A. & Shava, K. (2015). From whose perspective anyway? The quest for African disability rights. In A. de Waal (ed.) *Advocacy in Conflict: Critical Perspectives on Transnational Activism* (pp. 187–211). London: Zed Books.

Chataika, T. & McKenzie, J. A. (2016). Global institutions and their engagement with disability mainstreaming in the South: development and (dis)connections. In S. Grech & K. Soldatic (eds) *Disability in the Global South: The Critical Handbook* (pp. 423–436). Switzerland: Springer International Publishing.

Christian Blind Mission (2012). *Inclusion Made Easy: A Quick Program Guide to Disability in Development*. Bensheim, Germany: CBM. Retrieved from www.cbm.org/article/downloads/78851/CBM_Inclusion_Made_Easy_-_complete_guide.pdf on 15 September 2016.

Coe, S. & Wapling, L. (2010a). Practical lessons from four projects on disability-inclusive development programming. *Development in Practice* **20**(7). Retrieved from www.jstor.org/stable/20787356?seq=1#page_scan_tab_contents on 15 July 2017.

Coe, S. & Wapling, L. (2010). *Travelling Together: How to Include Disabled People on the Main Road of Development*. World Vision UK. Retrieved from www.worldvision.org.uk/travellingtogether on 10 September 2016.

Department of Economic and Social Affairs (2011). *Best Practices for Including Persons with Disabilities in All Aspects of Development Efforts*. New York: United Nations. Retrieved from www.un.org/disabilities/documents/best_practices_publication_2011.pdf on 16 April 2017.

Department of Economic and Social Affairs (2017). *Convention on the Rights of Persons with Disabilities*. New York: United Nations. Retrieved from www.un.org/development/desa/disabilities/convention-on-the-rights-of-persons-with-disabilities.html on 15 September 2016.

Department for International Development (DFID) (2000). *Disability, Poverty and Development*. Retrieved from www.make-development-inclusive.org/docsen/DFIDdisabilityPovertyDev.pdf on 15 April 2016.

Department for International Development (DFID) (2014). *Disability Framework: Leaving No One Behind*. London: DFID. Retrieved from www.gov.uk/government/uploads/system/uploads/attachment_data/file/382338/Disability-Framework-2014.pdf on 18 June 2016.

Department for International Development (DFID) (2015). *Disability Framework – One Year On: Leaving No One Behind*. Retrieved from www.gov.uk/government/uploads/system/uploads/attachment_data/file/554802/DFID-Disability-Framework-2015.pdf on 15 June 2017.

Deutsche Gesellschaft für Internationale Zusammenarbeit (GIZ) & Christian Blind Mission (CBM) (2012). *A Human Rights-Based Approach to Disability in Development: Entry Points for Development Organisations*. Retrieved from www.cbm.org/article/downloads/54741/A_human_rights based_approach_to_disability_in_development.pdf on 15 April 2018.

Groce, N. E. (2011). *Disability and the Millennium Development Goals: A Review of the MDG Process and Strategies for Inclusion of Disability Issues in Millennium Development Goal Efforts*. New York: United Nations. Retrieved from www.un.org/disabilities/documents/review_of_disability_and_the_mdgs.pdf on 15 August 2016.

Groce, N. E., Kembhavi, G., Wirz, S., Lang, R., Trani, J. F. & Kett, M. (2011). Poverty and disability: a critical review of the literature in low and middle-income countries. *Working Paper Series* 16. *London: Leonard Cheshire Disability and Inclusive Development Centre*. Retrieved from www.ucl.ac.uk/lc-ccr/centre publications/workingpapers/WP16_Poverty_and_Disability_review.pdf on 10 April 2018.

Hulme, D., Moore, K., Shepherd, A. & Grant, U. (2004). *Draft Knowledge Paper: How Can Development Reach and Assist the Poorest?* Chronic Poverty Research Centre, IDPM, Manchester University.

Kanter, A. S. (2015). *The Development of Disability Rights under International Law: From Charity to Human Rights.* London: Routledge.

Koistinen, M. (ed.) (2017). *Development for All: Experiences on Disability Mainstreaming in the Development Sector.* Helsinki: Disability Partnership. Retrieved from www.vammaiskumppanuus.fi/wp-content/uploads/2017/04/Development_whole_03042017_low.pdf on 10 April 2018.

Malawi Government (2012). *Disability*, Act No. 10 of 12.

Miller, C. & Albert, B. (2005). *Mainstreaming Disability in Development: Lessons from Gender Mainstreaming.* Retrieved from https://assets.publishing.service.gov.uk/media/57a08c5be5274a27b2001147/RedPov_gender.pdf on 15 September 2016.

Ministry of Education (2012). *Education Strategic Plan 2012–2016, Let's Learn! Building Competencies for Mozambique in Development.* Republic of Mozambique: Ministry of Education.

Mitra, S., Posarac, A. & Vick, B. (2013). Disability and poverty in developing countries: a multi-dimensional study. *World Development* **41**, 1–18. Retrieved from http://dx.doi.org/10.1016/j.worlddev.2012.05.024 on 15 September 2016.

Nordic Consulting Group (2012). *Mainstreaming Disability in the New Development Paradigm: Evaluation of Norwegian Support to Promote the Rights of Disabled People.* Oslo: NORAD. Retrieved from www.norad.no/en/toolspublications/publications/2012/mainstreaming-disability-in-the-new-development-paradigm-evaluation-of-norwegian-support-to-promote-the-rights-of-persons-with-disabilities/ on 15 April 2016.

Rohwerder, B. (2015). *Disability Inclusion: Topic Guide.* GSDRC, University of Birmingham, Birmingham.

Schulze, M. (2009). *Understanding the UN Convention on the Rights of Persons with Disabilities: A Handbook on the Rights of Persons with Disabilities.* Retrieved from www.hiproweb.org/uploads/tx_hidrtdocs/HICRPDManual2010.pdf on 10 April 2018.

Stone, E. (ed.) (2001). *Disability and Development: Learning from Action and Research on Disability in the Majority World.* Leeds: The Disability Press.

Swedish International Development Agency (2014). *Disability Rights in Mozambique.* Retrieved from www.sida.se/globalassets/sida/eng/partners/human-rights-based-approach/disability/rights-of-persons-with-disabilities-mozambique.pdf on 15 April 2018.

Thomas, P. (2004). *DFID and Disability: A Mapping of the Department for International Development and Disability KaR Knowledge and Research.* Retrieved from www.disabilitykar.net on 10 April 2018.

United Nations (2006). *The Convention on the Rights of Persons with Disabilities and Optional Protocol.* New York: United Nations. Retrieved from www.un.org/disabilities/documents/convention/convoptprot-e.pdf on 15 April 2016.

United Nations (2014). *United Nations Expert Group Meeting on Disability Data and Statistics, Monitoring and Evaluation: The Way Forward – a Disability-Inclusive Agenda Towards 2015 and Beyond.* Report to the Secretariat to the Convention on the Rights of Persons with Disabilities. Division for Social Policy and Development United Nations Department of Economic and Social Affairs in collaboration with United Nations Educational, Scientific, and Cultural Organization. Retrieved from www.un.org/disabilities/documents/egm2014/EGM_FINAL_08102014.pdf on 15 July 2017.

United Nations (2015). *Transforming Our World: The 2030 Agenda for Sustainable Development.* Resolution adopted by the General Assembly on 25 September 2015. Retrieved from https://sustainabledevelopment.un.org/post2015/transformingourworld on 25 September 2017

United Nations Children's Fund (UNICEF) (2012). *From Exclusion to Inclusion: Promoting the Rights of Children with Disabilities in Malawi.* Retrieved from www.unicef.org/malawi/MLW_resources_cwdreportfull.pdf on 21 September 2016.

United Nations Enable (2017). *Accessibility: A Guiding Principle of the Convention.* Retrieved from www.un.org/esa/socdev/enable/disacc.htm on 10 November 2016.

United Nations Relief and Works Agency for Palestine Refugees in the Near East (2013). *Disability Mainstreaming: Definition and Implementation.* UNRWA, *Disability Series* no. 3. Retrieved from www.unrwa.org/userfiles/file/disability/3_disability_mainstreaming.pdf on 18 September 2016.

van Veen, S. C. (2014). *Development for All: Understanding Disability Inclusion in Development Organisations.* Hertogenboscg: BOXPress.

Walton, O. (2012). *Economic Benefits of Disability-inclusive Development* (GSDRC Helpdesk Research Report 831). Birmingham, UK: GSDRC. Retrieved from www.gsdrc.org/docs/open/HDQ831.pdf on 10 April 2018.

Wiman, R. (2003). *The Disability Dimension in Development Action: Manual for Inclusive Planning.* Stakes for the UN. Retrieved from www.un.org/esa/socdev/enable/publications/FF-DisalibilityDim0103_b1.pdf on 15 April 2016.

Wiman, R. (2012). *Mainstreaming the Disability Dimension in Development Cooperation, Case Finland: Lessons Learned.* Presentation at the UN Commission for Social Development, 50th session (2.2.2012): Side-Event on Mainstreaming Disability in Development Policy and Programming, viewed on 15 April 2016. Retrieved from www.thl.fi/documents/189940/263914/Wiman_Mainstreaming_Disability_Dimension_CaseFinland.pdf on 23 November 2016.

World Health Organization [WHO] & the World Bank (2011). *World Report on Disability.* Geneva: WHO.

World Vision (2010). *Travelling Together: How to Include Disabled People on the Main Road of Development.* Retrieved from http://cdn.worldvision.org.uk/files/7813/8053/8460/About_the_Authors.pdf on 10 September 2016.

Yeo, R. (2001). *Chronic Poverty and Disability. CPRC Working Paper 4.* Frome: Chronic Poverty Research Centre, Action on Disability and Development.

3

REFLECTIONS ON THE DEVELOPMENT OF THE NATIONAL DISABILITY MAINSTREAMING PLAN IN LESOTHO

Nkhasi Sefuthi and Masekara Sekoankoetla

Introduction

Since the World Report on Disability estimates that disabled people constitute close to 15% of the world's population, with about 80% of these being located in low-income countries (World Health Organization [WHO] & World Bank, 2011), it becomes imperative to consider disability mainstreaming in development processes. Disabled people are often among the poorest in their communities and they are likely to experience discrimination and stigma (Grech, 2016). Yet, not much has been done despite the obvious link between disability and poverty. Many disabled people continue to be invisible in most family, community and national activities as disability mainstreaming tends to be a huge challenge to many countries, which seem not to recognise disability as a human rights, development and cross-cutting issue (Chataika & McKenzie, 2016).

In this chapter, we outline how the Lesotho National Federation of Organisations of the Disabled (LNFOD) was involved in the development of the country's National Disability Mainstreaming Plan (NDMP), which was adopted in 2015. Apart from being authors of this chapter, we are also in leadership positions in LNFOD; we also actively contributed to the development of the NDMP. Thus, we articulate what prompted the development of the plan, the level of participation of disabled people, challenges encountered and how the plan was adopted. We also discuss the challenges being currently faced as the country attempts to implement this plan in government policies, programmes and services, as well as how some of these challenges could be overcome. We then conclude by sharing lessons learned during the development of the plan, a process that can also inform others who are contemplating embarking on this route. However, before talking about the development of the NDMP, we provide the situational analysis of disabled people in Lesotho.

Situational analysis of disabled people in Lesotho

Lesotho is a small country, landlocked by the Republic of South Africa. Its population is estimated at around two million, 4% of which are recorded as disabled people ([Lesotho] Bureau of Statistics [BOS], 2006). However, after the 2006 census, LNFOD successfully advocated for the adoption of the Washington Group Questionnaire on disability statistics (Washington Group on Disability Statistics, 2014), as many disabled people doubted the statistics of the BOS (2006) report. This was because the first ever World Report on Disability reports that disabled people constitute about 15% of any country's population (WHO & World Bank, 2011) as indicated in the introductory chapter. As a result, Lesotho underwent a housing census in March 2016, where disabled people's organisations (DPOs) were fully involved in the development of the data-collection tools to ensure disability inclusion, using this questionnaire. Unfortunately, the United Nations Children's Fund (UNICEF) module for disabled children was not yet completed when the census was conducted in March 2016, and hence could not be tested to determine the impairments of children under the age of six years. It is expected that the 2016 census report will show the increased percentage of disabled people in Lesotho as the preliminary findings that are now available do not suggest otherwise.

Lesotho is a member state of the United Nations. She is also a state party to the United Nations Convention on the Rights of Persons with Disabilities (CRPD) (United Nations, 2006). Lesotho ratified the CRPD in 2008, only two years after its adoption. As a state party, Lesotho has undertaken several institutional and policy initiatives to address issues of disabled people, in line with the prescriptions of this treaty. Among other crucial policy measures undertaken by Lesotho in this regard is the adoption of the NDMP in 2015. With this plan, Lesotho undertook to mainstream disability in plans, programmes and policies of all ministries so that disabled people can meaningfully and equitably participate in all aspects of life.

Historically, disabled people in Lesotho have experienced severe discrimination and marginalisation (LNFOD, 2011). This is an unfair, unfavourable and prejudicial treatment where this group is regarded as least significant; thus, relegated to the periphery of the society. At the periphery, disabled people hardly participate in society due to various barriers, which include attitudinal, environmental and institutional barriers (Chataika, 2012). This treatment is thus attributed to negative societal attitudes rooted in cultural beliefs and norms passed down through generations through the socialisation process (French & Kayes, 2008). Barriers to the social participation and inclusion of this group in Lesotho are both attitudinal and institutional (Government of Lesotho, 2015). In many instances, there is minimal awareness of their diverse needs. This is reflected in the design and mode of delivery of services, laws and policies that are disability unfriendly (LNFOD, 2011). Such services, laws and policies continuously foster social exclusion of disabled people, who are unfortunately already disadvantaged in most aspects of life, such as education, healthcare services and employment (LNFOD, 2011).

Contrary to the CRPD, disabled people are under-represented in leadership and decision-making positions (United Nations, 2006). As a result, they do not actively participate when key decisions that affect them are made. Hence, disabled people are still considered objects and not agents of development in Lesotho. Thus, they hardly influence and direct developmental interventions that positively impact on their lives (Moore & Yeo, 2003). This has then caused impoverishment, abandonment, malnourishment, discrimination and extreme ill-health – aspects that demonstrate the need for interventions in disability issues in Lesotho (Government of Lesotho, 2011). It is against this background that the journey toward disability mainstreaming in all government ministries was embarked in Lesotho. In the next section we provide some background to the LNFOD.

Lesotho National Federation of Organisations of the Disabled

Lesotho National Federation of Organisations of the Disabled (LNFOD) is an umbrella body of DPOs in Lesotho, which was established in 1989. Its vision is to have a Basotho society that is inclusive of all people. LNFOD is fighting for a society where disabled people enjoy their social, economic and political rights on an equal basis with others and to reach their full potential (equity) in all aspects of development. Its mission is to advocate for, promote and defend the rights of disabled people and their families through provision of training, material and emotional support. It also presents disabled people's needs to government, development partners and the wider community. The membership of LNFOD consists of the Lesotho National Association of Physically Disabled, Intellectual Disability Association of Lesotho, Lesotho National League of the Visually Impaired Persons, and the National Association of the Deaf in Lesotho. Thus, it has a membership of four affiliate DPOs.

Interventions and policy environment for disability mainstreaming in Lesotho

It is against the above outlined situation of disabled people, that the need for intervention cannot be overemphasised. Lesotho ratified the CRPD on 2 December 2008. This followed immense advocacy by LNFOD and its member DPOs undertaken immediately after the adoption of this Convention by the United Nations General Assembly in 2006.

The CRPD seeks to promote, protect and ensure respect and enjoyment of human rights by all disabled people (United Nations, 2006). It does not create new specific rights, but couches the existing human rights into the context of disabled people (Kanter, 2015; French & Kayes, 2008). Its ratification was, therefore, a major milestone achieved by the Government of Lesotho, as our assumption is that it guides the country toward the promotion and protection of the rights of disabled people in Lesotho. The CRPD therefore became the basis for the strong advocacy for disability mainstreaming, inclusion and the protection and promotion of disability rights by LNFOD and its affiliate DPOs.

The ratification of CRPD by Lesotho also has united and strengthened the capacity of the disability movement in terms of advocacy for the elimination of discrimination and marginalisation of disabled people. Hence, disabled people are now taking a lead in domestication process of the CRPD. For example, LNFOD is acting as the technical expert in the drafting section of the Ministry of Law, Human Rights and Constitutional Affairs, which is responsible for drafting disability-specific legislation and the domestication of the CRPD. However, the CRPD is being domesticated at a very slow pace in Lesotho. The piece of legislation domesticating this convention has been in a draft form since 2012. This is because some of its drafters are of the view that disability-specific legislation might advantage disabled people at the expense of the non-disabled people (Sekokotoana, 2016, personal communication). They believe, for example, that if the legislation makes provision for a quota system, the public services might offer more job opportunities to disabled people, thus disadvantaging non-disabled people. They believe that equality requires the same treatment for both disabled and non-disabled people. However, this belief has been criticised as it does not take into account the diverse needs of disabled people, who are usually disadvantaged because of their access needs that are hardly addressed. These include access to information, education and decision-making processes (Bruce *et al.*, 2002). The CRPD thus takes an equitable approach. It requires that disabled people be treated in accordance with their needs and situations (United Nations, 2006). This approach further requires affirmative action be afforded to disabled people, who have been historically disadvantaged, so that they enjoy human rights on an equal basis with others (Bruce *et al.*, 2002).

Article 4 of the CRPD requires governments to adopt legislative, policy and administrative measures that are inclusive of and accessible to disabled people (United Nations, 2006). Hence,

Lesotho is required to enable disabled people to meaningfully participate in decision-making processes. Hence, the promotion of self-representation is required to ensure that the traditionally silenced disabled people's voices are also heard in decision-making processes. This is because disabled people's non-participation in decisions that affect them has denied them the right to influence and direct the course of such decisions. This has consequently fostered their discrimination and marginalisation. However, the challenge is that the provisions of Article 4 do not specify how the implementation should be done as this is entirely determined by states parties. It has therefore led to the long-term exclusion of disabled people in key decision-making processes in Lesotho, resulting in the provision of disability-unfriendly policies and services (LNFOD, 2011).

As a way of domesticating Article 4 of the CRPD, some countries have assigned one ministry as the disability focal point for proper coordination of disability mainstreaming within the government, and one example is Malawi. Lesotho also did the same four years after it ratified the CRPD. Before then, the small unit on disability was attached to the Ministry of Health and Social Welfare, whose functions were seriously hampered by allocating an insignificant budget for the implementation of its activities. Although the ratification of the CRPD by Lesotho was a major milestone, the domestication was challenging because of the delays in designating a disability coordinating ministry. As a result, disability remained invisible in ministerial plans, policies and budgets. This caused disability mainstreaming efforts in Lesotho to be fragmented, with little or no impact on disabled people's lives. In addition, disability mainstreaming within the government, was hampered by the fact that the Ministry of Health and Social Welfare was being informed by the ineffective medical model approach to disability. Such an approach believes that the problem lies within disabled people and not within the society (Chataika & McKenzie, 2016). It is based on the belief that limitations are caused by impairments as opposed to socially constructed challenges, which the proponents of the social model of disability believe are the problem (WHO & World Bank, 2011). This medical approach was therefore criticised by the disability movement as it was seen to be creating negative attitudes toward disabled people, where interventions would then focus on removing impairments as opposed to removing socially constructed barriers. Hence, it was and is still our conviction as LNFOD that the NDMP would direct the government's efforts toward a social model approach to disability mainstreaming in Lesotho.

Article 33 requires state parties to designate a focal point in government to coordinate the implementation of the CRPD (United Nations, 2006). Hence, the Government of Lesotho established a full directorate on disability social services (DSS) in 2012 within the Ministry of Social Development. This ministry, through the DSS, provides among other things assistive technology and vocational training to disabled people. However, this directorate is seriously understaffed, which has led to poor quality coordination of disability issues in Lesotho. Moreover, it is also worth noting that the effectiveness of its interventions has been compromised by the ministry's lack of presence at the grassroots level. However, the establishment of the DSS under the Ministry of Social Development instead of the Ministry of Health and Social Welfare, signals a positive change from the government perspective. Such understanding is in line with the CRPD, which recognises disability as a social rather than a medical disability issue. This approach puts disabled people at the centre of development. It also regards them as agents of development. Thus, with this new approach, our government is better positioned to enable disabled people to influence disability mainstreaming efforts. Also, the new approach shifts the focus from only viewing disabled people as people requiring medical intervention, to focusing on dismantling socially constructed barriers (WHO & World Bank, 2011). Thus, such shift has, to some extent, created an enabling environment for disability mainstreaming in Lesotho.

In addition to the establishment of the DSS, Lesotho devised a series of policy interventions, prompted by the advocacy for implementation of the CRPD. Among others is the

National Strategic Development Plan (NSDP 2012–17). With this policy, the government has committed to include disabled people into the mainstream society, with the aim of optimising social functioning and realising their full potential. To achieve this, the government committed to promoting and protecting the rights of disabled people and facilitating their access to adequate and equitable basic public services. Also, the government undertook to ensure that disabled people enjoy income security and empower them to become self-reliant. Again, the government pledged to promote the prevention and early identification of various forms of impairments and ensure accessibility of the physical environment to disabled people. Through the NSDP, government also has the duty to promote the participation of the disabled people in the national development process and ensuring their access to appropriate habitation and rehabilitation services (Ministry of Social Development, 2011a).

Despite the above good intentions of the NSDP, the government has not yet implemented any of the policy points. This could be attributed to lack of political will, poor coordination, lack of budget allocation, as well as the lack of capacity from respective government ministries. Also, minimal engagement of DPOs in the development of the NSDP has also contributed to the failure of this document to live up to its purpose. Moreover, focusing on integration instead of inclusion of disabled people is one of the flaws that have blocked this policy in guiding the government to achieving disability mainstreaming and, eventually, inclusion (Ministry of Social Development, 2011b).

Despite the minimal engagement, LNFOD, together with its membership, made efforts to advocate for their first-time participation and challenging the government to see disability as a cross-cutting issue that affects all the priorities set out by the NSDP. Among other provisions, this plan includes the training of teachers on inclusive education, making healthcare services and infrastructure accessible to disabled people and providing disability grants. Also, the plan covers issues on the engagement of disabled people in economic activities and provision of Sign Language interpreters for the inclusion of deaf people. LNFOD and its affiliates therefore worked hard to ensure that NSDP mainstreamed disability as a cross-cutting issue to be addressed by all government ministries depending on the role and mandate of each ministry.

Despite its participation in the development of NSDP, LNFOD could not participate in the development of the monitoring and evaluation of this document as it was given to a consultant to do it alone and submit it to the government for adoption. Hence, many stakeholders did not participate in the design of the monitoring and evaluation system, leading to the exclusion of disability-specific targets and indicators by the monitoring and evaluation system. LNFOD tried to influence the inclusion of disability-specific targets and indicators in the monitoring and evaluation system by holding several advocacy activities. However, the organisation did not achieve success with its advocacy work as the government argued that the plan was completed and it could not allow any editing for the sake of disability inclusion.

The consequence of the exclusion of disabled people in the monitoring and evaluation system of the NSDP is that it is, and will be, difficult for Lesotho to measure inclusion and the participation of disabled people in all priorities articulated in this plan. The evaluation report of this plan did not measure the inclusion of disabled people. As a result, Lesotho missed an important component in the implementation of the NSDP by failing to target disabled people. An inclusive evaluation report of this plan would have fully informed future interventions of the government toward disability issues. The attitudinal barriers emanating from the policy-makers therefore excluded disabled people from benefiting from the implementation of this important national document. It has transpired that during the revision of NSDP held from 19 to 23 July 2016, most of the government ministries did not mainstream disability into their ministerial plans because the monitoring and evaluation system of the NSDP did not incorporate inclusive targets. In addition, disability was put in a separate chapter entitled 'cross-cutting issue' but many ministries did not consider this chapter. As a result disability remained highly invisible in the implementation of NSDP by most of the government ministries (Government of Lesotho, 2015).

Lesotho has been able to theoretically mainstream disability within the NSDP which guides the strategic planning of government. It is evident, however, that despite that achievement much work still needs to be done to raise disability onto the national agenda. The Government of Lesotho, particularly the Ministry of Finance, should ensure that budget is allocated for the implementation of the disability-inclusive policies. It is imperative for LNFOD to advocate for the inclusion of disabled people in the upcoming NSDP so that it becomes visible in that plan. Also, the SDGs style of targeting disability (United Nations, 2015) should be adopted by the Government of Lesotho so as to ensure inclusion of disabled people within the strategic targets and indicators of the new NSDP. It is quite significant to mainstream disability in the NSDP so that it forms the basis for the inclusion of disabled people in the ministerial plans and that government can allocate budget for the implementation of the disability-related issues appearing in the plan. The NSDP defines the long-term goals of the government that are implemented by short-term national and ministerial policies and plans. If disability is embedded in the NSDP, all the relevant ministries shall therefore be inclined to mainstreaming disability into their plans and policies so that NSDP becomes a reality.

Despite the challenges aforementioned, the DPOs under the auspices of LNFOD successfully advocated for the development and adoption of the National Disability and Rehabilitation Policy (NDRP) in 2011. The purpose of this policy is to create an environment in which disabled people in Lesotho realise their full potential. Moreover, this policy's aim is that of eliminating all barriers facing disabled people in terms of job opportunities, social protection, education and physical access regarding infrastructure and information. Of most importance is the overarching objective that this policy is to be used as the guiding document for designing, implementing, monitoring and evaluating the generic public and specific policies for the meaningful inclusion of disabled people in Lesotho. The NDRP sets out the priority areas for disability inclusion, which the government will undertake to mainstream disabled people into society: these include access to inclusive education, job opportunities and access to physical infrastructure (Government of Lesotho, 2011).

Unfortunately, this policy was never implemented, particularly by other government ministries such as the Ministry of Health and that of Public Works. This was because the guidelines on the implementation of this policy were never developed by the Ministry of Social Development resulting in difficulties in implementing this policy. Moreover, there was no political will on the part of government to implement the policy. It is difficult if not impossible to come across a disability government policy and strategy on disability emanating from government initiatives. This is maybe due to negative perceptions or ignorance of the senior government officials that disability mainstreaming is burdensome and will be unnecessarily costly as the disabled people are the objects and not the subjects and agents of development (Yeo & Moore, 2003). This situation causes the senior government officials to neglect and ignore the implementation of the disability-related policies.

In LNFOD's advocacy for implementation of this policy, lack of disability policy, strategic action plan, and inadequate capacity to handle disability programming by government ministries were attributed as the contributing factors to the non-implementation of the 2011 NDRP. It was difficult for other ministries to implement the NDRP without the proper coordination and guidance from the Ministry of Social Development which equally lacked the requisite capacity to programme and budget for the disability framework of Lesotho. This is because the Ministry of Social Development was only established in June 2012 and was designated to be the disability focal ministry. However, disabled people continued to face deep inequalities in terms of access to social services, education, employment and justice, since the Ministry of Social Development did not act as the advocate of disabled people within the government. In addition, the ministry does not budget for the effective implementation of the disability-related policies despite robust advocacy on budget allocation for the disability-related framework by LNFOD and its affiliate DPOs. However, despite the above challenges, the NDRP remains an important advocacy tool for the promotion and protection of the human rights of disabled people, in the sense that it creates the basis for further disability advocacy for mainstreaming in Lesotho.

Through strengthening the social protection of vulnerable people, the Government of Lesotho, through the Ministry of Social Development, committed to assist LNFOD to publish and publicise the NDMP and improve the capacity of frontline officers, specifically those in charge of implementing rehabilitation within the Ministry of Social Development to deal with issues of disability. In addition, under this strategy, the government committed to work with LNFOD to review disability grants, copying neighbouring countries (e.g. South Africa, Namibia and Botswana). The government also committed to developing suitable mechanisms and procedures for the definition and classification of impairments, based on global best practice appearing in international frameworks such as the WHO's International Classification of Impairment, Disabilities and Handicaps. In addition, the government undertook to register all those defined as having severe impairments and chronic illnesses in the national information system database, on an on-demand basis, Moreover, the government will design and implement a disability grant for all those who are severely disabled above the age of eligibility for the infant grant and below the age of eligibility for the old age pension. Equally important also is that the government undertook to build linkages with other ministries, and with NGOs that work with disabled people to strengthen families, deliver assistive technology, reduce barriers to access issues and provide vocational training.

The above social protection strategy has attempted to mainstream disability by articulating on the actions to be undertaken to promote the inclusion and protection of disabled people in Lesotho. However, no budget has yet been allocated for its implementation to improve the social protection of disabled people. The only achievement regarding the implementation of the above-mentioned strategy is the adoption of the NDMP.

National Disability Mainstreaming Plan 2015

Building upon the above-stated initiatives on disability mainstreaming, Lesotho adopted the NDMP in 2015, which seeks to mainstream disability within all the government annual plans and programmes. Disability mainstreaming is a

> strategy for making the concerns and experiences of disabled people an integral dimension of the design, implementation, monitoring, and evaluation of policies and programmes in all political, economic, and societal spheres so that disabled people benefit equally.
>
> *(Handicap International, 2009, p. 5)*

Processes of mainstreaming disability in plans can be divided into five steps, namely; initiation, analysis, formulation, implementation, and monitoring and evaluation.

Initiation stage

This is where LNFOD and the Ministry of Social Development mapped the stakeholders to be involved in the development of the baseline survey and the NDMP. LNFOD and the Ministry of Social Development had regular monthly meetings in which they shared progress on the implementation of disability-related programmes on various aspects of development. It was in one of these progress meetings that LNFOD introduced the new project on disability mainstreaming, namely, Communities of Practice in Disability Advocacy for Mainstreaming (COPDAM). In Lesotho, this project was aimed at building the capacity of LNFOD to negotiate policies with government and other key development partners and to take the leading role in the development of the NDMP. One of the key activities envisaged in this project was the development of the NDMP intended to assist all government ministries to mainstream disability into ministerial plans. Considering the primary role of the Ministry of Social Development in the advancement of disability rights, LNFOD lobbied this ministry to develop the NDMP in consultation with all stakeholders to be involved in the implementation stage of the mainstreaming plan.

Formulation stage

At the formulation stage, the Ministry of Social Development and LNFOD agreed to conduct the baseline survey to determine the extent of disability inclusion in all government ministries so that the findings of the baseline study could fully inform the content of the NDMP. The overall purpose of the baseline study was to build a knowledge base through the production and dissemination of a report on the current status with regard to disability mainstreaming in the country (LNFOD, 2011). This was to support the development of the NDMP by government. It also assisted the government, DPOs and Civil Society Organisations (CSOs) to generate reliable evidence and to use the information for further planning and campaigning for inclusive policy development and implementation. In addition, the study established the extent to which existing legislation and programmes in Lesotho are disability inclusive.

The National Strategic Development Plan (NDSP) is a government document that highlights what ministries have already done and their intended plans for disability mainstreaming. It also highlights the gaps and challenges, thus providing research evidence meant to assist government ministries in their planning for disability mainstreaming. It will also assist DPOs to think through what they will prioritise for their advocacy, lobbying and awareness campaigns. Of course, one would perhaps say that this information was already known and that there was no need for a baseline. However, this information was known by few policy makers who usually file the documents in their drawers. It was extremely useful to bring it all together in one consolidated document.

The study was successfully conducted and validated by the stakeholders (see LNFOD, 2011). It was clear that there was lack of disability mainstreaming in government policies, programmes and services. This is because of lack of awareness and capacity for doing so from various stakeholders. Only the Ministry of Education and Training and that of Social Development were found to be dealing with disability even though most disability-related activities of these ministries were not government-funded. UNICEF was found to be the only United Nations agency providing the budget support for the education of children with disabilities. Another challenge was the absence of the disability focal persons in all government ministries to advocate for the participation of disabled people in the planning, implementation, monitoring and evaluation of national development processes. It was therefore found to be difficult to implement effective disability mainstreaming (LNFOD, 2011).

Finally, the study revealed that there was no strategic planning in disability mainstreaming to guide the implementation of the programmes and services of the government toward disability inclusion. Hence, it was recommended that the NDMP and the government ministries receive training on disability mainstreaming as the starting point for the meaningful inclusion of disabled people in the public sector services (LNFOD, 2011).

Informed by the baseline survey, LNFOD and the Ministry of Social Development found it worthwhile to engage other government ministries from the initial stage of the NDMP in order to enable each ministry to determine the actions to be undertaken in the mainstreaming processes. As a result, the Ministry of Social Development and LNFOD developed the terms of reference for the consultant who was to be engaged to assist with the writing up of the NDMP. It is crucial for countries to develop national disability mainstreaming plans to guide different ministries and departments on how to mainstream disability in their own plans, programmes and policies. A government ministry, department or unit responsible for coordinating disability issues in each country should be responsible for leading the development of the NDMP. The development should be done with inputs from different government ministries, national disability federations, DPOs and CSOs.

The NDMP includes targets and indicators for each government sector, which will then form part of their individual annual plans. In order to achieve this, the Ministry of Social Development successfully encouraged the appointment of the Disability focal persons from the ministries of Education and Training; Justice and Correctional Services; Health; Law, Human Rights and Constitutional Affairs; Communication, Science and Technology; Public Works and Transport; Energy; Trade and Industry; and Labour and Employment. In order to ensure that the disability focal persons become effective, it was proposed by LNFOD that persons to be appointed as focal persons should be senior government officials who are in the position to make decisions on behalf of their ministries. However, other government ministries did not honour the request from LNFOD and the Ministry of Social Development. Nevertheless, this negative response created the basis for further advocacy on the appointment of focal persons in the ministries in which they had not been previously appointed.

The ministerial disability focal persons have multiple roles in ensuring the disability mainstreaming within their respective ministries. They are responsible for conducting an analysis of legislation and policies, programmes and services of the government institutions to ensure effective disability mainstreaming. In addition, they have to facilitate capacity development of their respective ministries so that office bearers are able to account for disability inclusion, budgeting and planning. They are further granted responsibility to guide and support government ministries and institutions in providing accurate and timely information for the purposes of reporting to international treaties such as the CRPD. Facilitating performance agreements of senior managers to reflect developmental obligations for disability mainstreaming is also their crucial role. Equally important is that these focal persons provide support and guidance to government institutions and the private sector institutions as well as the CSOs in disability mainstreaming. Last, ministerial disability focal persons compel ministerial officials to submit quarterly and annual reports on the progress on the implementation of the departmental or ministerial programmes of action for the equalisation of opportunities for disabled people.

LNFOD and the Ministry of Social Development agreed to engage a consultant to lead the process of formulating the NDMP. There was a need to train the disability focal persons from the ministries so that they would be able to analyse their policies, programmes and services regarding the inclusion of disabled people. The understanding was that the training would enable the effective participation of these focal persons in the development of the NDMP. The training for the focal persons was organised by both LNFOD and the disability focal ministry in which the consultant was invited to start interacting with the ministerial disability focal persons. After that, the consultant began a series of consultative meetings with the focal persons and other senior government officials about how disability could be mainstreamed in their programmes. The consultation process took longer than expected because there was lack of interest in dealing with disability mainstreaming by other government ministries. In fact, some are still of the opinion that disability should be dealt with solely by the Ministry of Social Development.

The consultant developed the NDMP in consultation with the focal persons, DPOs, CSOs and leading commercial forum in Lesotho. He submitted reports to the Ministry of Social Development as a coordinating ministry and to LNFOD as the umbrella body of DPOs. LNFOD also had meetings where the inception, draft and final reports were reviewed and inputs and comments compiled and submitted to the consultant for his consideration. Sometimes the consultant would be part of the review meetings, depending on the magnitude of the comments provided by the stakeholders. The series of consultative meetings were held with the DPOs working in Lesotho to establish what they need to incorporate into the plan and determine their role in the implementation stage.

A validation workshop was conducted where all the stakeholders gathered to make a final review of the plan. The NDMP was adopted as the action plan of the government to inform the ministerial plans for the disability mainstreaming. Out of 22 government ministries, 12 were actively involved in the development of the NDMP. The plan seeks to mainstream disability in the areas of health, education, basic social services, access to infrastructure and information, recognition of people before and under the law, access to healthcare services, livelihoods, capacity building of the government officials, social protection, capacity building, and removal of disability discriminatory laws. The Ministry of Social Development launched the plan, to which all stakeholders were invited along with the development partners who were lobbied to support its implementation. It was at this launch that the NDMP was distributed among the disability focal persons, DPOs and other stakeholders.

Implementation stage

The NDMP was adopted in October 2015. This was immediately after the government ministries had prepared their budget paper. Hence, LNFOD launched the advocacy on the disability mainstreaming into the existing budget paper so that the implementation could start in the fiscal year 2016–17. As a result, the Ministry of Social Development, as the coordinating ministry, budgeted for the quarterly progress meetings in which all focal persons come together to discuss the progress and challenges facing the implementation of the NDMP. The first quarterly progress meeting was to be held in August 2016 in which the focal persons would share the disability-related activities to be undertaken from the master plan into the ministerial plan. This means that Lesotho is now in the implementation stage, which is the most critical stage for all the stakeholders involved in the implementation and the beneficiaries as well. The first quarterly meeting was meant to look into how the ministerial focal persons might work together with other departments from the same ministry to identify and mainstream disability activities into their upcoming annual ministerial plans. The quarterly meeting would have gone further to build the knowledge and understanding of the ministerial focal persons on how they can mainstream disability-related activities into their 2017–18 annual ministerial budgets. This is a crucial process of mainstreaming disability. However, none of these quarterly meetings were held and no explanation has been given by the Ministry of Social Development in this regard.

For effective implementation of the NDMP, there should be intensive undertaking of the capacity-building sessions which will assist the focal persons to advocate for effective disability inclusion within the ministries (Chataika *et al.*, 2011). The focal persons should be equipped with the various skills of imparting disability-related programming, which might help the ministries to meaningfully include disability in their daily activities. It is worth mentioning that the ministerial disability focal persons require more training on disability mainstreaming so that they can perform their disability-related functions effectively (ibid.). Nevertheless, they are not yet exposed to the international conferences on disability and programming, which could hinder effective operationalisation of disability mainstreaming. The ministerial focal persons should, as a matter of policy, undergo capacity development training on disability rights so that they can build their confidence and self-esteem in becoming the advocates of disabled people within their ministries. The government must also give out the directive to all the government ministries to mainstream disability through their ministerial plans informed by the NDMP 2015.

Monitoring and evaluation system of the National Disability Mainstreaming Plan

The monitoring and evaluation system of the NDMP is not yet developed because the Ministry of Social Development has communicated that it intends to incorporate the plan into their already existing ministerial monitoring and evaluation plan. However, LNFOD and its alliances are in the position to monitor the implementation of the NDMP through its advocacy strategy, which targets the implementation of national development activities, among other priorities.

Lessons learned

LNFOD as a civil society organisation has been working with the government through the Ministry of Social Development to develop the NDMP. The successful partnership between the two institutions marks a major achievement considering the nature of the relationship between the DPOs and the government. Disability activists and DPOs should be armed with the knowledge on disability mainstreaming in order to convince the government about the need to develop the NDMP (Wazakili *et al.*, 2011). Gone are the days when disabled people make disability their own agenda. In the process of disability mainstreaming, all stakeholders should be involved no matter how negative their attitude might be toward disability issues; hence the need for disability awareness raising.

Many senior government officials are not aware of disability issues and perhaps do not have enough time to learn about the disability inclusion and mainstreaming. Hence, the development of the disability mainstreaming plans might be delayed or hampered by the senior government officials fearing that they may not have the knowledge to deal with such processes (Wazakili *et al.*, 2011). The role of disability activists and DPOs is to convince the government of their full support toward the development of such a plan. Sometimes, when DPOs lobby for the development of the NDMP, governments may stop the advocacy by claiming that they lack the funds to commence such initiatives. The advocacy group should be able to mobilise the basic funds, which could enable the process of developing the plan. Second, it should be indicated from the very beginning that disability mainstreaming does not only require specialist expertise, but rather, political will (Chataika, 2013). In fact, the stakeholders can develop it alone if there are no funds to engage the consultant. Most importantly, the disability advocacy groups must understand disability as a human rights and development issue rather than a social welfare issue (WHO & World Bank, 2011). Thus, it requires intensive advocacy, lobbying and time to change the mindset of policy makers for them to view disability as a human right, cross-cutting and development agenda.

Reflective questions

1   What are the essentials of disability mainstreaming that you can draw from Lesotho's experience?
2   What are the major challenges of coming up with a disability mainstreaming plan that you have learned from Lesotho's experience?
3   How would you ensure meaningful participation of all the stakeholders in disability mainstreaming?

References

Bruce, A., Burke, C., Castellino, J., Kenna, P., Kilkelly, U., Quinn, U., Degner, T. & Quinlivan, S. (2002). *Human Rights and Disability: The Current and Potential United Nations Human Rights Instruments in the Context of Disability* (2nd ed.). Geneva: United Nations.

Bureau of Statistics (2006). *Lesotho Population and Housing Census Analytic Report IIIB.* Retrieved from www.bos.gov.ls/New%20Folder/Copy%20of%20Demography/2006_Analytical_Report_Volume_IIIB_Socio-Economic_Characteristics.pdf on 14 May 2017.

Chataika, T. (2012). Postcolonialism, disability and development. In D. Goodley & B. Hughes (eds) *Social Theories of Disability: New Developments and Directions* (pp. 252–269). London: Routledge.

Chataika, T. (2013). Cultural and religious explanations of disability and promoting inclusive communities. In J. M. Claassen, L. Swartz & L. Hansen (eds) *Search for Dignity: Conversations on Human Dignity, Theology and Disability* (pp. 117–128). Cape Town: African Sun Media.

Chataika, T. & McKenzie, J. A. (2016). Global institutions and their engagement with disability mainstreaming in the South: development and (dis)connections. In S. Grech & K. Soldatic (eds) *Disability in the Global South: The Critical Handbook* (pp. 423–436). Switzerland: Springer International Publishing.

Chataika, T., Mulumba, M., Mji, G. & MacLachlan, M. (2011). *Did What? Research Project in Brief: The African Policy on Disability & Development (A-PODD) in Uganda.* Dublin: The Global Health Press.

French, P. & Kayes, R. (2008). Out of darkness into light? Introducing the Convention on the Rights of Persons with Disabilities. *Human Rights Law Review* **8**, 1–34.

Government of Lesotho (2011). *The National Disability and Rehabilitation Policy.* Retrieved from www.lnfod.org.ls on 26 April 2018.

Government of Lesotho (2012). *National Strategic Development Plan 2012/13–2016/17.* Retrieved from www.gov.ls/gov_webportal/important%20documents/national%20strategic%20development%20plan%20201213-201617/national%20strategic%20development%20plan%20201213-201617.pdf on 17 March 2017.

Government of Lesotho (2015). *National Disability Mainstreaming Plan.* Retrieved from www.lnfod.org.ls on 26 April 2018.

Grech, S. (2016). Disability and development: critical connections, gaps and contradictions. In S. Grech & K. Soldatic (eds) *Disability in the Global South: The Critical Handbook* (pp. 3–19). Switzerland: Springer International Publishing.

Handicap International (2009). *Training Manual on Inclusive Development.* Retrieved from http://www.handicap-international.us/disability_rights on 24 April 2017.

Kanter, A. S. (2015). *The Development of Disability Rights under International Law: From Charity to Human Rights.* Milton Park: Routledge.

Lesotho National Federation of the Organizations of the Disabled (2011). *Living Conditions Among People with Disabilities: A National Representative Study.* Retrieved from www.lnfod.org.ls on 2 May 2017.

Ministry of Social Development (2011a). *National Disability and Rehabilitation Policy.* Retrieved from www.lnfod.org.ls on 17 March 2017.

Ministry of Social Development (2011b). *National Disability Mainstreaming Plan*. Retrieved from www.lnfod.org.ls on 17 March 2017.

Moore, K. &Yeo, R. (2003). Including people with disabilities in poverty reduction work: nothing about us without us. *World Development* **31**(1), 571–590.

United Nations (2006). *The Convention on the Rights of Persons with Disabilities and Optional Protocol*. New York: United Nations. Retrieved from www.un.org/disabilities/documents/convention/convopt prot-e.pdf on 15 May 2016.

United Nations (2015). *Sustainable Development Goals: 17 Goals that Sustains Our Lives*. Retrieved from www.un.org/sustainabledevelopment/sustainable-development-goals/ on 20 April 2017.

Washington Group on Disability Statistics (2014). *The Washington Group Short Set of Questions on Disability*. New York: United Nations. Retrieved from www.washingtongroup-disability.com/wp-content/uploads/2016/01/The-Washington-Group-Short-Set-of-Questions-on-Disability.pdf on 1 October 2018.

Wazakili, M., Chataika, T., Mji, G., Dube, A. K. & MacLachlan, M. (2011). The social inclusion of persons with disabilities in poverty reduction policies and instruments: initial impressions from Malawi and Uganda. In A. H. Eide & B. Ingstad (eds) *Disability and Poverty: A Global Challenge* (pp. 15–29). Bristol: Policy Press.

World Health Organization & World Bank (2011). *World Report on Disability*. Geneva: WHO.

Yeo, R. & Moore, K. (2003). Including disabled people in poverty reduction work: nothing about us, without us. *World Development* **31**(3), 571–590.

4

THEATRE FOR DEVELOPMENT

Bringing disabled students' hidden transcripts out of the closet

Nehemiah Chivandikwa

Introduction

In this chapter, I acknowledge and analyse the unrecognised (and private) resistive powers or 'hidden transcripts' (Scott, 1985, 1990) of disabled young people and how this power and agency can be nurtured and appropriated for transition into the public domain (resistive public transcript) in Theatre for Development (TfD) discourses. The hidden transcripts are in sharp contrast to the feigned respect, obedience and docility of oppressed people (public transcripts), when they are in the presence of their dominators (Scott, 1990). The hidden transcripts as resistance are necessary for the liberation and self-construction of disabled young people in publicly challenging their oppression and marginalisation. TfD is basically the use of participatory theatre in the service of holistic development that emphasises humanistic elements of growth – such as creativity, self-esteem, civic mindedness among target communities (Mda, 1993) – and how they are implicated in material and economic development (Baxter, 2009). TfD is largely inspired by Paulo Freire's (1970) liberatory pedagogy in which learners and communities are expected to be agents of their development/learning in transforming social situations that limit their humanistic growth.

I recognise that there is a need to appreciate the level of resistance and critical consciousness among disabled young people and not approach them as mere passive victims of impairment and social oppression, but rather as complex citizens with agency (Campbell, 2009). Yet this agency or knowledge is also limited (Campbell, 2008), and it might need to be complemented with outside knowledge from social scientists, critical art practitioners and critical disability activists and researchers. However, crucially, researchers and development facilitators need to respect the local knowledge of disabled participants (Rahman, 1993). In many cases, such resistive knowledge is hidden from the general populace; academics, policy makers and civil society (see Seda & Chivandikwa, 2014). The tendency is to treat disabled citizens as objects of study/charity or sites of medical attention (Campbell, 2009). Perhaps this is why it is rare to find TfD projects on disability in Zimbabwe (Chivandikwa & Muwonwa, 2013). Where they may occur, development partners are likely to treat disabled communities as objects and not subjects of development (Chivandikwa, 2016). Yet within an idyllic humanistic development perspective, no body develops another (Odhiambo, 2008). The outside animator/facilitator combines his/her external technical knowledge with the ontological knowledge of the disabled communities (Rahman, 1993). As a result, it is critical to access the ontological knowledge of disabled participants to use it as a foundation for their self-liberation. In this regard, it was important for me as a TfD facilitator to work with disabled communities to access their social, political and intellectual knowledge, as well as their ontological experience in order to learn from them and utilise them for their own advancement.

In light of the foregoing observations, I facilitated a TfD project with University of Zimbabwe students in which we wanted to explore, challenge and subvert the marginalisation and oppression of disabled people on campus and beyond. The details of the larger project are provided elsewhere (see Chinyowa & Chivandikwa, 2017; Chivandikwa & Muwonwa, 2013). In this chapter, my focus is on the preliminaries of the project in which I largely accessed the resistive power of disabled students. This approach was partly inspired by Thompson (2003, p. 34), who argues that in most cases, analyses of participatory theatre projects concentrate on artistic workshops and performances at the expense of surrounding events such as meetings, demonstrations and promotions leading and relating to the topic under investigation. It is in such encounters that I accessed hidden powers of disabled people that are not normally available in public spaces. In this chapter, however, I concentrate on the period before the theatrical performances, which largely functioned as 'raw materials' for constructing the theatrical performances that subsequently emerged. I analyse workshops, informal discussions in students' residences and private spaces and informal research processes as hidden transcripts (Scott 1985, 1990), which required my skills as the facilitator to enable their transition into public transcripts (resistive public dramatic performances). I pose the following questions: What forms of hidden transcripts exist among university disabled students? How might such hidden transcripts be accessed and nurtured to facilitate their transition into the 'resistive public transcript'?

Participatory theatre for development and critical disability perspectives

Over the years there has been a growing recognition and appreciation of the use of theatre in development projects and programmes in the developing world (Manukonda, 2013). This interest is largely predicated on two major considerations, namely, that theatre is an effective tool in enhancing development communication, and that it has the capacity to motivate target communities into participating and making sound decisions on issues, programmes and projects relating to their own development (Mda, 1993). Disabled people are generally excluded from participating in development practice and theory (Breeden, 2008).

I use the term disability in this chapter to refer to the social oppression of people with impaired bodies (see Breeden, 2008; Oliver, 2004). I share the view that impairment is a legitimate and unique bodily or corporeal human characteristic that is, however, considered 'defective' by normative culture (see Cameron, 2010). Although sometimes considered as a 'touchy' term (ibid.), impairment is a biological, physical and cognitive feature/condition or mechanism of the human body parts which might not perform specific 'typical' functions (Harris & Enfield, 2003). Regrettably, normative society generally considers anything that is not 'typical' as deficient and abnormal (Breeden, 2008). However, since oppression happens on and through the body (Campbell, 2009); impaired bodies can also be referred to as disabled bodies. In the larger project from which this research derives (see Chivandikwa & Muwonwa, 2013; Chivandikwa, 2016), I focus on how TfD might be a site to validate the disabled body in order to recognise and celebrate it as a unique and legitimate human characteristic.

Given that the disabled body is the site for disability oppression (Hamilton, 2008), I realise that the body is implicated in development discourse much more than TfD scholarship has acknowledged. By extension, TfD and its participatory aspirations, has to engage in disability and development. Critical disability perspectives recognise disability oppression as the complex interrelationship between impairment, individual response and the social environment (Hosking, 2008). Most relevant to TfD discourse are three major characteristics of critical disability perspectives. The first is that critical disability theory raises critical questions about access, participation, inclusion and exclusion. The second aspect is that critical disability perspectives are concerned with matters of liberty, equality, belonging, agency identity and distribution (Hosking, 2008). All these issues are directly implicated in participatory human-centred development – a key theme in TfD discourse and practice (see Mda, 1993). Hence, critical disability perspectives challenge notions of normalcy and deviance (Hosking, 2008). In this regard, just like TfD, critical disability perspectives challenge taken for granted power-laden discourses (see Plastow, 2014). Last, just like TfD critical disability perspectives are forms of praxis (Freire, 1970), because they combine and try to balance between theory and practice (Hosking, 2008). In the same manner, TfD is simultaneously an ideology, an intervention and a methodology (Odhiambo, 2008). TfD specifically seeks to subvert hegemonies that limit opportunities and access to participation, leading to critical consciousness and the practical removal of barriers to development (Manukonda, 2013). Therefore, TfD resonates with critical disability and wider development discourses in ways that are yet to be fully acknowledged and this means there is need for more TfD projects on disability.

Preliminaries, surrounding events, hidden transcripts

This section discusses aspects of TfD work that are often overlooked by scholars of participatory applied theatre work (Thompson, 2003). Participatory applied theatre is an interdisciplinary field that adopts works and strategies from other disciplines (Mda, 1993). To this extent, what happens before and after a rehearsal, performance or artistic workshop is critical to understanding the transformative and ideological function of TfD projects. When 'trespassing' into unfamiliar territories, it is therefore important to take into account 'non-theatrical' activities and contexts that inevitably impact on the 'actual' theatre work. Thompson (2003, p. 34) highlights the importance of surrounding events such as meetings, planning sessions and promotions before the performance and he argues that they actually take more time than the rehearsals and performances. I consider the preliminaries and surrounding events as inseparable from the context and discourses surrounding disability. They are part and parcel of the project and not 'mere' preliminaries. The meetings, discussions, seminars and formal research processes that the students participated in constitute part of hidden transcripts on disability politics among disabled students. They enabled me to appreciate the nature and complexity of resistance to normalising discourses and practices among disabled students.

When power is exerted, complex responses and reactions become possible and these responses include resistance to dominating power relations (Foucault, 2001, p. 240). Foucault's observation links with Scott's (1990) theory on hidden transcripts and public transcripts, which essentially refer to the fact that dominated people are not always passive pawns in the power 'game'. Rather, they oscillate between subservience and resistance. In this regard, Scott (1990) argues that the oppressed publicly feign respect and obedience to their oppressors or dominators. They pretend to be very docile and loyal to those in authority. This feigned obedience and respect is what is referred to as the 'public transcript'. In private, however, oppressed people engage in various forms of 'power performances' (Mbembe, 1992, p. 3) which challenge and mock their oppressors, and these private forms of resistance are what Scott (1990) refers to as 'hidden transcripts'. They include humour, self-assertion, slander, pilfering, sabotage, evasions, disobedience, laughter, mockery, anger and bitter criticism (Scott, 1990, p. 78). The next sections examine the manifestations and nature of hidden transcripts in the project under study. I will describe and discuss how we collectively made attempts to use these hidden transcripts as sites of unmasking invalidating and oppressive discourses and strengthening the critical abilities of disabled students to celebrate their identities.

'Accidental' access into hidden transcripts

I 'accidentally' accessed private forms of students' 'rebellion' against ableist marginalisation on 6 March 2008, as I was waiting for my TfD students in my office. My office is located in a building that has three floors – the ground floor, the second floor and the third floor. The ground floor immediately below my office houses the Disability Resource Centre (DRC), where disabled students meet for various academic, personal and recreational activities and services (see Chataika, 2007). On that particular day, the 'noise' that came from the centre made it very difficult for me to concentrate and frustrated me immensely. As I was about to 'descend' on the 'noisy' students, my attention was drawn to the content of the 'noise' and I found myself intrigued by the discussion presented in Box 4.1.

While at times critically and humorously appropriating the language of the 'oppressor', such as *chirema* (cripple), the disabled students discussed their marginalisation very freely in private. They linked all forms of marginalisation to their bodies. Their discussion, while intriguing, revealed the complexity of the identities of disabled students that I had taken for granted. What

---

Box 4.1   Accidental access into hidden transcripts

Student 1: *Iwe shamwari hazviite kuti ndidanane nemunhu ari* non-disabled. (My friend I can't possibly go out with a non-disabled person!)

Student 2: *Zvinoita vakawanda vamwe vanenge vachitokuda but imi vanhu vari* disabled *ndimi munongotyira kure* (But you can! They are so many non-disabled people who want to go out with disabled people. The problem is that you disabled people are very timid) (noise, laughter and interjection).

Student 3: No *Shaz*, (my friend), love is blind (laughter and injections).

Student 1: No. I know that, but the problem is that relatives and friends might pressurise the girl or boy who might be genuine.

Student 2: *Imi vanhu vane madisability ndimi dambudziko* (you disabled people are the problem because you look down upon yourself) (noise).

Student 4: Some people are not genuine. They want to use disabled people. I don't believe that there can be genuine love between a non-disabled person and a disabled one.

Student 1: It's not easy. Because your chances . . . of getting a job are slim and this makes it difficult especially, if you are a boy – you are expected to be a breadwinner. The girl will say; *Chirema changu ndinochida* (I love my crippled boyfriend), the parents will say: *unochidii chirema chisingashandi* (of what use to you is a crippled boyfriend without a job?)

Student 3: No. Such parents are both ignorant and stupid.

Student 2: They are no different from University of Zimbabwe workers who treat us as if we should be grateful for coming to university.

Students 1: Don't blame them, some of them are frustrated because they could not manage to pass even their 'O' Levels. So they are angry because they think they failed to do what the disabled can do.

Student 4: You are right; some of them have children with big bodies who cannot spell their names, and you think they will be happy to see a little boy in a wheelchair doing Law? No ways!!!!

Student 3: Now I think you are talking about big *dhara* (old man) (laughter).

---

struck me right from the start was how critical the students were of discourses and practices that 'othered' their bodies. This 'private' discussion was a form of hidden transcript in which the students mocked and challenged their oppressors, namely non-disabled officials and fellow students in particular, and non-disabled people in general. From this initial encounter with disabled students, I was therefore disabused of the common notion that subordinated groups of people are perpetually compliant (see Scott, 1985; Foucault, 1980). The private discussion I overheard among disabled students was laced with jokes, rumours and insults. Non-disabled bodies were simultaneously 'admired', mocked and insulted. These subversive attitudes appeared to be an expression of disabled students' struggles (see Mbembe, 1992, p. 3). As an aspiring facilitator, therefore, I was going to be an agent of an already existing hidden transcript, unlike some TfD projects which purport to create 'awareness' on issues that are presumably unknown by the local target community (Baxter, 2009).

Having 'accidentally' accessed hidden transcripts, I was encouraged to deliberately search (ethically and systematically) for means in which to encourage disabled students to reveal what they usually say in the absence of oppressive able-bodied people in general. I organised a meeting in which I asked them to consider participating in a project to research and challenge the marginalisation of disabled people. In this project, they would work together with my TfD students. I therefore involved them in various forms of research and informal conversations to achieve this objective.

Searches for hidden transcripts

The above was a major eye opener to the existence of forms of resistance among disabled students. It was important to identify more spaces and strategies for accessing private performances of power which are critical in the crafting of complex identities of disabled students in order to enrich the theatrical content of the project. The complication was that by their very nature, hidden transcripts are meant to be private. Subsequent sections will show how I tried to solve this paradox.

As will be explored in subsequent sections, informal and semi-formal discussions provided space in which disabled students could make remarks about previous experiences, revealing some of the 'guerrilla' tactics they used to critically and disrespectfully talk about non-disabled bodies and 'powerful' people in general. My casual engagements with participating disabled students in private spaces such as students' rooms were occasions in which hidden transcripts came out spontaneously. I encouraged participating non-disabled theatre arts and disabled students to mingle freely and sociably with different disabled students in different forums so as to increase the chances of accessing as much 'dissident' behaviour as possible. Generally it is not easy for disabled people to create common bonds, giving rise to organised hidden transcripts at group level (Oliver, 2004). I therefore argue that it is the duty of facilitators in sociopolitical projects on disability to create forums in which disabled people can spontaneously or deliberately express dissent. However, if this becomes difficult, informal research processes with individuals are also helpful. As a result, participating students visited colleagues and used informal discussions to determine the nature and manifestations of hidden transcripts among disabled students.

The above-mentioned processes revealed the following manifestations of hidden transcripts:

- satirical drawings of lecturers and administrators;
- verbal mimicking of patronising pastors;
- biting and bitter criticism of university middle managers;

- mocking non-disabled people's fear of disabled bodies;
- ascribing nicknames to 'helpers';
- exuberant celebrations with music and dance in the DRC library.

The above forms of hidden transcripts became the foundational basis for the construction of plays that publicly challenged the marginalisation of disabled students. Clearly, the 'power performances' or 'practices of freedom' (Foucault, 1988) of disabled students remain largely unrecognised. However, Scott (1985, 1990) notes that these hidden transcripts are more spontaneous than organised. They occur largely at personal levels and/or they are shared among very close friends. Yet researchers and TfD facilitators can deploy strategies such as sustained and continuous encounters with disabled people to learn from them and also to encourage them to reveal what they usually say in private. This is what the students who participated in the project under consideration did (Chivandikwa, 2016). Yet to an extent, this research confirms Scott's theory. In most cases, visually impaired students engaged in subversive activities among themselves, while physically impaired students generally did the same. However, there were students with different types of impairments who also engaged in hidden transcripts in small groups. Although these transcripts were significant, they were hidden from the public realm. Such forms of resistance are drowned out by grand narratives of overt power relations in normative politics, and because of this preoccupation with grand narratives, TfD scholarship on power tends to miss multiplex and sophisticated dimensions of localised power struggles (see Foucault, 1988). The following paragraphs show how sustained encounters might enable facilitators to access and publicly celebrate resistive hidden transcripts within the public TfD performance context.

Hidden transcripts become public transcripts when the dominated group manages to convey the message of rebellion in an unambiguous manner in a public forum (Scott, 1985). However, this is usually difficult to achieve if the community is not sufficiently organised in socio-political terms. I realised that preliminaries and surrounding events in participatory TfD processes are important sites in which to prepare disabled people for a direct confrontation with their dominators without facing serious personal and group risks. However, since disabled people did not have a coherent political movement, it was difficult to convince them to openly challenge their 'oppressors'. Consequently, the facilitation process played a significant role in psychologically, socially and intellectually preparing disabled students to negotiate the transition from hidden transcripts to resistive public transcripts.

In the following section, I describe how I facilitated the transition by organising preliminary meetings to establish a working relation with the community. Together with the disabled students, we christened the first big meeting: the Great *Indaba*. I will explore how I managed to motivate the students to take interest in disability politics by narrating to them two stories to explain my unforgettable encounters with disabled students when I was still a university student. I will use the narratives to show complexities surrounding hidden transcripts and public transcripts in the context under consideration. I will argue that there is a need to appreciate the complexities surrounding hidden transcripts and public transcripts in disability contexts in order to successfully negotiate the transition from private resistance to public resistance. In the case of TfD, this simply means the transition from private and isolated rebellious conversations into collectively expressing resistance in a public theatre forum.

The Great *Indaba*: hidden transcripts–public transcripts dialectics

The Great *Indaba* took place at 2.15 pm on 5 April 2010 at the University of Zimbabwe's Beit Hall. Thirteen Honours and 12 Bachelor of Arts (BA) General Students attended, as did

89 students from DRC, which was more than 98% of the total disabled students registered at the centre. Three professionals from DRC (including the coordinator) also attended the meeting. Initially, there was tension before we started the meeting because the disabled students were generally suspicious of non-disabled researchers and 'well-wishers' (see Chivandikwa & Muwonwa, 2013, p. 56). However; I realised that such situations demanded honesty, transparency and sensitivity. I made a 'speech' that I considered the turning point in the project. I transcribed this speech, presented in Box 4.2, not only because it marked the beginning of a good relationship between disabled students and myself, but also because the speech was strategically laced with body-based humorous elements, which provided the thematic content of the project – body politics.

Before looking at responses to the speech, I want to briefly analyse Taurai and Kuda's narratives in terms of the hidden transcript-public transcript dialectic. On one hand, the two

---

Box 4.2   The Great *Indaba* speech

Good afternoon ladies and gentlemen (complete silence) . . . mmm as you would know, my name is Mr Nehemiah Chivandikwa. I am a lecturer here. I have three children and one legitimate wife (laughter). My totem is Soko . . . and I wonder how many of you are my relatives in that regard (five disabled students excitedly raise their hands followed by inaudible interjections).

There was one visually challenged young man – let us say his name was Kuda. He was funny, and very charming (cheers from disabled male students) and perhaps controversial. In one student union meeting where aspiring candidates for the union leadership were campaigning, he really undressed one candidate, by using what I call vulgar language. (Some students demand from me the exact words that Kuda spoke.) Well the words were so crude that I am embarrassed to repeat them. But in essence, his insult involved some sensitive parts of the human anatomy (laughter and inaudible interjections). And you know as Africans we do not usually pronounce some parts of the human anatomy especially in public (some students shout to urge me to continue without verbalising the exact words spoken by Kuda).

A student sitting next to me challenged Kuda in Shona and said '*Kuda haunyare here kutaura zvinonyadzisa pakazara vanhu*' (Kuda are you not ashamed of speaking such vulgar language in the presence of so many people?). His response was in Shona. He said, 'Ndinonyara ndinoona here? (How can I be ashamed? Do I have eyes to see anyone?') (raucous laughter) Okay! Okay! Second story. In 1996, I was doing my fourth year Bachelor of Arts Honours Degree in Theatre Arts. So on this day, as cadres, we were preparing for a demonstration in protest against the low grants that we were given as students. As usual, some students are always reluctant to participate in demonstrations. The student union leadership called one young man, let's call him Tendai. He was physically impaired and he shouted: '*Ahoyi* comrades' (students respond with a vociferous '*Ahoyi!!*'). I see we have cadres here (laughter).

Tendai continued: 'Comrades, as you can see I have one arm. But when it comes to the issue of demonstrating for my grants, I develop 13 more arms' (laughter). Good people, I wonder what we can learn from these stories about society and disabled people. Anyway before that, currently, do we have such characters at DRC? (students respond with a thunderous 'yes'). I am also wondering how such issues can help us to make good plays without offending anyone. Is it possible to perform such issues from such stories? So there we are, let us brain storm (wild applause).

disabled students used insults, ridicule and humour ['powers of the weak'] (Scott, 1985), which are associated with private spaces of the marginalised. Yet students' meetings at the University of Zimbabwe are not purely private, since they are attended by both government officials and representatives of the university executive, albeit in disguised identities for security reasons. In any case, a 'pure' hidden transcript in this case would not have involved non-disabled students. So while Kuda and Taurai's 'performances' were admirably brave resistive public transcripts, which deployed forms of power usually associated with hidden transcripts, the two 'performances' lacked the coherent political organisation that is imperative in fostering successful resistive public transcripts. This simply means the 'performances' from the two students were individual exploits that did not reflect the level of community organisation among disabled students.

The two 'performances' also provide interesting dialectics from the point of view of the power dynamic between non-disabled and disabled students. On the one hand, Kuda and Tendai subverted normative expectations of disabled students, who are not expected to be proud of their bodies. Kuda seemed to be suggesting that he was entitled to 'benefits' of being visually impaired, in this case the 'benefit' of being exempt from social censor with regard to codes of propriety. At the same time, Tendai argued that where student activism was concerned, he was 13 times stronger than the average non-disabled student. Yet the two students might have unwittingly reinforced negative identities of 'lesser people'. In discussions on the two performances, Samanyanga (a Philosophy student with physical impairment) rightly noted that perhaps Kuda and Tendai provided 'entertainment' to the larger student body. In other words, their bodies were some form of 'spectacle' (see Sandahl, 1999). This to me would deny them full status as university citizens with complex, fluid and dynamic identities.

Given the above, there was still urgent need to provide space to relocate disabled students at the centre of university public life. I am proposing that successful transition from hidden transcripts into public transcripts necessarily involves understanding and contextualising some of the above hidden transcripts-public transcripts dialectics. I now briefly turn my attention to how participants responded to my speech and the implication of that response to both access and strengthening of hidden transcripts.

Creating the context for reflections on disability politics

I recognise the theoretical contention that hidden transcripts are not 'pure', since they also contain elements of oppressive 'public' transcripts' (Scott, 1985, 1990). I propose, therefore, that it is important for TfD facilitators to equip disabled participants with critical tools from emancipatory discourses. Subsequent sections of this chapter focus on the discussions and research processes in which the participants formally and informally discussed discourses and practices that marginalise them. This is significant, because participatory theatre is supposed to be thoroughly researched (Thompson, 2003). One of the major reasons for engaging in research on participatory theatre is to ensure that dramatic scenarios hold resonance with participants. Unfortunately, most researches and critical discussions seem to be held by 'experts' and facilitators outside the context of intended beneficiaries of target groups (Oliver, 2004). In the case of disabled people, researches are carried out by medical and social science experts (Campbell, 2003). In the project under consideration, I tried to challenge this trend by making sure that disabled students were exposed to 'expert' medical and academic discourses on disability and subjected these discourses to interrogation. In addition, I created spaces to enable disabled students to examine and unravel knowledge that emerges from their everyday experiences.

Unravelling myths about impaired bodies

The first session held on 15 May 2010 at the University of Zimbabwe Beit Hall was a seminar on myths about disabled bodies. The students had conducted some interviews with both non-disabled and disabled students to find out common myths about disabled people. The session explored the individual and societal implications of these myths. Sinyoro (male Law student with visual impairment) chaired the first meeting, suggesting that we start with the common myth that disabled people are asexual. The students expressed the view that the myth limits the choices of disabled people in finding marriage partners. Manyoni (female Political Science student with a short limb) specifically noted that this myth explains why disabled people tend to marry among themselves. This discussion was also marked by humorous moments. Dismissing the myth, Samanyanga (male Philosophy student with a physical impairment) joked that the fact that his leg could not walk did not mean that his 'third' leg (penis) was immobile (impotent), drawing much laughter and applause from the rest of the group. The discussions focused on sexuality and the importance of medicine in mitigating any pain that is associated with body impairments. However, my advice was that, as agreed, no knowledge was sacrosanct. I posed a question: are we saying that body impairments are 'diseases' which should be cured? This was certainly a difficult question for all the participants. There was no unanimous response to the question. What was critical, however, was that students discussed the issue openly and extensively. I challenged them to go and do further researches, fully aware that the research would challenge facts that society usually takes for granted. As the session was drawing to a close, Sinyoro, remarked:

> Good people, what are we saying here? Are we saying all myths about disabled people are baseless? Are they not based on scientific research? Do you know that visually impaired men have an electrical romantic touch? Research has proved this to be true. It's simple. We make up for lack of sight with a powerful sense of touch. So ladies there you are. Make wise choices.
>
> *(Chivandikwa, 2010 personal journal)*

The students infused the humorous remark above (a typical and powerful form of hidden transcript) in *Visionaries* – a play production on disability and sexuality (Chivandikwa & Muwonwa, 2013), which seeks to validate the sexual desires of young people with visual impairments. This discussion prompted me to encourage students to read on relevant topics to deepen their knowledge about the politics of the body. A critical academic working on disability challenged them to think more complexly about disability, and would hopefully inform the play-building process.

I deliberately started with cognitive thinking on the body in order to give the participants pedagogical grounding so that the performance space would not be a site where they would be manipulated. I encouraged the participants to do research on models of disability and submit their findings in four weeks. In the next section, I discuss how the research by students on models of disability strengthened their theoretical knowledge about disability politics and how this was crucial in giving focus and impetus to hidden transcripts (see Seda & Chivandikwa, 2014). I will argue that the 'new' knowledge was ultimately part of the solid base from which to assert the worth of their impaired bodies. I was hoping that this knowledge would strengthen and give focus and impetus to hidden transcript as a transition in order to give them confidence to perform their resistance in a public theatre forum.

Musings on disability models

After four weeks, students had done sufficient research, and the excitement that the findings generated was well beyond my expectations. The students engaged the traditional and charity models of disability in the context of their own lives. The traditional and charity models of disability regard disabled people as tragic victims of impairment arising from a curse or misfortune (Harris & Enfield, 2003). As a result, the students noted that the traditional model of disability was one of the most oppressive discourses and associated it with most pervasive myths about disability. Of particular interest to me was Samaita's (BA male student with a visual impairment) observation that even supposedly progressive Western countries, were still grappling with dismantling traditional views on disability. Students started to express how their marginalisation was based on retrogressive discourses and practices that emanated from traditional views on disability. Mhofu (male Engineering student with physical impairment), for example, noted that he never enjoyed outdoor life like other children, because his grandmother would refuse to let him go out even to herd cattle on the grounds that he was a 'special' child of God. Mhofu revealed that this was very frustrating and his home was like a prison.

The students noted that the charity model of disability was most perverse among modern Pentecostal churches. They highlighted two trends that struck me. One was the fact that once charismatic preachers set their eyes on a disabled person, the first thing they think of is to 'deliver' or 'heal' him/her. Mukanya (male Political Science student on wheelchair) said that this was clear even on popular television gospel programmes where, in his view, popular charismatic preachers seem to be obsessed with wheelchair users. Addressing me directly, Mukanya remarked, 'Sir, tell the Pentecostal pastors that we come to church to worship God, for crying out loud! We do not come to be delivered!' (Chivandikwa, 2010, personal journal). The second trend among churches was that they sometimes invited disabled students to their meetings without having organised a 'meaningful' programme. The disabled students would just be given plenty of food and left to eat, while the church members engaged in their own programmes. In short, the experience of disabled students in churches suggests that the sight of disabled bodies in churches evokes images of pity, sympathy and charity, which largely dehumanise them. For example, the assumption that human beings, especially disabled communities, need nothing beyond food, clothes or wheelchairs is dehumanising. The churches related to disabled students at the level of consumption, although the distinguishing feature of the human race is not consumption, but the creative ability (Mda, 1993). Such creativity is intellectual, political, scientific, artistic and spiritual in nature. The TfD processes recommended in this chapter might help to unleash such creativity among disabled young people in order to counter dominant theories and practices on development, which reduce human beings to levels of materialism and consumption (see Rahman, 1993).

To achieve the above levels of creativity among disabled students, I had to introduce to them major concepts and political practices of the social model of disability. Engagement with the social model of disability generated intense excitement. Although the students had not heard about the social model of disability, they felt that it resonated with their views on oppression. They felt that there was need to educate the wider society using the social model of disability since 'many people – including proffers are ignorant about it' (Manyoni, 2010, personal interview). Clearly, critical disability theories sharpened their consciousness of oppression and enhanced their clarity in articulating their embodied oppression. More importantly, the students saw the need to go beyond discussions and engage in practical activism to correct misconceptions about their bodies. Mukanya aptly said that the social model does not blame 'our bodies, but social attitudes and processes' (Mukanya, 2010, personal interview).

Above all, the students insisted that in line with the social model of disability, plays and post-performance activities should focus mainly on attitudes that discriminate against impaired bodies. In emphasising this point, Maphiri (female Administration student with a visual impairment) read the quote that says the problem is not in 'the individual with an impairment, but societal structures' (Harris & Enfield, 2003, p. 17).

Through her observation, Maphiri, like other students, convinced me that the students had grasped the basics of the major hegemonic and radical discourses on disability. In the early stages, the students were more celebratory than they were critical of the social model of disability. However, two years later (2012), I began to sensitise them on the limitations of the social model of disability. One of the limitations of the social model of disability that I alerted the students to was that by its sustained emphasis on social structures that limit the participation of disabled people, the social model of disability unwittingly marginalises the material disabled body (see Cameron, 2008). By the time *Visionaries* (2011) was devised, the students were aware of some of the limitations of the social model. However, this model remained a significant source of motivation and inspiration for the practical activities that the students undertook during and after the devising period.

Evidently, students were becoming sufficiently critical of social and academic discourses that marginalised disabled people. Their active participation in formal and subversive informal discussions and research processes created spaces in which they were no longer compliant bodies or passive objects of 'stare' (Sandahl, 1999).

The process of engaging and challenging mainstream social and academic discourses that marginalised disabled people was, however, also laden with ambiguities and contradictions. Box 4.3 captures such ambiguities and contradictions. It is an excerpt of an informal discussion among four students in a *kombi* [mini bus] on our way to Ruwa (20 kilometres from the capital) to attend a performance on disability and mental health.

In the above excerpt, my interest is on Shumba's remarks about the mindset and attitudes that enable one to achieve, rather than the limitations of one's physical condition and social context. Shumba's remarks present three dangers, even if they reflect a high level of self-esteem and positive mental state. First, such attitudes can easily lead disabled people to

---

Box 4.3 Informal discussion of four disabled students

Maphiri: Shumba, next year, you will be a parent. Please bring us cash.

Murehwa: (in response) Shaz (my friend) I wish I could. It's not that easy. People do not want to employ disabled people.

Mukanya: *Taura zvako mudhara* (You can say that again, my man). It's a jungle there in the industry. These are the things we should talk about in our plays.

Muendamberi: But hey guys!!!! Let's get into the shoes of the employer. In your case, Murehwa, the employer will think of constructing special facilities for your thing for you . . . Your . . . wheelchair (laughter). It's damn expensive! Who will do that *nyika yakatodhakwa zvayo iyi?* (Who can afford that in this economically depressed country?).

Shumba: No, no guys. I always say the problem is with us disabled people. Focus on your disabilities [impairments], then you are destined nowhere. But focus on what you can do best; your capabilities, then you can be whatever you want to be. It's the mindset that is important.

celebrate their minds at the expense of their physical bodies, which could be a reflection of the influence of mind–body dualism. Second, however progressive it might be, such a position often overlooks the fact that there are certain impairments that make it difficult if not impossible for disabled people to carry out specific tasks (Hamilton, 2008). During the course of the project, for example, it became apparent to students that certain theatre games were difficult for them to take part in, regardless of their mental attitudes (Chivandikwa, 2016). Third, an over-celebration of the mindset (itself based largely on the American dream of individual triumph), could unwittingly suggest that individuals are responsible for their 'misfortunes'. In the context of disability, this is not very different from the traditional and medical views on disability, which posit that the problem is with the individual body and not society-induced barriers that limit the academic, social, physical and economic participation of disabled people (see Cameron, 2010). In the excerpt above, Shumba was almost absolving (unwittingly) employers and government from any sense of responsibility by emphasising the issue of a positive mindset. This gives credence to Foucault's (2001) thesis that resistance is a continuous battle of part subordination and part subversion. It takes time and effort, therefore, to separate resistive hidden transcripts from internalised 'subordinate' public transcripts (see Scott, 1985, 1990). In simple terms, this means disability oppression is complex because it also occurs among relatively liberated and agentive disabled people. This means oppression coexists with conscious resistance. Yet on the whole, the advantages of a positive mindset seem to supersede the limitations, because it is possible to challenge a young disabled person with a positive self-esteem, and they are able to critically look at their views and change positively.

In summary, I want to reiterate the fact that successful transition from hidden transcripts into public transcripts involves exposing marginalised communities to radical power-laden disability discourses in order to equip participants with intellectual and 'expert' knowledge from outside to complement their ontological knowledge and skills. I suggest that engaging participants in participatory TfD before the actual performances in sustained intellectual and socio-political discourses on critical disability can avert the common danger of having corporeal movements and gestures that are devoid of critical consciousness (see Odhiambo, 2008; Baxter, 2009; Mushangwe & Chivandikwa, 2014).

Conclusion

My experience in this project prompts me to propose that given the complexity of disability oppression, it is important for facilitators to inspire, motivate and challenge disabled participants intellectually in order to access and engender forms of radical resistance that can give them the skills and confidence to challenge grand 'truths' at the public level. This challenging of 'grand truths' can happen in preliminary and surrounding events such as meetings, workshops and informal research processes that I have conceptualised as 'restricted public transcripts'.

First, it is important to gain the trust and confidence of disabled participants in order to access what goes around at the 'backstage'. Second, the activities and events (meetings, social interactions, informal discussions and participatory research processes) that take place before the 'actual' theatre work are valuable sites in which to access and nurture coherent and organised forms of private resistance. Third, since hidden transcripts are not 'perfect' (because they are also contaminated by oppressive public transcripts), it is important for the facilitator to expose disabled participants in TfD to radical disability discourses to equip them intellectually and socio-politically for the public confrontation with power-laden dominating discourses and practices that denigrate their embodied lived experiences. To a large extent, this transitional phase, or 'restricted public transcript', equipped disabled students to come up with ideologically, intellectually, aesthetically and socio-politically engaging public theatre productions which defiantly challenged disability oppression on and beyond the University of Zimbabwe campus.

Reflective questions

1 How might a TfD project unearth the hidden transcripts among disabled university students?
2 What forms might such hidden transcripts assume?
3 How might the TfD facilitator provide impetus to the transition from hidden transcripts to resistive public transcripts?
4 What complications if any might emerge in the transition from hidden transcripts to resistive public transcripts in a TfD context?

References

Baxter, V. (2009). *The Aesthetics of Participatory Theatre*. Unpublished PhD Thesis, University of Winchester, Winchester.

Breeden, L. J. (2008). *Transformative Occupations: Life Experiences of Performers with Disabilities in Film and Television*. Unpublished DPhil Thesis, University of Southern California, California.

Cameron, C. (2008). Further towards an affirmation model. In T. Campbell, F. Fontes & C. Till (eds) *Disability Studies: Emerging Insights and Perspectives* (pp. 14–30). Leeds: The Disability Press.

Cameron, C. (2010). *Does Anybody Like Being Disabled? A Critical Exploration of Impairment, Identity, Media and Everyday Experience in a Disabling Society*. Unpublished PhD Thesis, Queen Margaret University, Edinburgh.

Campbell, F. K. (2003). *The Great Divide: Ableism and Technologies of Disability Production*. D.Phil Thesis, Queensland University of Technology, Queensland.

Campbell, F. K. (2008). Exploring internalized ableism using critical race theory. *Disability and Society* **23**(2), 151–162.

Campbell, F. K. (2009). *Contours of Ableism: The Production of Disability and Ablebodiness*. London: Palgrave Macmillan.

Chataika, T. (2007). *Inclusion of Disabled Students in Higher Education in Zimbabwe: From Idealism to Reality – a Social Ecosystem Perspective*. Unpublished PhD Thesis, University of Sheffield, Sheffield.

Chinyowa, K. C. & Chivandikwa, N. (2017). Subverting ableist discourse as an exercise in precarity: a Zimbabwean case study. *Research in Drama Education: The Journal of Applied Theatre and Performance* **22**(1), 50–61.

Chivandikwa, N. (2016). *Engendering Body-Validating-Community Participation in Theatre for Development (TfD): A Reflective Investigation into Selected TfD Projects in Zimbabwe*. Unpublished DPhil Thesis, University of Zimbabwe, Harare.

Chivandikwa, N. & Muwonwa, N. (2013). Forum theatre, disability and corporeality: a project on sexuality in Zimbabwe. *Platform: The Journal of Theatre and Performing Arts* **7**(1), 55–66.

Foucault, M. (1980). *Power/Knowledge: Selected Interviews and Other Writings*. New York: Knopf Doubleday Publishing Group.

Foucault, M. (1988). Technologies of the self: a seminar with Michel Foucault at the University of Vermont, October 1982. In L. H. Martin & G. T. Huck (eds) *Technologies of the Self: A Seminar with Mitchell Foucault* (pp. 16–49). Amherst: University of Massachusetts Press.

Foucault, M. (2001). *Fearless Speech*. New York: Semiotext.

Freire, P. (1970). *Pedagogy of the Oppressed*. New York: Continuum.

Hamilton, A. (2008). Corpo-reality: personal history, disability and the queering of the American ideal, *Seminar Paper*, Department of Women & Gender Studies University of California, California, 6–8 March 2008.

Harris, A. S. & Enfield, F. (2003). *Disability, Equality and Human Rights: A Training Manual for Development and Humanitarian Organisations*. London: Oxfam.

Hosking, D. (2008). Critical disability theory. A paper presented at the *4th Biennial Disability Studies Conference*, Lancaster University, Lancaster, United Kingdom, 2–4 September 2008.

Manukonda, R. (2013). Theatre-communication that captivates and enchants. *Global Media Journal* **4**(2), 2249–2260.

Mbembe, A. (1992). The banality of power and the aesthetics of vulgarity in the post colony. *Public Culture* **4**(2), 1–30.

Mbembe, A. (2001). *On the Postcolony*. Los Angeles: University of California Press.

Mda, Z. (1993). *When People Play People: Development Communication through Theatre*. Johannesburg: Witwatersrand University Press.

Mushangwe, H. & Chivandikwa, N. (2014). Aspects and dimensions of community participation in theatre for development: the case of the University of Zimbabwe's Manfred Hudson hall sanitation project (2004). *Applied Theatre Research* **2**(2), 119–135.

Odhiambo, C. J. (2008). *Theatre for Development in Kenya: In Search of Appropriate Procedure and Methodology*. Bayreuth: Bayreuth African Studies.

Oliver, M. (2004). The social model in action: if I had a hammer. In C. Barnes & G. Mercer (eds) *Implementing the Social Model of Disability: Theory and Research* (pp. 18–31). Leeds: The Disability Press.

Plastow, J. (2014). Domestication or transformation? The ideology of theatre for development in Africa. *Applied Theatre Research* **2**(2), 107–118.

Rahman, A. M. D. (1993). *People's Self-Development: Perspective on Participatory Action Research*. London: Zed Books.

Sandahl, C. (1999). Ahhhh freak out! Metaphors of disability and femaleness in performance. *Theatre Topics* **9**(1), 11–30.

Scott, J. C. (1985). *Weapons of the Weak: Everyday Forms of Peasant Resistance*. New Haven, CT: Yale University Press.

Scott, J. C. (1990). *Domination and the Arts of Resistance: Hidden Transcripts*. New Haven, CT: Yale University Press.

Seda, O. & Chivandikwa, N. (2014). Power dynamics in applied theatre: integrating the power of the university-based TfD facilitator. *Research in Drama Education: The Journal of Applied Theatre and Performance* **19**(2), 143–158.

Thompson, J. (2003). *Applied Theatre: Bewilderment and Beyond*. Winchester, New York: Peter Lang.

5

BUILDING SUSTAINABLE COMMUNITIES

Why inclusion matters in the post-conflict environment

Rebecca Irvine

Introduction

> Disabled people have not benefited from charity, because charity is not part of the development process. It is not part of national socio-economic development. Disabled people want to be treated as equal citizens, with rights. They want to be treated equally and participate as equal citizens in their own communities. To achieve this, one needs political and social action to change society.
>
> *(Malinga, cited in Coleridge, 1993, pp. 53–54)*[1]

Charity is neither sustainable nor desirable as a way to improve the quality of life for disabled people.[2] What is needed instead is the recognition that they are full and equal citizens and should be treated as such. Since colonisation, disability has largely been viewed by African states as an issue of social welfare, focused on care and charity (ideas exported and perpetuated by colonial powers). As charity is focused on addressing the needs of an individual, it has limited the recognition of people with disabilities as a minority group deprived of their full rights of citizenship (Coleridge, 1993). Joshua Malinga[3] (see quote above) is not alone in his assertion that disabled people have been denied citizenship as a result of negative attitudes and discriminatory practices (see Drake, 1999; Dwyer, 2003; Morris, 2005; Lister, 2007). This argument has been at the heart of the global disability rights movement for decades; however, it is now, not only a matter of recognising human rights (which has often delivered policies and legislation but failed to foster the political will to see through the implementation), but also one of sustainability for the state in social and economic terms.

The global population of people with disabilities continues to increase (from 10% to 15%) as a result of advances in medical treatments, improved data collection methods and the presence of large-scale terrorism and modern warfare (WHO & World Bank, 2011). During civil conflicts, those directly involved (both combatants and civilians) can experience various forms of inhumane acts (e.g. intimidation, killings, amputation of limbs and disfigurement of bodies, rape and property destruction). These experiences are likely to increase the number of people that have impairments in a post-conflict environment. As a result, more attention needs to be given to how people with disabilities are included within their communities. This chapter seeks to explore the relationship between the inclusion of disabled people and sustainable communities by focusing on the experiences of societies that have undergone conflict transformation in southern Africa. Countries emerging from conflict have been selected to represent circumstances in which the potential for change is heightened, as new policies are developed at unprecedented rates in order to address historic inequalities and create a new post-conflict identity (Irvine, 2015a).

What is a sustainable community?

Sustainability can be defined as: 'society's ability to achieve economic development and improve the standard of living of the people without compromising that of future generations' (Awuah-Nyamekye, 2015, p. 227). The concept of improving the quality of life of residents while also considering the environmental impact has encountered challenges when applied to global development strategies. One of the critiques of sustainable development is that it has failed to consider what it might mean for others in different cultures and times (Redclift, 2000; Ukaga, 2005). For example, the 'African concept of community is predicated on the belief that public interest takes precedence over private interest' (Afoaku, 2005, p. 49), a belief in opposition to some development 'partners' from the global North. This difference, it has been argued, is what lies at the heart of the global North's failed attempts to 'develop' Africa (Mawere & Awuah-Nyamekye, 2015).

The African perspective of development has traditionally considered sustainability, as Africans have tended to take a more holistic approach than the nations from the global North. Mawere and Awuah-Nyamekye (2015, pp. xvi–xvii) argue that:

> [I]n Africa, cultural knowledge and other such skills are profoundly interwoven in the mantra of sustainable development. It is this complex equation of the African conceptualisation and understanding of the matrix of sustainability that eludes many elites. African political leaders and policy makers who are still trapped at the edge of colonialism and neo-colonialism such that they remain holding fast onto Western ideologies and approaches in their bid to address African problems.

Okechukwu Ukaga also argues, 'Africa's problems will never be solved by non-stakeholders' and that 'grassroots efforts, good domestic leadership, and an enhanced continental ability to negotiate with other participants in the global economy' are what is needed to address the issues of poverty and development (2005, p. 5). 'Indigenous knowledge' should not be underestimated in this process (Awuah-Nyamekye, 2015, p. 221).

The recent introduction of the Circles of Sustainability approach has been heralded as a better way forward, with a number of studies piloted around the world in partnership with United Nations Habitat. Originally conceived as part of a wider project entitled Circles of Social Life, sustainability is considered alongside other social conditions such as resilience, adaptation, innovation, and reconciliation, in order to address complexities, which had previously been ignored in discussions about sustainable communities (James, 2015). Under the Circles of Sustainability approach, there are four major headings: economics, ecology, politics, and culture. Each of these headings includes a number of factors that are considered when determining the overall sustainability of a given location. Although the approach is intended to be flexible, examples of the core components considered might include: organisation and governance; law and justice; dialogue and reconciliation; health and well-being; gender and generations; labour and welfare; wealth and distribution; and constructions and settlements. Each component is scored on a nine-point scale ranging from vibrant to critical, and providing an overall picture of the sustainability of the area.[4] Although this newer, more holistic approach to determining sustainability has primarily been used in urban areas, it can also be a useful tool for considering the long-term development of post-conflict communities, since both urban and rural areas undergo significant development following civil conflict.

Sustainable communities are about empowering citizens and political leaders to consider the long-term impact of policies on the environment, economy, and society. A sustainable community is, therefore, about equipping the state and society to prepare for the future by considering the needs of not only the current generation, but also anticipating the needs of generations to come. As the number of people with disabilities continues to increase, considering their needs becomes ever more important in the development of communities. The shift from the traditional charity model of supporting the individual to viewing disability as an issue that impacts on society as a whole, is needed to ensure that disabled people are able to experience 'full and effective participation in society on an equal basis with others' (United Nations, 2006, Article 1).

Why does the inclusion of people with disabilities matter?

If we consider citizenship to be about determining a common identity rooted in a recognition of a set of rights and responsibilities in order to share the 'benefits and burdens of social life' (Faulks, 2000, p. 5), then the denial of citizenship will limit participation. In theory, citizenship offers members an equal status within the political public regardless of any social and economic inequalities that might exist (Marshall, 1950; Young, 1990); however, in practice, various forms of marginalisation and hierarchies have developed that reinforce the power of the majority (Turner, 2016). Drake (1999) argues that using a citizenship framework based in equal recognition of social, political, and civil stature among members of a community, is a powerful tool to combat discrimination and create a positive change in the daily experiences of people with disabilities.

In order to understand the barriers that people with disabilities face in exercising full citizenship, it is helpful to consider inclusion from a historical perspective. During many of the earliest civilisations, communities were closely bound to one another and each person had a role within it. People with impairments were usually included in some aspect of the production process and therefore were considered valued members of society (Finkelstein, 1980). Oliver (1999) argued that it was actually the transition to industrialised economies that led to the exclusion of disabled people from mainstream society. He claimed that capitalism allowed for some people to accumulate surpluses, allowing them to care (or to hire professional carers) for other family members who were unable to earn for themselves. The change to outcome-based productivity in factories also disadvantaged the contribution that many people with disabilities could make to the rigid expectations of many capitalist business owners, contributing to their marginalisation and exclusion. This theory is clearly developed in the context of the global North or, in some cases, it might also be relevant to people with high social standing and affluence in the global South, but it is not transferable more broadly. Many societies in southern Africa continue to be based on agricultural or subsistence farming and informal labour markets, yet despite this link to 'more traditional community structures' (Meekosha & Soldatic, 2011, p. 1388), disabled people still face significant exclusion in their communities.

It is also worth noting that the concept of human rights is not universal and is contested in many communities in the global South (Meekosha & Soldatic, 2011). Despite the frequent use of human rights frameworks at the national and international levels, the concepts often fail to 'trickle down' into people's everyday lives. For example, despite Uganda's progressive legislation rooted in human rights, people with disabilities still remain isolated within their communities.

It is also argued that the increased political participation of disabled people as a result of quotas has failed to 'significantly change the provision of services to people with disabilities, or their quality of life' (Hedström & Smith, 2013, p. 29). Similar findings have also been reported under the introduction of quotas for disability representation in Kenya.[5] It is therefore argued that resources must be invested in changing social attitudes at a community level, in addition to the introduction of policies of inclusion, in order to facilitate real social change. The importance of raising disability awareness is highlighted by the prominence it receives in the Convention on the Rights of Persons with Disabilities (CRPD), following only after general principles and obligations (Articles 3 and 4), equality and non-discrimination (Article 5), women with disabilities (Article 6), and children with disabilities (Article 7). Article 8 of CRPD explicitly states that State Parties have a responsibility to raise disability awareness and 'foster respect for the rights and dignity of persons with disabilities', to 'combat stereotypes, prejudices and harmful practices relating to persons with disabilities', and 'to promote awareness of the capabilities and contributions of persons with disabilities'.

Challenging society to recognise that all people have the ability to 'contribute to humanity' and that social structures should aim to empower individuals to achieve their potential is necessary to overcome the historic inequalities that people with disabilities have experienced (Quinn & Degener, 2002, p. 18). It should be recognised that investments to improve access to education and employment, as well as a change in public perceptions of the abilities of people with disabilities, is what is needed to improve the social and economic inclusion of people with disabilities. In the best-selling book, *The Spirit Level*, Wilkinson and Pickett (2009) argue that a more equal society will not only result in a better quality of life for all citizens, but that it will also have additional benefits in the development of a more sustainable economic system.

The inclusion of people with disabilities is something that should be considered when discussing the development (or redevelopment) of an economic system. The historic welfare state structure is facing challenges in its ability to meet the needs of modern societies and many countries that had previously subscribed to the neo-liberal concepts, are reviewing their systems of resource distribution. There are signs of this in the United Kingdom, where austerity measures have been found by the United Nations Committee on the Rights of Persons with Disabilities to disproportionately affect disabled people, constituting 'grave or systemic violations of the rights of persons with disabilities' (United Nations Committee on the Rights of Persons with Disabilities, 2016, p. 20). This reconceptualising of redistribution is likely to have a substantial impact on the way international agencies work with communities in the global South broadly and with disabled people more specifically (Stone, 1999; Groce *et al.*, 2011). It also has implications for countries in the global South, which might have attempted to develop a welfare system (sometimes as a result of international pressures), but which was never able to fully develop in practice.

It is worth noting that the relationship between poverty and disability is cyclical, as disability both leads to and results from poverty, resulting in an over-representation of people with disabilities among the poorest people in the world (WHO & World Bank, 2011). The inability to access education or employment results in a poverty trap for many disabled people, with women with disabilities particularly vulnerable because of double marginalisation: (1) being a woman and also (2) being a disabled person (Chataika, 2013). According to Mike Oliver, households with a disabled family member in countries in the global North and South 'experience conditions of life far inferior to the rest of the population' (Oliver, 1999, p. 15). Poverty can be linked to poor health resulting from malnutrition, poor living conditions, or an inability to access health care. The World Disability Report also stated that 'children in the poorest three quintiles of households in most countries are at greater risk of disability than others' (WHO & World Bank, 2011, p. 40) and poor people are also at greater risk of acquiring impairments as a result of living in undesirable or dangerous environments or working in hazardous jobs (e.g. mining or factories without safety standards).

Addressing issues related to poverty in the global South is a major concern, as many countries are resource poor and unable to provide adequate support to improve the quality of life for their citizens. Despite the widespread recognition that people with disabilities are among the poorest of the poor, they have largely been invisible in poverty-reduction strategies (Bonnel, 2004). The failure to include people with disabilities is not just an issue related to poverty reduction, but is often the case in the development of social policy more broadly. This exclusion at a policy level creates additional barriers to facilitating social and economic inclusion in practice. Banks and Polack (2014, p. 1) posit that 'not making efforts to promote inclusion is arguably more costly', as there are 'significant economic costs associated with the on-going exclusion of people with disabilities'. They provide the example that the exclusion of children with disabilities from education is likely to result in a loss of job opportunities for the individual, as well as their family carers, and a substantial loss of potential earnings for the household.

The economic and social costs of having impairments are difficult to quantify, but important to study. Understanding the direct and indirect consequences of impairments will have an impact on the development of policies and services that can best address the needs of people with disabilities and their families. We also know that 'disability does not just affect the individual, but impacts on the whole community' (Department for International Development [DFID], 2000, p. 4). Programmes aimed at poverty reduction, therefore, must include strategies for the inclusion of people with disabilities in order to be successful (European Disability Forum, 2002). In fact, it was largely agreed that one of the factors contributing to the inability to meet the Millennium Development Goals targets was the failure to include people with disabilities within their indicators (Astbury, 2008), an issue that has been rectified, at least to some extent, within the post-2015 Sustainable Development Goals (Brolan, 2016).

Finally, since 'environmental problems bear down disproportionately upon the poor' (Agyeman, Bullard & Evans, 2003, p. 1) and people with disabilities are disproportionately represented among the poor, incorporating social, economic, and ecological components should be considered when aiming to improve the quality of life. For example, linking the experiences of disabled people to the Circles of Sustainability demonstrates the relationship to:

- poverty, as it relates to labour and welfare (as an indicator of economics);
- the environment (as poor living conditions can contribute to the development of various forms of impairments and the poverty often associated with disability leads to living in undesirable or dangerous environments);
- the lack of political representation can mean that the concerns of disabled people are not represented in policymaking; and
- people with disabilities often experience discrimination in areas of engagement and identity (or citizenship) (an indicator of culture).

When considering the experiences of disabled people in relation to the Circles of Sustainability, it becomes clear to envision why the inclusion of people with disabilities could contribute to more sustainable communities. Without efforts made to develop inclusive communities, resources will continue to be spent on maintaining exclusion and perpetuating the status quo, and as the inequalities gap continues to grow, disabled people will continue to be left behind. Developing sustainable communities offers an alternative to the 'way things have always been done' by encouraging people to consider the long-term impact of policies and programmes on the community as a whole for generations to come. It encourages planning for a population that continues to increase in life expectancy and of the prevalence of people with disabilities and how to improve their well-being.

Why focus on post-conflict societies?

Since the 1970s, southern Africa has witnessed many wars, with most of them taking place primarily between citizens of the same country and within the boundaries of a single state. Considering that war destroys life, health, law and order, livelihoods, and the economy, and weakens social capital (Baker, 2006, p. 31), the process of conflict transformation offers the opportunity to rebuild (Miles, 2013). The post-conflict context of development implies a sense of urgency that is not always present in other developmental contexts. Although usually faced with financial constraints similar to those facing other countries in the global South, the often weak or inexperienced post-conflict government must successfully navigate the timing and sequencing of policies in an environment that is deeply divided and undergoing significant transitions (Jeong, 2002). The legacy of the conflict might include poverty, destruction of social dynamics and political structures; but it can also provide an unprecedented opportunity for change (Collier *et al.*, 2003). These opportunities for change can be maximised by considering the long-term impact of policies on the economy, environment, and society and the ways in which the needs of the new or redeveloping state can be met. This might include addressing the post-conflict problems of high levels of migration (particularly of skilled labourers), poverty and environmental destruction. In addition, the erosion of the traditional social fabrics, which results from conflict, also creates opportunities to challenge traditional views of disability and gender, which might have previously reinforced practices of exclusion.

New governments are more likely to introduce policies that promote change in order to differentiate themselves from the past. Recognising that 'violent conflict is more likely to arise in areas where economic, social, political, and cultural status inequalities occur simultaneously and where some groups are deprived across every dimension' (Langer, Stewart & Venugopal, 2012, p. 7), many new governments will understand that '[e]conomic development and political arrangements that simply reproduce divisions will not build peace or prevent conflicts from re-emerging in the future' (Hillyard, Rolston & Tomlinson, 2005, p. 208). If the new government is to demonstrate their leadership and unite a divided society, they will need to introduce 'just and transparent political, social, and economic systems that are inclusive and participatory' (Colletta & Cullen, 2000, p. 91). A nation emerging from civil conflict is fragile and will need to consider the best approaches to building social and economic capital among its citizens and make the necessary investments to achieve peace and stability. Addressing historic inequalities will require a sustained effort that will run beyond a single election cycle, and needs a firm commitment from the government and international community to challenge 'structurally ingrained forms of deprivation' (Langer *et al.*, 2012, p. 9). States, therefore, need to build communities that are stable, safe, and sustainable in order to move forward and maintain peace. In fact, there may be no more important time to focus on building communities that empower citizens and political leaders to consider the long-term impact of policies, as the potential of relapsing into war is often a strong motivator.

If the potential for social change is to be capitalised upon at the end of a civil conflict, the inequalities must be addressed as part of the peace-building process. Pugh (1995, p. 24) argues that the 'benefits of peacebuilding should be distributed unequally to assist the most vulnerable sections of society'. Giving extra attention to facilitating the inclusion of the most marginalised groups' participation in the peace-building process will ultimately include people with disabilities, as they are inevitably among the most marginalised citizens in any post-civil conflict society. It is important to remember that participation can take many forms, including membership in civil society organisations, community activism, or holding political office. As such, 'attention needs to be paid to the degree to which the distribution of seats in the legislature and the composition of the executive provides representation for all social groups, especially marginalised and war-affected groups' (Baker, 2006, p. 36). Not only should the political representation be representative, but they should also aspire to 'governance that is effective, participatory, transparent, accountable and equitable, and that promotes the rule of law' (United Nations Development Program, 1999). This is directly in line with the rallying cries of the Disability Rights Movement (DRM), 'nothing about us without us'.

Lessons from southern African examples

While international agencies have traditionally viewed peace and development as separate entities, much like they have tended to view sustainability in isolation, the 'African perspective sees peace and development as intimately related' (Hansen, 1988 cited in McCandless & Karbo, 2011, p. 7). Again, similar to the claims regarding sustainability made by Ukaga (2005) and Awuah-Nyamekye (2015), Pearce (1999, p. 86) advocates for recognition of the differences in views regarding peace-building between the global North and South, 'learning from [local people's] experiences and building on their capacities, rather than introducing quick-fix solutions dreamed up by outsiders, may be a longer path to peace, but a more sustainable one'. As more participatory approaches to conflict transformation continue to grow in popularity, it is worth reflecting on what has come before and the lessons that can be drawn upon in moving forward.

Southern Africa provides an excellent sample of different experiences related to building inclusive communities following civil conflict. Four southern African countries (Mozambique, Namibia, South Africa, and Zimbabwe) experienced armed liberation campaigns against colonialism in order to gain their independence, in which socialist rhetoric was employed (Bauer & Taylor, p. 2011). This link, however vague, to socialist ideals, suggests a commitment to social justice and inclusive principles. Bauer and Taylor (2011, p. 7) also make the case that 'southern Africa is politically and socially interconnected and interdependent', a fact that extends beyond the traditional political and economic actors to also include interconnectedness between disability rights activists within the region. This section acknowledges that disability in Africa is often reduced to 'homogenisation, simplification and generalisation' (Grech, 2011, p. 89) and warns against oversimplification. However, it aims to highlight how experiences within southern African countries could contribute to our understanding about how to capitalise on opportunities presented during conflict transformation.

Building sustainable communities requires the expressed intent to recognise the rights and responsibilities of citizens in order to increase participation. The following section seeks to explore where opportunities were seized (or in some cases, missed) to 'build back better' by creating more inclusive communities in the aftermath of civil conflict. Examples are drawn from four southern African countries: South Africa, Angola, Mozambique and Zimbabwe as highlighted earlier. It is important to note that space restrictions do not allow for a thorough analysis of each country's experience, but, rather, a small sample of where lessons might be learned. It will focus on the participation of people with disabilities during conflict transformation (primarily in influencing political decisions) and the impact that the resulting policies and legislation have had on creating inclusive societies.

Post-conflict South Africa and disability

South Africa expressed unequivocally their commitment to overcoming past injustices during the post-apartheid redevelopment. Nelson Mandela is famously quoted as saying, 'The new South Africa we are building must be accessible to all' at the opening of the first junior wheelchair sports camp in 1995. With this one statement he gave hope to people with disabilities that they would be included in the new South Africa. In the early stages of conflict transformation, South Africa introduced progressive policies (heavily influenced by international standards) that set out to improve the quality of life for people with disabilities. However, despite progress in the representation of disabled people in positions of influence (namely as politicians and board members of statutory agencies), the policies have largely gone unimplemented. Speaking at the 2011 Disabled People International Conference in Durban, the then Minister for Women, Children, and People with Disabilities declared that 'people with disabilities face more barriers to social and economic inclusion than any other section of the community'.

South Africa was in a unique position at the end of apartheid,[6] in that it had managed to maintain a strong civil society presence throughout the period of political violence. Building on links that had been made with disability rights activists in Zimbabwe, Disabled People South Africa (DPSA) was formed in 1984 as a multi-racial and pan-disability activist group. DPSA coordinated the disability movement in South Africa. However, it should not be confused with the South African Disability Rights Movement, as many other organisations also played important roles in the advancement of disability rights during the 1980s and 1990s.

Since its inception in the early 1980s, the South African DRM had maintained strong links with the movement in Zimbabwe from whom they often sought advice. The Zimbabwean DRM (one of the first in Africa) included many disabled veterans from the struggle for liberation[7] and had been very political. As a result of the close working relationship between the two DRMs, the South African activists often made decisions based on the experiences of their 'comrades'[8] in Zimbabwe. The Zimbabwean movement, having already experienced the transformation process, warned South African activists to be prepared for chaos and ready to be in the centre of it (Rowland, 2004, p. 146). The South African leadership listened to the advice of their neighbours and managed to find their place in the transition process.

The South African disability movement decided to prioritise the mainstreaming of disability issues in their approach to influencing social and political change. In doing so, it identified a subject specialist on each particular issue in order to include the disability perspective in all policy discussions. The approach required careful planning and a great deal of trust that each specialist was representing the interests of disabled people broadly while allowing activists to integrate themselves into different areas and build strategic partnerships. In regard to the mainstreaming approach in a post-conflict context, Berghs (2015, p. 753) has claimed, 'mainstreaming disability during and post conflict can enable and create a more equitable society and change the conditions that fostered violence and conflict in the first place, but these conditions remain enclosed within neoliberal settings'. She warns that an emphasis on health and rights reinforces the perspectives of the global North and fails to consider how more inclusive and sustainable societies could be developed to meet the needs of the population affected, drawing upon local skills and priorities.

Post-conflict Zimbabwe and disability

As mentioned earlier, Zimbabwe has a long history of disability rights activism. However, 'disabled activists have expressed disenchantment at the lack of gains for disabled people after the armed struggle for political independence' (Barnes & Mercer, 1995, p. 40). One of the reasons that has been suggested for the failure of the Zimbabwe DRM to improve the quality of life of people with disabilities is the failure of the elites to support the equality agenda and, instead, using disability rights as a way to 'ensure access to debt relief' (Chataika *et al.*, 2015, p. 197). They argue that Zimbabwean policies might recognise disability, but the lack of political will inhibits social change. Chataika *et al.* (2015) discussed seven challenges to true inclusion and respect for disability rights in Zimbabwe, as proposed by disability rights activist and lawyer, Abraham Mateta. The seven challenges are: gatekeepers of financial resources; failure to consult and involve disabled people; lack of funding, training, and understanding of resources needed and allocated; specialised charity mentality; superficial mainstreaming in development aid; rights not connected to realities; and lack of legislative and regulation frameworks. Failing to confront these challenges limits the potential to develop inclusive and sustainable communities.

In order to increase participation of people with disabilities in society, it is often necessary for a shift in public attitudes. In Angola, it was the view that disability was not the state's responsibility but should be dealt with by the family and charities. In response to a question about the level of disabled veterans forced to beg, the minister responded that 'this was principally a concern for Angolan disability groups and not the state' (Angoflash, 2004 cited in Power, 2008, p. 183). Without challenging the ideas that people with disabilities have the capacity to contribute meaningfully to the redevelopment of post-conflict societies, it will be difficult to make significant advances. The weak civil society within Angola has meant that disability organisations only began to form in the 1990s. Similar experiences have been reported in Mozambique, with disability organisations beginning around the same time and political leadership shifting responsibility for supporting people with disabilities from the state to the family (Power, 2008). By focusing on the responsibilities of families or charities, states deflect their role in delivering a high quality of life for all citizens on an equal basis, and fail to provide the funding necessary to deliver the services needed to build sustainable communities. For example, a recent report on the physical redevelopment of Angola's capital, Luanda, fails to mention any accessibility accommodations that might have been made to ensure equal access by people with disabilities (Croese, 2016). Building the capacity of people with disabilities and their organisations is essential to challenging public attitudes on capacity and capabilities to contribute to the community and to challenge states for the recognition of equal citizenship. It is also important to remember that the physical redevelopment should also consider how to best meet the needs of all current and future citizens.

The traditional beliefs associated with the causes of impairments are particularly important when considering disability within many southern African societies, as disability is often seen as a punishment and thus, shameful. A 2010 study by RAVIM and Handicap International Mozambique found that these negative beliefs about disability were deeply imbedded in popular culture and transcended social class, though they were most prominent among people who had lived in rural areas for long periods of time. Many people with disabilities have little contact with people outside of their immediate families, as they are often confined to the home, either by the family's fear of being ostracised within the community, or because the services that could facilitate social integration for people with disabilities are not available. On visits to Mozambique in 2010 and 2011, the visibility of disabled people seemed to be improving when compared with other older accounts of Mozambican life. This is not to imply that their lives were equal to other Mozambicans, but it does suggest a shift in the practice of keeping disabled family members hidden and without outside stimulation. Worrying reports about treatment of children with disabilities were heard, however, and specific campaigns to address the mistreatment and social isolation of disabled children were planned following significant international investment (personal interview, August 2012).

The view that disability was not taken seriously at the policy level is substantiated by a number of different reports on the accessibility of social services for people with disabilities. The National Poverty Assessment in 2010 showed that although there had been 'significant improvements in access to basic social services', inequalities still existed for people with disabilities in accessing those services (United Nations, 2012, p. 11). Other recent reports found that specialised services aimed at addressing the needs of people with disabilities were rare, and the few that did exist were not accessed because of a lack of awareness of their availability, or because they were often based in Maputo (Lang, 2008; Eide, 2009). These findings indicate that little has changed since the end of the war, as a 1994 study reported similar findings and stated that 'service provision was rare, and when it did exist, it was overstretched and primarily based in Maputo' (Miles & Medi, 1994, p. 286).

Another important aspect of participation is the inclusion of people with different life experiences working together for the advancement of rights and inclusive societies for all. Partnership working between disabled veterans and victims can also play an important role in promoting social inclusion. When resources are limited, the competition between groups for recognition can be destructive. For example, Angola and Mozambique both experienced exceptionally high numbers of landmine victims and found that many international agencies prioritised resource allocation to landmine victims over other people with disabilities (Irvine, 2015b; Power, 2008). In Angola, the divisions go beyond just disabled victims, veterans, and people with disabilities perceived to be unrelated to the conflict, as they also distinguish between former combatants involved in the liberation struggle and the civil war.[9] Power (2008, p. 191), however, argues that the initial focus on former combatants as the voice of disability has shifted and that disability movements in both Angola and Mozambique continue to become more inclusive. This is in contrast to the South African model, which aimed to be more inclusive from the start (though they have been criticised for failing to include people with intellectual or psychosocial impairments [personal interview]).

Lessons for building sustainable communities in post-conflict contexts

The experiences highlighted on the participation and inclusion of people with disabilities in post-conflict societies in southern Africa, have highlighted a number of findings in relation to building sustainable communities. Four key similarities have been identified in the experiences of conflict transformation in southern Africa: the role of the DRM in challenging the status quo, the importance of participatory decision-making; the need to build capacity for not just people with disabilities, but also for their families, organisations, communities, and decision-makers; and that introducing policies is not enough to ensure the realisation of equal rights. In fact, all four countries have constitutions that specifically acknowledge people with disabilities as rights holders. However, they have received criticism of the barriers that disabled people still face to being recognised as full and equal citizens in practice.

The importance of the national DRM cannot be underestimated. The role that they have played in the transition process is widely documented (Charlton, 1998; Rowland, 2004; Irvine, 2014; Chataika *et al.*, 2015). However, in all of the case studies considered, the organisation of disability rights activists had a distinct impact on the political recognition of disability within the redevelopment of state and society. Participation, as a key component of building sustainable communities, 'puts emphasis on persons with disabilities as partners in charge and as key stakeholders who can hold governments, the private sector, NGOs, and other development actors accountable' (Lockwood & Tardi, 2014, p. 436). Investment needs to be made in developing the capacity of people with disabilities to be able to participate in meaningful ways in order to develop better and more inclusive policies and programmes.

There are areas of building sustainable communities in which little evidence of consideration to the promotion of participation of disabled people has been found. For example, environmental concerns are rarely connected to the DRM and there is broadly a failure to plan for not just the current needs of citizens with disabilities, but also the future needs. There has been some improvement in the recognition that disabled people are more likely to live in poverty, but fewer acknowledgements about meeting their basic needs.

Overall, we still need to do better at building more inclusive post-conflict communities, as none of the experiences demonstrated a clear, sustainable model. Despite the opportunities for change located within policy and legislative reform, there seems to be a failure to capitalise on the opportunities for implementation. Limited financial resources, international pressures, national tensions, and competing interests, are all given as reasons why it is not being done. Hence, we need to think more creatively about how we can build sustainable communities that can thrive, and these need to be inclusive of people with disabilities as full and equal citizens.

Reflective questions

1   What are the primary challenges faced when building sustainable post-conflict communities that are inclusive of disabled people?
2   What are the primary benefits to including disabled people in building sustainable post-conflict communities?
3   How can we use the previous examples in southern Africa to improve future outcomes and build more inclusive communities?

Notes

1 Joshua Malinga is a former chairperson of Disabled People International & Secretary General of the Southern Africa Federation of the Disabled.
2 The author uses the terms 'disabled people' and 'people with disabilities' interchangeably in order to respect the differences of opinion on the preferred terminology within the broad disability community.
3 Joshua Malinga is regarded as one of the founders of the disability rights movement in Africa, though his connections with the current ruling party administration later brought his reputation into disrepute.
4 For more information on the Circles of Sustainability approach see James (2015).
5 Unpublished interviews conducted by the author with disability rights activists in Nairobi, April–May 2015.
6 Apartheid was a system of racial segregation introduced by the National Party in South Africa in 1948 and legislated for the promotion of the minority rule of Afrikaners. It was ended through a series of negotiations during the early 1990s and culminated in the first free election in 1994 in which Nelson Mandela was elected President.
7 The Zimbabwe War of Liberation (1964–1979) ultimately ended white minority rule of Rhodesia and granted Zimbabwe independence in March 1980.
8 The term 'comrade' was often used among activists but was not linked to communist associations.
9 The national liberation struggle against Portugal took place between 1961 and 1975. The civil war began following Angolan independence in 1975. It is argued that veterans of the civil war should receive preferential treatment since more people acquired disabilities as a result of the long-term violence and excessive use of landmines (Power, 2008).

References

Afoaku, O. G. (2005). Linking democracy and sustainable development in Africa. In O. Ukaga & O. G. Afoaku (eds) *Sustainable Development in Africa: A Multifaceted Challenge* (pp. 23–56). Trenton, NJ: Africa World Press.
Agyeman, J., Bullard, R. D. & Evans, B. (2003). Joined-up thinking: bringing together sustainability, environmental justice and equity. In J. Agyeman, R. D. Bullard & B. Evans (eds) *Just Sustainabilities: Development in an Unequal World* (pp. 1–18). London: Earthscan Publications.

Astbury, V. (2008). *Not on the Guest List: Disabled People and the Millennium Development Goals (MDGs)*. West Sussex: Sightsavers.

Awuah-Nyamekye, S. (2015). Indigenous knowledge: a key factor towards Africa's sustainable development. In M. Mawere & S. Awuah-Nyamekye (eds) *Harnessing Cultural Capital for Sustainability: A Pan Africanist Perspective* (pp. 221–242). Bamenda, Cameroon: Langaa RPCIG.

Baker, B. (2006). Post-settlement governance programmes: what is being built in Africa? In O. Furley & R. May (eds) *Ending Africa's Wars: Progressing to Peace* (pp. 31–45). Hampshire: Ashgate.

Banks, L. M. & Polack, S. (2014). *The Economic Costs of Exclusion and Gains of Inclusion of People with Disabilities: Evidence from Low and Middle Income Countries*. London: London School of Hygiene & Tropical Medicine.

Barnes, C. & Mercer, G. (1995). Disability emancipation, community participation and disabled people. In G. Craig & M. Mayo (eds) *Community Empowerment: A Reader in Participation and Development* (pp. 33–45). London: Zed Books.

Bauer, G. & Taylor, S. D. (2011). *Politics in Southern Africa: Transition and Transformation*. Boulder, CO: Lynne Rienner Publishers.

Berghs, M. (2015). Radicalising 'disability' in conflict and post-conflict situations. *Disability & Society* **30**(5), 743–758.

Bonnel, R. (2004). *Poverty Reduction Strategies: Their Importance for Disability*. Cornell University ILR School, Retrieved from http://digitalcommons.ilr.cornell.edu/cgi/viewcontent.cgi?article=1444&context=gladnetcollect on 3 January 2017.

Brolan, C. E. (2016). A word of caution: human rights, disability, and implementation of the post-2015 Sustainable Development Goals. *Laws* **5**.2(22), 1–18.

Charlton, J. (1998). *Nothing About Us Without Us: Disability Oppression and Empowerment*. Berkeley and Los Angeles: University of California Press.

Chataika, T. (2013). *Gender and Disability Mainstreaming Training Manual*. Disabled Women in Africa: GIZ Sector Initiative Persons with Disabilities on behalf of BMZ. Retrieved from www.diwa.ws/index.php?option=com_phocadownload on 2 October 2017.

Chataika, T., Berghs, M., Mateta, A. & Shava, K. (2015). From whose perspective anyway? The quest for African disability rights activism. In A. De Waal (ed.) *Advocacy in Conflict: Critical Perspectives on Transnational Activism* (pp. 187–211). London: Zed Books.

Coleridge, P. (1993). *Disability, Liberation and Development*. Oxford: Oxfam.

Colletta, N. J. & Cullen, M. L. (2000). *Violent Conflict and the Transformation of Social Capital: Lessons from Cambodia, Rwanda, Guatemala, and Somalia*. Washington, DC: International Bank for Reconstruction and Development & The World Bank.

Collier, P., Elliott, V. L., Hegre, H., Hoeffler, A., Reynal-Querol, M. & Sambanis, N. (2003). *Breaking the Conflict Trap: Civil War and Development Policy*. Washington, DC: The World Bank.

Croese, S. (2016). *Urban Governance and Turning African Cities Around: Luanda Case Study*. Partnership for African Social & Governance Research Working Paper 018. Retrieved from www.pasgr.org/wp-content/uploads/2016/11/Urban-Governance-and-Turning-African-Cities-Around_Luanda-Case-Study_.pdf on 11 January 2017.

Department for International Development (2000). *Disability, Poverty and Development*. Retrieved from http://hpod.org/pdf/Disability-poverty-and-development.pdf on 18 April 2018.

Drake, R. F. (1999). *Understanding Disability Policies*. London: Macmillan.

Dwyer, P. (2003). *Understanding Social Citizenship: Themes and Perspectives for Policy and Practice*. Bristol: Polity Press.

Eide, A. H. (2009). Discussion. In A. H. Eide & Y. Kamaleri (eds) *Living Conditions among People with Disabilities in Mozambique* (pp. 84–94). Oslo: SINTEF Health Research.

European Disability Forum (2002). *Development Cooperation and Disability*. EDF Policy Paper. Doc. EDF 02/16 EN.

Faulks, K. (2000). *Citizenship: Key Ideas*. London: Routledge.

Finkelstein, V. (1980). *Attitudes and Disabled People*. New York: World Rehabilitation Fund.

Grech, S. (2011). Recolonising debates or perpetuated coloniality? Decentring the spaces of disability, development and community in the global South. *International Journal of Inclusive Education* **15**(1), 87–100.

Groce, N., Kett, M., Lang, R. & Trani, J. F. (2011). Disability and poverty: the need for a more nuanced understanding of implications for development policy and practice. *Third World Quarterly* **32**(8), 1493–1513.

Hedström, J. & Smith, J. (2013). *Overcoming Political Exclusion: Strategies for Marginalized Groups to Successfully Engage in Political Decision-Making*. Stockholm: International Institute for Democracy and Electoral Assistance.

Hillyard, P., Rolston, B. & Tomlinson, M. (2005). *Poverty and Conflict in Ireland: An International Perspective*. Dublin: Institute of Public Administration & Combat Poverty Agency.

Irvine, R. (2014). Getting disability on the post-conflict agenda: the role of a disability movement. In D. Mitchell & V. Karr (eds) *Crises, Conflict and Disability: Ensuring Equality* (pp. 161–167). Oxon: Routledge.

Irvine, R. (2015a). Prioritising the inclusion of children and young people with disabilities in post-conflict education reform. *Child Care in Practice* **21**(1), 22–32.

Irvine, R. (2015b). *The Other Minority: Disability Policy in the Post-civil Conflict Environment*. Unpublished PhD Thesis, Queen's University Belfast, Belfast.

James, P. (2015). *Urban Sustainability in Theory and Practice: Circles of Sustainability*. Oxon: Routledge.

Jeong, H. W. (2002). *Approaches to Peacebuilding*. Basingstoke, NH: Palgrave Macmillan.

Lang, R. (2008). *Disability Policy Audit in Namibia, Swaziland, Malawi and Mozambique: Final Report*. London: The Leonard Cheshire Disability and Inclusive Development Centre.

Langer, A., Stewart, F. & Venugopal, R. (2012). Horizontal inequalities and post-conflict development: laying the foundations for durable peace. In F. Stewart, R. Venugopal & A. Langer (eds) *Horizontal Inequality and Post-Conflict Development* (pp. 1–27). Basingstoke: Palgrave Macmillan.

Lister, R. (2007). Inclusive citizenship: realizing the potential. *Citizenship Studies* **11**(1), 49–61.

Lockwood, E. & Tardi, R. (2014). The inclusion of persons with disabilities in the implementation of the 2030 Agenda for Sustainable Development. *Development* **57**(3–4), 433–437.

Marshall, T. H. (1950). *Citizenship and Social Class and Other Essays*. Cambridge: Cambridge University Press.

Mawere, M. & Awuah-Nyamekye, S. (2015). Cultural capital, social security and sustainability in conversation: an introduction. In M. Mawere & S. Awuah-Nyamekye (eds) *Harnessing Cultural Capital for Sustainability: A Pan Africanist Perspective* (pp. 1–32). Bamenda, Cameroon: Langaa RPCIG.

McCandless, E. & Karbo, T. (2011). *Peace, Conflict, and Development in Africa: A Reader*. Switzerland: University for Peace.

Meekosha, H. & Soldatic, K. (2011). Human rights and the global South: the case of disability. *Third World Quarterly* **32**(8), 1383–1398.

Miles, S. (2013). Education in times of conflict and the invisibility of disability: a focus on Iraq? *Disability & Society* **28**(6), 798–811.

Miles, S. & Medi, E. (1994). Disabled children in post-war Mozambique: developing community based support. *Disasters* **18**(3), 284–291.

Morris, J. (2005). *Citizenship and Disabled People: A Scoping Paper Prepared for the Disability Rights Commission*. Retrieved from http://enil.eu/wp-content/uploads/2012/07/Citizenship-and-disabled-people_A-scoping-paper-prepared-for-the-Disability-Rights-Commission_2005.pdf on 18 April 2018.

Oliver, M. J. (1999). Capitalism, disability and ideology: a materialist critique of the Normalization principle. In R. J. Flynn & R. A. Lemay (eds) *A Quarter-Century of Normalization and Social Role Valorization: Evolution and Impact*. Retrieved from www.independentliving.org/docs3/oliver99.pdf on 1 June 2016.

Pearce, J. (1999). Sustainable peace-building in the South: experiences from Latin America. In D. Eide (ed.) *From Conflict to Peace in a Changing World: Social Reconstruction in Times of Transition* (pp. 72–87). Oxford: Oxfam.

Power, M. (2008). War veterans, disability, and postcolonial citizenship in Angola and Mozambique. In D. Cowen & E. Gilbert (eds) *War, Citizenship, Territory* (pp. 177–198). New York: Routledge.

Pugh, M. (1995). *The Challenges of Peacebuilding*. Plymouth: University of Plymouth Press.

Quinn, G. & Degener, T. (2002). *Human Rights and Disability: The Current Use and Future Potential of United Nations Human Rights Instruments in the Context of Disability*. New York and Geneva: United Nations.

RAVIM & Handicap International Mozambique (2010). *People with Disabilities in the Suburban Areas of Maputo and Matola*. Maputo: RAVIM & HI Mozambique.

Redclift, M. (2000). Introduction. In M. Redclift (ed.) *Sustainability: Life Chances and Livelihoods* (pp. 1–14). London: Routledge.

Rowland, W. (2004). *Nothing About Us Without Us: Inside the Disability Rights Movement of South Africa*. Pretoria: UNISA Press.

Stone, E. (1999). *Disability and Development: Learning from Action and Research in the Majority World*. Leeds: The Disability Press.

Turner, B. S. (2016). The erosion of citizenship. *British Journal of Sociology* **52**(2), 189–209.

Ukaga, O. (2005). Sustainable development in Africa: a multifaceted challenge. In O. Ukaga & O. G. Afoaku (eds) *Sustainable Development in Africa: A Multifaceted Challenge* (pp. 1–6). Trenton, NJ: Africa World Press.

United Nations (2006). *Convention on the Rights of Persons with Disabilities*. New York: United Nations.

United Nations (2012). *United Nations Development Assistance Framework for Mozambique, 2012–2015*. New York: United Nations.

United Nations Committee on the Rights of Persons with Disabilities (2016). *Inquiry Concerning the United Kingdom of Great Britain and Northern Ireland Carried Out by the Committee under Article 6 of the Optional Protocol to the Convention*. CTRPD/c/15/r.2/Rev.1. New York and Geneva: United Nations.

United Nations Development Program (1999). *Governance Foundations for Post-conflict Situations: UNDP's Experience*. New York: UNDP.

Wilkinson, R. & Pickett, K. (2009). *The Spirit Level*. London: Penguin.

World Health Organization and World Bank (2011). *World Report on Disability*. Geneva: World Health Organization.

Young, I. M. (1990). *Throwing Like a Girl and Other Essays in Feminist Philosophy and Social Theory*. Cloomington & Indianapolis: Indiana University Press.

6

EXPERIENCES OF DISABLED PEOPLE IN USING INFORMATION AND COMMUNICATION TECHNOLOGY IN MOZAMBIQUE

Jorge Manhique and Anthony G. Giannoumis

Introduction

Scholars have examined the accessibility of information and communication technology (ICT) as a mechanism for participation in society (Giannoumis, 2016). The United Nations Committee on the Rights of Persons with Disabilities considers accessibility as a precondition for enjoying all other substantive rights (United Nations, 2014). The right to access is established within international law and framed strongly as a component of disability rights in the United Nations Convention on the Rights of Persons with Disabilities (CRPD) (United Nations, 2006). In addition, the United Nations has published the Sustainable Development Goals (SDGs), part of the Agenda 2030, which urges states to, among other things, 'significantly increase access to information and communications technology and strive to provide universal and affordable access to the internet in least developed countries by 2020' (United Nations, 2015). The SDGs also explicitly call attention to disability in relation to inclusive education, employment, social, political and economic participation. The SDGs' first year of implementation was 2016, thus making it possible for governments to begin to develop action plans for their operationalisation at national and local levels. A crucial part of that process includes decisions about the priority areas on which the country should focus. Mozambique ratified the CRPD in 2012, and has yet to submit its initial State Report to the responsible committee, which was due in 2014. Mozambique's economic and political situation poses particular constraints on the way interest groups engage in the policy-making process (Gaster *et al.*, 2009; Giannoumis *et al.*, 2017). Partnership and collaborative work between major stakeholders is crucial to implement both the CRPD (Article 4.3) and the Agenda 2030 (United Nations, 2006, 2015). In this chapter, we examine the experiences of persons with disabilities in relation to ICT accessibility in Mozambique.

Conceptualising and analysing ICT

In this chapter, we define ICT accessibility as a measure of the extent to which a product or service can be used by disabled persons as effectively as it can be used by non-disabled persons

(Narasimhan, 2010). However, accessibility of ICT products or services is not only determined by the level of usability (as a feature of the product or service). Instead, it also depends on the ability of the person to operate or use the technology. In this way, ICT accessibility relates to the 'relational model of disability' as enshrined in the CRPD and the World Health Organization's International Classification of Functioning, Disability and Health (Bickenbach *et al.*, 1999). Thus, another important element of accessibility is assistive technology, which is a technology, product, device, equipment used to maintain, or enhance the functional capability of individuals with disabilities, and facilitate interaction with ICTs (G3ict and ITU, 2014). Therefore, accessible ICT has to be understood in the continuum of interactions between a person, their environment and the technology that they use. Giannoumis (2016) relates the concept of ICT accessibility with universal design, which is the *use* of ICT by *everyone*, which necessitates both access to ICT for persons with disabilities and *compatibility* with assistive technology. While this chapter focuses on ICT accessibility, issues of access to and use of assistive technology are vital. Therefore, this chapter adopts a holistic approach to examining ICT accessibility.

Laws and policies are seen as critical tools to address the digital divide and enhance ICT accessibility (Giannoumis, 2014b). Previous studies have documented the impact of different regulatory approaches, given varying legal traditions and socio-political constraints on ICT accessibility in different countries and regions (Myhill & Blanck, 2009; Halvorsen, 2010; Easton, 2013; Samant *et al.*, 2013). Drawing from the experience of low-income countries, Samant *et al.* (2013) argue that the acquisition and wide use of ICTs for disabled people is dependent on several aspects. These include the political, legislative, climatic, nature of government supports, availability of financial assistance and facilitation of access to appropriate assistive technology.

Halvorsen (2010) has shown how the redistributive approach of the Nordic countries to ICT accessibility increased the access to ICT for persons with disabilities in terms of availability, but had limited impact in terms of accessible services, products and goods. The author also showed that the social regulation approach (use of procurement to achieve social goals) used in the United States has resulted in more accessible services, products and goods for Americans with disabilities, but limited impact in terms of availability of ICT services, products and goods. Based on a case study of the European Union, Easton (2013) illustrated the problem of the piecemeal approach to regulating ICT accessibility. The author further argues for a more coherent and comprehensive approach, which has procurement as a tool for securing a Europe with accessible services, products and goods for persons with disabilities.

Critics of the social regulation approach have pointed out that one of the weaknesses of such an approach is lack of guidance on how to achieve accessibility through the public procurement system, especially in a context of a heavy and complex bureaucracy system (Jaeger, 2008). For instance, Busuulwa, reflecting on the Uganda case, has pointed to a potential conflict that arises from applying both social inclusion criteria and cost criteria to the procurement process. The author argues that projects targeting persons with disabilities are typically expensive, because of the cost for procuring assistive technologies and specialised training (Busuulwa, 2015).

Participation and inclusivity in the design of ICT accessibility law and policy is a crucial element. For instance, Jaeger argues that the involvement of multiple stakeholders – industry, regulators, experts, and persons with disabilities – in the formulation of public procurement standards in the United States of America (USA), was crucial to promoting ICT accessibility (Jaeger, 2008). However, it becomes difficult to reach a consensus, since different stakeholders sometimes pursue divergent interests (Giannoumis, 2014b). Thus, the ability to find a proper balance between various interest groups, while upholding and respecting the rights of persons with disabilities, is crucial.

Accessible ICT as a human rights and development issue

The CRPD's Article 9 calls upon State Parties to proactively promote the design, development, production and distribution of accessible information and communication assistive technology and systems (United Nations, 2006). This is linked with the concept of universal design, articulated in Article 3 of the CRPD. The assumption is that ICT becomes accessible (in terms of affordability, and flexibility for adjustments), if 'born accessible', rather than adjusted later. Scholars have argued that ICT is an important tool for realising the SDGs (Tjoa & Tjoa, 2016; Sachs *et al.*, 2016). Specifically, it is enabling the transformation of the most expensive public services such as education and healthcare, as well as advancing low-income countries' economies in agriculture, trade/e-commerce and transportation (Sachs *et al.*, 2016).

Mozambique ratified the CRPD and its Optional Protocol in 2012. The Optional Protocol is a side agreement to the CRPD that allows for individual complaints to be submitted to the CRPD Committee by individuals, groups of individuals, or a third party. The first State Report to the CRPD Committee was scheduled for January 2014, but as of the writing of this chapter, has not yet been submitted. A draft State Report was developed with limited participation of persons with disabilities, and is still under review by the Ministry of Gender, Children and Social Affairs – the government body in charge of disability issues.

The Mozambican government is also committed to implementing the SDGs. To date, Mozambique is preparing for the domestication of the SDGs in national development programmes. The Government's Five Year Plan 2015–2019 (*Plano Quiquenal do Governo*), is composed of three main pillars, which include the SDGs' economic, social and environmental dimensions. At the sectoral level, there is an ongoing process of mapping, which aims to develop: (1) medium- and long-term sectoral plans consistent with the SDGs; (2) a database of indicators, targets and other sources of data collection to report on the SDGs; and (3) internal and external existing financing sources to support policy measures related to the SDGs' implementation. The Ministry of Economy and Finance is responsible for implementation of the SDGs, while the Ministry of Earth and Environment is the government focal point for the SDGs.

SDGs are not a binding instrument. As such, citizens cannot claim and or prosecute their government for not fulfilling a given goal. On the contrary, the CRPD is binding, and gives Mozambican citizens' rights and mechanisms to hold governments accountable in regard to the legal obligations assumed under this convention. It is therefore important that persons with disabilities and their representative organisations understand and participate meaningfully in the implementation of the CRPD and SDGs at national level, taking into account accessibility of ICT.

ICT legislation in Mozambique

Article 35 of the Mozambican Constitution states that all citizens are equal before the law, and they shall enjoy the same rights and be subject to the same duties. The right to access is recognised under the constitution of Mozambique. Article 125, paragraph 4.d, explicitly recognises the right to access public places as a matter of policy action. In this regard, the Policy for Persons with Disabilities, which was approved in 1999, among other things, recognises the right to access for persons with disabilities, based on the principle of non-discrimination emanating from the constitution, to 'social services, to grounds or venues, transport (public and private)'. However, the conceptualisation of the right to access embedded in both instruments focuses only on physical access. ICT accessibility is not addressed, resulting in regulations and standards that do not address accessibility in every dimension.

The ICT policy was introduced in 2000. It aims to establish a framework for the harmonious and sustainable development of information in society. Thus, the ICT policy serves as the basis upon which all the efforts to promote ICT will be built. The ICT policy defines the following priority areas: education, development of human resources, health, universal access, infrastructure, and governance.

In 2002, the Implementation Strategy (*Estratégia de Implementação da Política de Informática*) was approved. With this strategy, the government intends to (1) expand the availability and access to contents and applications, (2) promote an environment favourable to expansion of innovative activities in ICT by the private sector; (3) promote the use of ICT inside governmental institutions and civil society organisations. Despite these commitments, the reality shows that the initial investments were centred among state institutions. Innovation in ICT remains, to a large extent, unexplored, and Mozambique, as other developing countries, remains a recipient of technologies.

To implement projects related with universal access, the Telecommunication Law established a Universal Access Fund (Fundo de Acesso Universal), hereinafter UAF, with the purpose of financing the cost of providing services in the framework of the obligation of providing universal access services, and special tariffs to specific categories of users, in order to ensure accessibility to services. Article 39 of the Telecommunication Law defines the terms of provision of universal access services. The Telecommunication Law tasked the government agency responsible for telecommunications to develop projects that ensure access to telecommunication services for persons with various forms of impairment and other diverse needs. Universal service is a concept promoted by the International Telecommunication Union (ITU), to ensure that 'telecommunication services are accessible to the widest number of people (and communities) at affordable prices'. Although specifically conceived to promote telecommunication services, with technological developments, which might lead to the convergence of different technologies, the UAF has the potential to extend its scope to other technologies such as internet.

Despite the above initiatives, the Mozambican government has yet to fully address issues of ICT accessibility for persons with disabilities in laws and policies. Although the current reform process of the Telecommunication Law and related regulations points to some improvements, namely the introduction of unified licence regimes, substantive measures, such as broadening the concept of access to include ICT accessibility for persons with disability, among others, have yet to be introduced. Further, there are still areas such as accessible websites, which remain unregulated. The study focused especially on web accessibility including hardware (cell phones, computers) that support access to it. Recent studies have supported the idea that Mozambican citizens are increasingly relying on the internet to access information (Mabila, 2013).

Methodology

We utilised a qualitative approach where we used gathered data using focus group discussion and semi-structured interview as data collection methods. Data were collected from a Disabled People's Organisation (DPO) in Mozambique. Since a DPO is an organisation led by and made up of people with some form of impairment/s, this implies that all participants were persons with disabilities (Waldschmidt *et al.*, 2014).

The DPO was purposively selected for the focus group discussion and interview as it is a recognised actor on disability issues, including ICT accessibility, with a good representation of people with various forms of impairments in Mozambique. The participants had a range of impairments including those with sensory and physical impairments.

A purposive sample of 13 persons with disabilities was deliberately recruited to provide information on ICT accessibility as they experience it. As indicated earlier, participants were selected because they were members of an established DPO in Mozambique and had experience working with ICT. The focus group discussion was composed of persons with physical, hearing and visual impairment. We conducted a semi-structured interview with the director of the DPO. Twelve persons with disabilities also participated in the focus group discussion. We designed an interview schedule and a focus group discussion schedule that covered a broad range of questions related to the participants' experiences in using ICT in Mozambique. The focus group discussion took place in Maputo in November 2015 and lasted approximately two hours.

We obtained informed consent from participants prior to beginning the interview and focus group discussion. While the participants were not offered financial compensation, they were informed that one benefit of their participation was the opportunity to contribute to ICT accessibility, with implications for policy and practice in Mozambique. The participants were also informed that there would be minimal risk and that they could refuse to answer any questions without any justification. They were also informed that they were free to stop the interview or withdraw from the study at any time. Data were retained digitally on encrypted and password protected media. Participants were also assured that data would be anonymised in order to protect their identities.

We conducted a thematic analysis of the interview and focus group data (Miles & Huberman, 1994). The findings are presented based on the salient topics presented during the focus group. While the analysis did not focus on any specific type or types of ICT, the results revealed the relevance of different types of ICT for persons with disabilities in Mozambique.

Findings

The results revealed three broad themes regarding the experiences of persons with disabilities in using ICT in Mozambique: the experiences of persons with disabilities using ICT, the barriers experienced by persons with disabilities using ICT and the opportunities that accessible ICT provides for persons with disabilities to participate in society.

ICT usage

The results revealed two principal themes related to the use of ICT. Persons with disabilities in Mozambique typically use technology as a source of information and entertainment and as a tool for communication. First, most participants reported that they use television (TV) and radio to access information on current local, national and international events. For example, one participant stated, 'I use TV and radio to find out what is going on in my country as well as international news'. Several other participants confirmed this statement. Another participant commented: 'I use TV for entertainment – sports, especially athletics and I watch the news too'. Another participant said: 'I use TV and radio to get news about my country and other countries around the world'. These results suggest that persons with disabilities in Mozambique rely on ICT for accessing relevant information and for enjoying their leisure time. In addition, several participants used internet-connected computers to access information and research. One participant explained: 'I use internet to research issues related to inclusive education . . . but I also research matters related to psychology'. This implies that persons with disabilities rely on the internet to access educational and other information.

Most participants also reported that they use mobile phones as a means for communication. One participant commented, 'I use the mobile phone to communicate, sending and receiving messages'. Other participants cited their use of mobile phones in different contexts. For example, a deaf participant stated, 'I am deaf and I can't use the phone to speak; I use it for sending and receiving messages'. Another participant said, 'I use my mobile phone to communicate with family members', while another indicated that he uses a telephone to exchange messages with colleagues and relatives. Also, one of the participants indicated his mobile phone usage: 'I use the mobile phone for exchanging information with my family; I tell them where I am, what time I will be back home and so on'. The participant further articulated the role of the mobile phone in relation to communicating their personal safety:

> I avoid asking people to call or send a message on my behalf. I would rather prefer asking for a couple of airtime minutes from someone and call home personally. Hearing my voice, I make sure that they don't get worried about the situation I am involved in.

These results suggest that persons with disabilities rely on mobile phones to communicate and access information in a variety of contexts and with a variety of aims. Participants also reported using mobile phones to connect to the internet as indicated by one of them: 'I use the mobile phone as a tool of communication, entertainment and to access internet'.

Some participants reported using mobile phones to communicate through social media. Such media refers to a variety of software applications that include Facebook, Twitter and WhatsApp, which allow users to create and share content. Participants indicated that they use social media to communicate with family and friends, as well as for business purposes. However, participants noted usage as presented in the sub-heading.

Barriers to communication technology usage

The results revealed three principal themes related to the barriers that persons with disabilities experience using technology and these are accessibility, access, and ICT and law and policy.

Accessibility of ICT

Most participants acknowledged that the design of ICT can act as a barrier to use for persons with disabilities. One participant explained the barriers experienced:

> Technology tools are not barriers to people who aren't blind and have both hands. But they become barriers for someone with a visual impairment. Generally, the information comes in written form; visually impaired people may use a software system with voice [text-to-speech] to get the same information but as audio as an alternative and not in a written form.

Another participant similarly identified the barriers they experience when using ICT:

> There are many people with disabilities who face great difficulties using ICT. There are some people who think that ICT is only used to say hello, use Facebook and WhatsApp. Our greatest difficulty is accessibility and the equipment itself. Most of us have a mobile phone; our phones don't have enough programmes to be exploited. We can just speak.

Another participant further confirmed the accessibility barriers experienced by persons with disabilities:

I have a problem and I think most of us have the same problem. There is no doubt that these new smartphones are very good. It is difficult for us to use smartphones. It's complicated for us to use them. I can't use even 5% of the phone's capacity, it is worse for a person with a visual impairment. I can't even access the internet on my smartphone. The instructions are in English, and as a result, I don't know how to change the language into Portuguese; that's where the problem starts. So, I can hardly use most of the applications and functions in the phone.

Participants further suggested that inaccessible ICT limits access to education. One participant noted:

In Mozambique, it is quite complicated for people like me to study. Deaf people don't use the telephone much because they communicate through sign language. Because they face great difficulties in [accessing] professional training, an interpreter or translator is needed . . . Deaf people use computers through sign language but there are gaps in the software. Some instructions are in English and they don't understand anything.

These results suggest that persons with disabilities experience barriers using ICT due to its design, which limits the individual's ability to communicate and fully utilise the functions. Such barriers have implications on the individual's ability to use various from of ICT as educational tools.

Access to ICT

Many participants cited financial barriers as limiting access to ICT. One concerned participant commented, 'Everyone wants to access the internet but the price is very high . . . accessibility in terms of internet and technology devices cost'. Another participant discussed experiences using Skype (a software application that enables users to communicate over the internet using voice and video):

My daughter is deaf. There is Skype, which makes it easy for deaf people to communicate among each other . . . to access Skype is very expensive, you need too many megabytes . . . Skype is the best service for deaf people but it is very expensive.

Here, the participant suggests that while Skype might be freely available and optimal for deaf persons to use, the indirect costs of using Skype, in the form of internet subscription fees, limits it usage. Some participants cited disparities in geographical access as a barrier to ICT use. According to one participant, disparities exist between accessing ICT in urban and rural settings: 'Information gets to me . . . [but] what about for the people in the countryside? . . . Some of them might have a smartphone, but they have no idea how [to] take advantage of the phone'. Another participant highlighted the disparities among low-income and high-income communities.

The internet price in Maxaquene neighbourhood [a low-income community in Maputo city] should be cheaper than Sommershield neighbourhood [a high-income community]. There are significant differences among the people who use internet; there is a difference between a person with visual impairment and a person with a motor or physical impairment. The standard of living of each social class and how the internet is accessed should be taken into account.

The results suggest that persons with disabilities can experience barriers in accessing ICT due to disparities in urban versus rural and high-income versus low-income communities.

Some participants cited the lack of financial resources and skills as limiting access to ICT. One participant commented: 'I don't have the skills to use a smartphone as well as money to purchase one'. Another participant further articulated the relationship between access to ICT and knowledge of ICT:

> The acquisition of technology means import and acquisition, they [ICT] are materials that can only be bought out of the country . . . it is necessary to train human resources who can be able to use such equipment. The two items have never matched; when we get the equipment, we lack trained people to operate and vice versa . . . In fact, there has never been a combination of material acquisition and qualified human resources. Therefore, we should import the material and have qualified people.

Thus, the results suggest that persons with disabilities might experience barriers in accessing ICT due to lack of knowledge and training in the use of ICT.

Legislation

Many participants cited legislation as a barrier to using ICT. One participant commented: 'In Mozambique, there is no official planning in order to develop such [accessible] applications'.

Another person related barriers to using ICT for persons with disabilities with law and policy:

> At the bank, a deaf person can pick up the ticket number but will not hear when the teller calls for him. We find same situation at the hospital and cash points too. Deaf people and persons with visual impairment go through such difficulties. Nothing is clear in government policy.

Another participant confirmed the above view: 'There is no clear government policy on how to make digital inclusion. Any existing policy is on paper and has never been implemented'. Lack of clarity regarding ICT accessibility in law and policy was also noted by another participant:

> Government policy reforms should be clear concerning information technology . . . if the technology is going to serve the Mozambican people, the policy must be clear on that. After the reform, the implementation stage should take place. If there are inclusion reforms and implementation . . . the changes should be directed to an inclusion system.

The results suggest that the lack of clarity concerning ICT accessibility in law and policy has acted as a barrier to persons with disabilities using ICT. Similarly, another participant suggests that law- and policy-related barriers might limit access to ICT due to a lack of sustainability:

> They [an educational institution] have allocated . . . equipment for people with visual impairment. There is a computer with voice system for people with visual impairment, a scanner and a Braille printer. There is also a machine called text Braille. With this machine we can write while reading what we are writing. The project is there, no one . . . has ever been trained to help the users. The specialist came, installed the equipment and left. Myself as a student I wasn't trained to use the machine. So, the machine is just sitting in the library. We lack skills to operate the machines.

The participant suggests that laws and policies aimed at providing accessible ICT to persons with disabilities should also provide the competencies necessary for training and maintenance.

ICT as an enabler

The participants were asked about the relevance of ICT for their political participation. The results revealed that in several contexts, ICT has enabled persons with disabilities to participate politically. One participant discussed political participation in the context of sharing information:

> It was through internet that I found out that it was possible to share information about the rights of people with disabilities with people all over the world. It was through internet that I found about other types of technology that assist people with disability. I have also come across several documents that promote the rights of persons with disabilities. Moreover, I managed to get to a number of links where we share documents. So, it was through internet that we have made improvements in getting information. What we have accomplished so far is thanks to the Internet.

Another participant discussed ICT in relation to participation in local elections:

> Our organisation participated in the latest local municipal elections. In these elections, we managed to be . . . one of the most dynamic activist groups in the elections process. We would not reach such position without the help . . . and the support of Facebook and other social media tools . . . This performance had never been achieved before in the history of people with disabilities.

Other participants confirmed this view as noted by one of them: 'we were the ones who used information technology for our campaign . . . the response was excellent'. The results suggest that accessible ICT has a useful role in promoting political participation for persons with disabilities in Mozambique. In addition to political participation, participants suggested that accessible ICT enables persons with disabilities to take part in sports, culture and education. In relation to sports, a mother of a disabled child had this to say:

> I was once invited to a programme on TV as a mother of a person with disability. I went there with my daughter to share ideas with other Mozambicans on how to make improvements [for persons with disabilities]; it was discussed how people with disabilities could participate in sports. As a result, some people with disabilities started participating in sports and some families who had not sent their kids to school did so.

In relation to culture, one participant indicated that ICT enabled them to take part in an intercultural exchange programme:

> We [participated] in a cultural international exchange programme with other groups in Africa and overseas through internet; we met people from other African countries for cultural activities. We were also invited to go to Norway; myself, a colleague of mine and other African group members visited Oslo and another city . . . In Norway, we paid a visit to a visual impairment association.

In relation to education, one participant cited learning conducted over the internet (e-learning) as a component of education: 'I used to do lessons with a teacher abroad and have debates with students around the world . . . it was a good experience for me'. The results suggest that in addition to political participation, ICT accessibility can enable persons with disabilities to participate in sports, culture and education.

Discussion

This chapter has examined the experiences of persons with disabilities accessing ICT in Mozambique and has used as a point of departure, the implementation of the CRPD and the SDGs as cardinal points. The results provide an in-depth exploration of how, and to what extent, persons with disabilities in Mozambique use and experience ICT as a facilitator or barrier to social participation. The results suggest that persons with disabilities in Mozambique largely use ICT as a source of information, entertainment and to communicate. As such, persons with disabilities in Mozambique use ICT in much the same ways as people throughout the world. However, the results suggest that despite a common approach to using ICT, persons with disabilities experience challenges in accessing ICT, which has been caused, in part, by its design. This finding confirms research that has examined the design of ICT as a barrier to active citizenship (Giannoumis & Kline, 2015; Blanck, 2014). In other words, persons with disabilities in Mozambique are not able to use ICT on an equal basis with others – an experience directly addressed by the CRPD in Article 9. The results also suggest that a lack of accessible ICT has limited access to education for some persons with disabilities in Mozambique.

While research in ICT accessibility has typically focused on how the design of ICT creates usage barriers, it has yet to fully examine the relationship between the accessibility of ICT and access to ICT. This chapter provides initial evidence for this relationship and shows that ICT accessibility is connected with access to ICT. The results show that persons with disabilities experience disparate access to ICT due to financial, geographical and knowledge barriers. Specifically, persons with disabilities experience barriers to accessing ICT due to high relative cost. In addition, persons with disabilities experience barriers accessing ICT due to their place of residence – in particular rural versus urban and low-income and high-income communities. Article 9 of the CRPD specifically obligates States Parties to provide access to ICT in both rural and urban areas. However, it is unclear what the requirements for providing equal access in both rural and urban areas means in practice. Persons with disabilities in Mozambique also experience barriers accessing ICT due to the lack of knowledge capacity within ICT service providers.

The results further show that persons with disabilities experience policy barriers in accessing ICT. While this chapter shows that the Mozambican government has yet to fully address ICT accessibility in law and policy, there is an obligation under the CRPD to 'adopt all appropriate legislative, administrative and other measures' to support its implementation (United Nations, 2006). The findings have largely confirmed that the Mozambican government has yet to substantively enact ICT accessibility law and policy aimed at remediating accessibility and access-related barriers. In addition, the data suggest that this policy gap acts as a barrier to ensuring access to ICT on an equal basis with others.

The results confirm that ICT has enabled persons with disabilities to participate in society. First the results have shown that ICT enables persons with disabilities in Mozambique to participate politically. Article 29 of the CRPD guarantees persons with disabilities the right to participate in political life and specifically provides for persons with disabilities' right to form and participate in DPOs (United Nations, 2006). The results suggest that accessible ICT might act as a necessary precondition for fully realising the right to political participation in Mozambique. Second, the results have shown that ICT has enabled persons with disabilities to participate in sports and culture. Article 30 of the CRPD requires that persons with disabilities have the right to participate in cultural life and sporting activities. Thus, accessible ICT might act as a necessary precondition for realising these rights. Third, the results have shown that ICT has enabled persons with disabilities to participate in education. Article 24 of the CRPD requires that persons with disabilities have the right to inclusive education. Hence, it becomes important to ensure accessibility for all with reference to ICT (Tjoa & Tjoa, 2016), if the goal of education is to be realised in Mozambique.

The results confirm previous research evidence on ICT accessibility, which suggests that the design of ICT poses a barrier to its use by persons with disabilities (Giannoumis, 2016). This view has been enshrined in the CRPD and in national and international legal frameworks (United Nations, 2006). It is from this understanding that persons with disabilities in Mozambique have experienced several barriers to using ICT.

While ICT accessibility conventionally refers to the use of ICT by persons with disabilities, these definitions typically only refer to the *accessibility of* ICT and not *access to* it. The results have suggested that, in practice, accessibility of ICT and access to ICT are two phenomena that are inextricably linked. We argue that the relationship between the design of ICT and the opportunity to use ICT (i.e. the relationship between accessibility of and access to ICT), provides a useful basis for examining ICT accessibility legislation. Research has revealed that ICT accessibility legislation typically adopts a social regulation approach to ensuring that persons with disabilities have access to and use of ICT (Giannoumis, 2014a, 2014b). These laws and policies typically focus on influencing market actors to ensure that persons with disabilities can use ICT by changing its performance of ICT as an outcome of the ICT development process. However, research differentiates regulatory policies for ICT accessibility from redistributive policies for ICT accessibility (Halvorsen, 2010). Redistributive policies aim to promote ICT accessibility by providing resources such as financial incentives, equipment or training to persons with disabilities. Thus, the results suggest that, while research has largely focused on ICT accessibility legislation from a social regulative approach, research on ICT accessibility law and policy could include a holistic examination of both regulative and redistributive laws and policies aimed at ensuring persons with disabilities can use ICT. The results also suggest that reframing research on ICT accessibility to include redistributive legislation could provide a useful basis for ensuring sustainability in ICT accessibility.

Conclusion

Article 9 of the CRPD calls State Parties to promote the design, development, production and distribution of accessible ICT (United Nations, 2006). In the framework of the SDGs, ICT is viewed as an important tool to achieve the transformation to sustainable development by 2030. We have examined the experience of persons with disabilities in Mozambique in relation to CRPD and the SDGs. It is clear in this chapter that ICT is an important tool for the social inclusion of persons with disabilities in Mozambique. However, the results also suggest that the design of, and access to, ICT prevents persons with disabilities in Mozambique from using it, with implications for their participation in public life. In addition, the current approach to ICT legislation has yet to address ICT accessibility for persons with disabilities in Mozambique. We therefore propose a holistic approach to examining ICT accessibility, which combines an investigation of both social regulations and redistributive policies if persons with disabilities are to fully participate in national development in Mozambique.

Reflective questions

1 How can persons with disabilities build capacity as social innovators and developers of accessible technology in Mozambique?
2 To what extent can government, industry and civil society in Mozambique form partnerships to support the implementation of the CRPD?
3 How can pan-African organisations, including governmental and quasi-governmental organisations, aid organisations and advocacy organisations, support policy innovations in Mozambique?
4 What lessons can be drawn from this chapter to ensure maximum use of ICT among disabled people?

References

Bickenbach, J., Chatterji, S., Badley, E. M. & Ustün, T. B. (1999). Models of disablement, universalism and the international classification of impairments, disabilities and handicaps. *Social Science & Medicine* **48**, 1173–1187.

Blanck, P. (2014). *Equality: The Struggle for Web Accessibility by Persons with Cognitive Disabilities*. New York: Cambridge University Press.

Busuulwa, A. (2015). *From Disparity to Parity: Understanding the Barriers to Inclusion of Persons with Visual Disabilities in the Digital Revolution of Uganda*. Enschede: Universiteit Twente.

Easton, C. (2013). Website accessibility and the European Union: citizenship, procurement and the proposed Accessibility Act. *International Review of Law, Computers & Technology* **27**, 187–199.

G3ict & ITU (2014). *Model ICT Accessibility Policy Report*. Geneva: G3ict.

Gaster, P., Cumbana, C., Macueve, G., Domingos, L. N. C. & Mabila, F. (2009). *Inclusão Digital Em Moçambique: Um Desafio Para Todos*. Maputo: Ciuem.

Giannoumis, G. A. (2014a). Regulating web content: the nexus of legislation and performance standards in the United Kingdom and Norway. *Behavioral Sciences & The Law* **32**, 52–75.

Giannoumis, G. A. (2014b). Self-regulation and the legitimacy of voluntary procedural standards. *Administration & Society* **49**, 1–23.

Giannoumis, G. A. (2016). Framing the universal design of information and communication technology: an interdisciplinary model for research and practice. *Studies in Health Technology and Informatics* **229**, 492.

Giannoumis, G. A. & Kline, J. (2015). *Active Citizenship through the Use of New Technologies: The Experiences of Three Generations of Persons with Disabilities*. Oslo: Discit.

Giannoumis, G. A., Nthenge, M. & Manhique, J. (2017). The pivot model of policy entrepreneurship: an application of European ideas in the global South. In M. Stein & J. Lazar (eds) *Global Inclusion: Disability, Human Rights, and Information Technology* (pp. 227–243). Philadelphia: State College, University of Pennsylvania Press.

Halvorsen, R. (2010). Digital freedom for persons with disabilities: are policies to enhance e-accessibility and e-inclusion becoming more similar in the Nordic countries and the US? In L. Waddington & G. Quinn (eds) *European Yearbook of Disability Law* **2**, 73–75.

Jaeger, P. (2008). User-centered policy evaluations of Section 508 of the Rehabilitation Act: evaluating e-government web sites for accessibility for persons with disabilities. *Journal of Disability Policy Studies* **19**, 24–33.

Mabila, F. (2013). Understanding what is happening in ICT in Mozambique: a supply- and demand-side analysis of the ICT sector. *Policy Paper 10*, Research ICT Africa.

Miles, M. B. & Huberman, A. M. (1994). *Qualitative Data Analysis: An Expanded Sourcebook*. Thousand Oaks, CA: Sage Publications.

Myhill, W. & Blanck, P. (2009). Law & Policy Challenges for Achieving an Accessible Information Society in the EU: Lessons from America. *2009 Mid-Term Conference of the Nordic Centre of Excellence in Welfare Research (Ncoe) 'Reassessing the Nordic Welfare Model'*, Oslo.

Narasimhan, N. (2010). *E-Accessibility Policy Handbook for Persons with Disabilities*. Retrieved from http://g3ict.org/resource_center/e-Accessibility%20Policy%20Handbook on 27 April 2018.

Sachs, J. D. *et al.* (2016). *ICT & SDGs: How Information and Communications Technology Can Accelerate Action on the Sustainable Development Goals.* Retrieved from www.ericsson.com/assets/local/news/2016/05/ict-sdg.pdf on 12 August 2016.

Samant, D., Matter, R. & Harniss, M. (2013). Realizing the potential of accessible ICTs in developing countries. *Disability and Rehabilitation: Assistive Technology* **8**, 11–20.

Tjoa, A. M. & Tjoa, S. (2016). The role of ICT to achieve UN Sustainable Development Goals (SDG). In *ICT for Promoting Human Development and Protecting the Environment: Proceedings of the 6th IFIP World Information Technology Forum* (pp. 3–13). Springer.

United Nations (2006). *Convention on the Rights of Persons with Disabilities and Optional Protocols.* New York: United Nations.

United Nations (2014). *Convention on the Rights of Persons with Disabilities Committee General Comment No. 2 (2014) Article 9: Accessibility.* New York: United Nations.

United Nations (2015). *Sustainable Development Goals.* Retrieved from www.un.org/sustainabledevelopment/sustainable-development-goals/ on 27 April 2018.

Waldschmidt, A., Karačić, A., Sturm, A. & Dins, T. (2014). *A Comparative Analysis of Disability Rights Activism – with Reference to the Concept of Active Citizenship.* Working Paper. Making persons with disabilities full citizens – new knowledge for an inclusive and sustainable European Social Model. DISCIT.

PART II

Access to education

In Part II, authors discuss issues of access to education of disabled people from early childhood to secondary education, with more bias toward deaf learners, an aspect that has not received much attention in southern Africa.

7

PERSONAL REFLECTIONS OF DISABLED WOMEN ON ACCESS TO EARLY CHILDHOOD EDUCATION IN ZIMBABWE

Christine Peta

Introduction

While several measures can be taken to prevent impairments from occurring among children, the number of children with disabilities across the world has remained high. About 10% of the world's young people have either congenital or acquired impairments, with more than 80% of them living in low-income countries (UNICEF, 2014). The same author reports a high number of children who for example, in 2009, were dying before they turned five, at an unprecedented rate of one child every three seconds. The irony of the matter is that such children lose their lives due to factors that can be avoided, such as a lack of obstetric assistance, pneumonia, malnutrition, measles, tuberculosis, Acquired Immune Deficiency Syndrome (AIDS), accidents and lack of access to clean water. UNICEF (2014) states that those who survive such calamities often struggle to thrive as they acquire poverty-related forms of impairments, which include physical, intellectual, sensory and developmental impairments. In addition, such children also lack experiences of other essentials, such as early childhood education as further discussed below.

Compared to their non-disabled counterparts, children with disabilities are usually excluded from, among other things, educational services, and they are more vulnerable to violence, abuse and exploitation (Philpott & McLaren, 2011). Yet, high-quality inclusion in early childhood education (ECE) can enable children to benefit in both short-term and long-term ways, with some of the benefits manifesting later on in life (William, Henninger & Gupta, 2014). Furthermore, children who gain access to ECE settings, experience immense growth, acquire abilities, skills and knowledge in numerous overlapping spheres; thus, physical, emotional, social and self-help skills, which include aspects such as communication, language and being able to dress oneself. It therefore follows that denying children with disabilities access to ECE settings is tantamount to thwarting their potential to attain full growth; a scenario that is in direct contradiction with various treaties seeking to secure the rights of children with disabilities.

Treaties that pay attention to the realisation of the rights of children with disabilities include: The Convention on the Rights of the Child (1989), the first human rights legal instrument that made an explicit reference to disability (Article 2 on non-discrimination) and a separate article (23) solely devoted to the rights and needs of children with disabilities. The African Charter on the Rights and Welfare of the Child (1990) contains articles on the rights of children with disabilities.

The Convention on the Rights of Persons with Disabilities gives direction on ways through which discrimination can be overcome (United Nations, 2006). It also suggests how the right to full participation of children with disabilities can be recognised in schools, homes and communities, health care services, recreational activities and in all other aspects of life (Philpott & McLaren, 2011). Nevertheless, in spite of such treaties, the early childhood years have not received much attention or investment from governments in most nations.

Philpott and McLaren (2011) have attributed the above scenario to the fact that political determination does not automatically mean the availability of appropriate knowledge regarding disability or adequate capacity and budgets. Prior to 2005, ECE was primarily offered by private institutions, who charged fees that were way beyond the reach of many and such institutions were scarce in rural areas. Early childhood development (ECD) was officially integrated into the mainstream education system in 2005 as indicated in the Director's Circular Minute No. 12 of 2005 (Ministry of Education, Sport, Arts and Culture [MoESAC] (Zimbabwe), 2005). Thus, ECD became annexed to existing primary schools. Such education comprises of the first two years, plus an additional two years that are embedded in Grades 1 and 2 (the four years are known as infant school); junior school comprises of Grades 3–7 and secondary education comprises of Forms 1–6. Zimbabwe has not yet had a comprehensive ECD policy other than Permanent Secretary and Directors' circulars and statutory instruments spanning from 2004 to 2014 (Makokoro, 2017). Furthermore, due to the prevailing economic decline in the country, the ECD sector is grossly underfunded and a large amount of education funds are directed to salaries, leaving less than 3% for infrastructure and professional development (ibid.). The same author states that the ECD sector has about 427,800 learners taught by 4,000 teachers; with 5,800 more qualified teachers required. Only 21.6% of children aged 36–59 months are attending an ECD programme.

This chapter is informed by data that are emerging from ongoing case study research among persons with disabilities in Zimbabwe; on their access to ECE in their formative years, over the past three decades. While the main study from which this chapter is emerging is broader, in this chapter I specifically discuss four disabled women's personal experiences of access to ECE in Zimbabwe.

Marginalisation of disabled women

Considering that this chapter is focusing on access of disabled women to ECE, it is imperative to point out the double discrimination of women and girls with disabilities. According to Chataika (2013, p. 8) 'women and girls with disabilities face double discrimination due to their impairments and womanhood; hence relegating them into chronic poverty when compared to women without disabilities and men with disabilities'. Women are generally regarded as substandard beings, particularly in patriarchal contexts which esteem masculinity and denigrate femininity (Peta, 2017). The situation is worse for women with disabilities, as evidenced in part by reports of low literacy and narrow employment opportunities among the women (Chataika, 2013). As disability adds a rung of disadvantage to the personal development of girls and women with disabilities, disabled men are twice as likely to secure educational and employment opportunities compared to their female counterparts.

However, that is not to say that I intend to assume an additive, one-plus-one approach, which adds one social life attribute to the other (gender to disability). Rather, I acknowledge the simultaneous interaction of the various social lives' attributes in shaping the experiences of access to ECE of persons with disabilities in Zimbabwe. In any case, while disability is closely interconnected with gender, it is also interrelated with other identity markers such as poverty, sexuality and nationality; a scenario that is apparent in the accounts that are discussed in this chapter. Nevertheless, the intersection of different identity markers, that include disability and gender in the experience of access to ECE of women with disabilities, imply that such experiences do not present a clear-cut picture, but a complex and multidimensional terrain.

Methodology

A case study represents an empirical inquiry that allows the contextual exploration of a phenomenon, thereby enabling the researcher to select a small geographical area or limited number of participants (Gray, 2009). In this study, I am using the case study approach to explore the past experiences of access to ECE of persons with different kinds of impairments in Zimbabwe. A non-probability snowball sampling approach is being used to draw participants aged between 18 and 30, with different kinds of impairments who are currently living in Harare, the capital city of Zimbabwe. According to Gray, in snowball sampling, the researcher allows participants to identify others within the population of interest, thereby enabling access to those who are 'hidden'. In this chapter, I draw quotes from case study accounts of four women who form part of the study, and who among them have deafness, albinism and partial visual impairment as well as physical impairment (wheelchair user). A sign language interpreter was used to facilitate communication with deaf participants.

Although case studies have been criticised for providing limited basis for scientific generalisation due to the small number of participants that are usually involved, the focus of qualitative research is not on generalisation. Rather, the rich and detailed qualitative accounts that are arising from the case study accounts enhance the illumination of the complexities that surround real-life experiences of access to ECE by disabled persons, which might not be captured by laboratory quantitative experiments. Due to its focus on numbers, a quantitative approach might not be able to illuminate some of the phenomena that disability researchers are attentive to, such as experiences; hence a qualitative case study approach was chosen.

A thematic analysis approach is being used to analyse data for this study. Data is initially coded, and recurring elements are noted and grouped together into themes, drawing out similarities and differences among the case accounts. Thematic analysis has been criticised for its flexibility, which threatens to constrain the researcher in selecting elements of focus. However, Allan and Skinner (1991) argue that it is a principled approach, which is generally accepted by the research community. Each theme drawn from the cases is discussed separately. In the end, the interconnectedness of the themes and how they interrelate is finally drawn out.

This study ascertains that all participants are not lacking in decisional capacity. Informed consent is obtained after explaining to each participant what the study involves. Such consent is obtained in the language of the participant's preference, between Shona (one of the main local Zimbabwean languages) and English. The researcher is fluent in both languages. The letter of information was translated to Shona, and also printed in Braille to accommodate blind participants. A sign language interpreter is used to facilitate communication with deaf participants. The principle of non-maleficence is upheld by ensuring that participants are not exposed to any kind of physical harm. For confidentiality purposes, any information that identifies the participant is kept in the strictest of confidence and pseudonyms are used to reduce the possibility of identifying participants. In terms of beneficence, this study is making a contribution to the existing body of knowledge.

Findings and discussion

I draw direct quotes from the case accounts of participants, thereby illuminating their experiences of access to education or lack thereof in their early childhood and in some instances the resultant outcome. The quotes are intercepted with literature and my own perspectives, in an effort to offer a meaningful analysis of the ECE experiences of the participants. The main theme of ECE is presented and discussed below, under two subheadings: (1) lack of ECE and (2) quality of ECE programmes.

Lack of ECE

Taita is a 23-year-old woman who is deaf from birth. She was raised by her grandmother in her maternal village in Masvingo. Following the death of her grandmother, she moved to the city to live with her mother and stepfather at the age of 16. Box 7.1 provides Taita's views on her access to ECE.

Box 7.1 Taita's early childhood education experiences

My father died just after I was born and my mother went to look for a job in Harare and left me in the care of my grandmother. I didn't go to crèche or anything like that, because the crèche was in town where my mother lived, but I could not live with my mother because my mother had married a man who did not like me because I am deaf. My grandmother also said the crèche doesn't matter because it's not real education, so I should just wait for primary school, which is the real school which has more value, the crèche would just be an unnecessary problem for me because I am deaf. She also said that men don't want to marry disabled women, but if I am lucky, I may just get a deaf man to marry me and to look after me, when I grow up, so I should not worry much. I was 8 years old when my grandmother said I should start learning. She took me to a primary school which is close to our village and I started Grade one. I could not hear what the teacher was saying or what other school children were saying, but I could see that they were just talking and laughing. I spent one month going to that school and no one could talk to me like my grandmother did. One day my teacher asked my grandmother to stop bringing me to school because I was not hearing anything or talking to anyone. After that my grandmother did not try to send me to another school but I just stayed at home. When my grandmother died, my mother had no choice but to take me to the city to live with her and my stepfather, I was 16 years old at the time.

According to UNESCO (2006), learning begins before a child walks through the door of a classroom. The child's early learning experiences form the foundation upon which later education can be grounded. While Taita's earlier learning could have been informally fostered by her caring grandmother, there is evidence that her grandmother was of the understanding that Taita's valuable education would begin when she started primary school at the age of 8. Devoid of prior access to earlier good educational programmes, which according to UNESCO are provided in kindergartens, pre-schools and nurseries, Taita was reportedly 'thrown' into Grade 1 (mainstream primary school), so that she could 'start' learning along with other children of her age if not younger.

One could argue that both the school and Taita's grandmother were taking an inclusive approach, which sought to allow Taita to have access to the same range of educational services as other children of her age. However, the definition of inclusion proffered by Moore, Symes and Bull (2013), calls for not just access to the same environment, but also to meaningful participation of children with disabilities. To buttress that point, the same authors state that participation is more than a cosmetic presence of a disabled child in a classroom, but the child must be able to actively participate in a scenario where the child's contribution and participation are not only valued by others involved, but also by him or herself.

Spending a month 'attending classes' in a school that does not cater for the needs of children with disabilities, all in the name of 'inclusive education' could actually be traumatising for a young child who is unable to participate in class activities due to communication barriers. In any case, UNESCO (2006) reported that inclusive educational programmes ought to respect children's linguistic diversity. Perhaps efforts could have been made to use a sign language interpreter or, if that was not possible, to arrange a transfer of the child to another school that caters for her needs, depending on such school's availability. But perhaps such mitigation strategies were not easy for Taita's grandmother to arrange, given her socio-economic status and lack of appropriate knowledge about issues of disability.

Either way, the narrative of Taita raises questions about the school curriculum, staffing and family involvement and ability to address the educational needs of children with disabilities. One might wonder if the situation could have been different if Taita had been given an opportunity to enrol in pre-primary education; perhaps her transition to primary school education could have been easier. The entrenchment of early childhood learning in mainstream primary schools in Zimbabwe began only about a decade ago. Literature shows that such education was officially introduced in 2005 (Makokoro, 2017), and many early educational learning institutions were of a private nature and predominantly located in the urban areas. Taita could not access such centres as she was unable to live with her mother and stepfather in the city because her stepfather resented her on the grounds that she is deaf.

Although there was an ECE centre in her grandmother's rural village, Taita states that her grandmother thought that such formal early childhood programmes were not valuable because 'real' education starts at Grade 1 in primary school. In addition, the grandmother thought that the 'lesser' value of such early childhood programmes would just be an unnecessary burden for Taita because she is deaf, and also if she is lucky, she could find a deaf man who would marry her and look after her in her adult years, hence she did not need to worry much about education. Taita's grandmother felt that it was best for her to wait and focus on 'real' education, which begins in primary school. Such an understanding provides evidence of a lack of awareness of the value of ECE. One therefore wonders if Taita's grandmother would have enrolled her on such an ECE programme if it was available within the rural area where they lived, alongside also the gendered perspective of the grandmother toward education and marriage. The importance of ECE was emphasised by the former President of the United States of America, Barack Obama, in his 2013 state of the union address:

> Study after study shows that the sooner a child begins learning, the better he or she does down the road . . . And for poor kids who need help the most, this lack of access to preschool education can shadow them for the rest of their lives . . . Every dollar we invest in high-quality early education can save more than seven dollars later on.
>
> *(Obama, 2013)*

Articulating what she perceives as the outcome of her lack of ECE and ensuing education, Taita said:

> I started thinking that if I was educated I could do what other girls of my age where doing; I saw them going for teaching and nursing training and living on their own. When I was 18 years old, I met a non-disabled man who said he loved me and he wanted to marry me. I thought this was my chance of escaping my horrible stepfather. I agreed to sleep with him, I got pregnant and the man ran away. I later gave birth to a son and my stepfather accused me of stubbornness and he kicked me out of the house

into the streets. Deaf men did not want to marry me, so I saw that my grandmother was wrong and I decided to become a prostitute, because I don't need education to do that. Now I am sick with HIV and I see that my life has become worse and I can die and leave my son.

As previously noted, ECE lays a strong foundation upon which later education can be constructed, thereby creating an avenue through which people can escape vulnerability to abuse and poverty (UNESCO, 2006). Such an assertion resonates with the narrative of Taita, which indicates that in her later years in life, she could not access professional training as a nurse or as a teacher as per her wish. She lacked prior education from early childhood, through to primary and secondary level. Consequently, Taita became vulnerable to sexual abuse as she sought to escape the guardianship of her resentful stepfather; she was impregnated by a non-disabled man who purported to love her and she bore a son, whom she also began to raise in poverty. Taita's narrative again brings to the fore part of the statement made by Barack Obama, who stated that ECE is likely to reduce, among other things, teen pregnancies, and in addition:

> studies show students grow up more likely to . . . graduate high school, hold a job, and form more stable families of their own. So let's do what works, and make sure none of our children start the race of life already behind. Let's give our kids that chance.
>
> *(Obama, 2013)*

UNESCO (2013) established that children from poor families, living in rural areas, are most likely to drop out of school. Nevertheless, the preliminary findings of this study indicate that disability adds another rung to the ladder of disadvantage, in a scenario where disability, gender, class, poverty and sexuality intersect to frame the oppression of girls and women with disabilities, thereby narrowing their chances of accessing ECE and, ultimately, professional opportunities. In this instance, disability intersects with Taita's socio-economic class to deny her access to early childhood learning and, ultimately, leading to her dropping out of primary school. Hence, this increased her vulnerability to sexual abuse in the later years of her life, resulting in a teenage pregnancy. In her quest to shoulder her responsibilities of motherhood, she became a commercial sex worker; a livelihood option which, in her own words, 'does not require any form of educational qualifications, save for my femininity'. Although the sex work industry seems to be profitable and it employs millions of people across the world (Hakim, 2015; Spice, 2007), it might not always be the best option as it can put individuals at sexual risks. As a young single mother raising her son, Taita bemoans the fact that she has been infected with HIV. Taita's livelihood options were evidently limited by her lack of education, which began in early childhood. The mitigation measures she adopted in trying to lessen the negative impact of a lack of education, appear to be far more costly than the provision of timely ECE, which transcends into primary and secondary education and beyond. This does not imply that persons who experience early childhood learning are immune to sexual abuse or that they do not get infected with HIV, but Taita's vulnerability was worsened by her lack of education in a context of poor family relations that resulted in her teenage pregnancy, early motherhood and HIV infection.

Quality of ECE programmes

Maidei is a 19-year-old woman with albinism. She attended a boarding ECE institution located in a city, which is about 400 kilometres from her home. Maidei shares her story in Box 7.2.

Box 7.2   Maidei's early childhood education experiences

I was 6 years old and my parents said it was time to go to crèche so that I can prepare to start Grade 1 at the age of 7. However, they saw that the crèches near us had no disabled children. So they did not want to send me there. My aunt said there was a crèche in Masvingo for disabled children, and I could fit in well. I was sent to Masvingo thinking that I was going to live with my aunt, but when I got there I realised that I was going to live in a boarding school. In fact, I can't call it a school; let me just call it a boarding house because it was a house not a school. I would only see my aunt when she came to pick me up when the 'school' closed. I liked that we were drawing things on paper with my pencil and colouring those things. Also, I had friends but I was not very happy. I was thinking about my mother, father, brother and sister, and I would cry when I started missing home. When I cried, I would be beaten up by the lady. We were not allowed to choose food; what she gave us is what we ate. Even if you were hungry, the lady would shout at you if you told her. I started wishing I was at home, where I could ask for food from my mother. I don't like brown bread but we were forced to eat it, we were forced to clean the house, water the garden and to do a lot of work that made me very tired. When I have my own children, I will never send them to a boarding school. The truth is I did not learn anything, except to draw pictures and to colour. Most of the time, we were just playing, working or sleeping. But the day when our families were coming to collect us, the lady would smile and be nice to us all and our parents and relatives would think she is nice, but I don't think she cared about us.

There is evidence that the enrolment of children in ECE institutions, which are of a boarding nature, denies them the opportunity to grow up in family environments (UNESCO, 2006). It is therefore not surprising that Maidei reported that while she liked the idea of 'schooling', her concentration was in part obstructed by the fact that she was missing her family. A study carried out in South Africa, revealed that while most children liked the idea of going to school, finding an appropriate learning environment is not an easy task, because challenges that include special schools that are far away from home are encountered (Philpott & McLaren, 2011). Furthermore, in some instances a high number of parents and guardians resort to just keeping their children with disabilities at home, after experiencing challenges in finding a proper ECE centre.

Considering Maidei's memories of her pre-primary 'education' as quoted in her narrative above, it becomes debatable to send a child to an ECE centre that is far away from home. It is clear that in such situations, the problem is not the impairment itself, but it is the daily life issues, which are attitudinal, social and physical in nature that can present more challenges (Philpott & McLaren, 2011). Although Maidei was only 6 years old when she attended the boarding house in Masvingo, she vividly remembers the neglect, negative attitudes and heavy workloads assigned to her by the founder of the institution. The reported workloads represent what the International Labour Organisation (n.d.) in part calls child labour, which deprives children of schooling or requires them to attempt to combine school attendance with heavy workloads, to the detriment of their physical and mental well-being.

For children with or without disabilities, the nature and quality of their contextual key relationships contributes greatly to their development and formation of secure attachments (Moore, 2012). The same author states that positive attachments arise from responsive and warm caregiving, thereby establishing a secure basis for future development and learning. The absence of good-quality relationships and care can compromise the learning and development of the child.

Oblivious of such perspectives, and the knowledge that children with disabilities might give subtle cues as opposed to initiating activity or interaction, the teacher may have sought to use forceful directives (Moore, 2012), resulting in children being exhausted with physical work. There is a possibility that the ECE teacher at Maidei's school might not have received adequate training or she was just bent on cashing in on parents who were determined to ensure that their children with disabilities acquire ECE.

The above perspective resonates with the fact that, historically, the concept of ECE in Zimbabwe was framed around a community development approach, which underpinned the roll out of ECD centres under the National Early Childhood Development (NECD) programme (Makokoro, 2017). The same author also noted that limited attention was paid to criteria and there was generally a lack of capacity to make valuable contributions, within a context where ECE activities and facilities were offered in diverse ways. The national review of the education system in 2004 made a significant contribution by making recommendations for the integration of ECD in mainstream education structures, instead of leaving all ECE programmes to run parallel to the conventional system.

One can therefore argue that the government's 2005 introduction of ECD as a compulsory practice, which is embedded in schools, is significant. However, as noted in the introductory section of this chapter, Zimbabwe does not have an adequate number of professionals who are trained in ECD. According to Makokoro (2017) there is need for the government to train 5,800 more qualified teachers and at the moment only 21.6% of children aged 36–59 months are attending a mainstream ECD programme. Of notable concern is that such statistics are silent on the number of ECD teachers who are trained to cater for the educational needs of children with disabilities.

In another example, Rufaro who is 18 years old said:

> I have a little brother who has albinism like me, so I told my parents that the boarding school in Masvingo was not nice for me. So this year (2017) my little brother, who is 4 years old, has started going to a nearby crèche, which has children who are not disabled. But the teacher does not care about my disabled little brother. Sometimes he is not allowed to wear his hat. Direct sun can damage his skin and he can have cancer. The teacher sometimes tells everyone not to wear their hats, including my brother; what kind of thinking is that? My brother's eyesight is also poor because of albinism but he is not allowed to sit very close to the writing board and he is also not allowed to hold a paper or book very close to his eyes. He tells me that the teacher says 'there are no favours in class, put your book down'. Even when other children are laughing at my little brother about the colour of his skin, the teacher does not say anything. Surely, what kind of teaching is that? This teacher does not understand disability issues and he needs to learn.

Writing from a teacher's perspective, Palmer (2015) argues that one of the key elements of ECE is to teach children the value of respecting not only others, but their belongings and immediate and global environments. On her blog, Palmer (2015) argues that 'there is no better place to learn this virtue than in a hectic pre-school environment, where everything is shared and civility and manners are taught and learned organically'.

The teacher's insensitivity to Rufaro's brother and his indifference to the aspect of other children teasing him on the grounds of his condition raises concern. A study carried out in Zimbabwe revealed that it is common for early childhood learning to be conducted by untrained staff (para-professionals) (Makokoro, 2012). However, such a practice could hinder the attainment of good-quality education. While Nhaka Foundation (an NGO) is working with the Government of Zimbabwe to ensure that para-professionals provide quality care and education to children; of notable concern is that the initiative is silent on children with disabilities (Makokoro, 2017).

It is indisputable that Zimbabwe's attitude toward education is that of valuing high-quality standards of education (Makokoro, 2017). The Medium Term Strategic Plan, 2011–2015, enhanced the professional status of teachers by setting expected standards and providing a diversity of opportunities for professional development (Government of Zimbabwe, 2011). In turn, every child has a right to access and participate in ECE activities. Thus, denying children with disabilities such access is a violation of their human rights. But drawing from the findings of this study, perhaps the idea should not just be about enrolling children with disabilities in early childhood learning centres, for the sake of achieving inclusion. Rather, both parents and the Ministry of Primary and Secondary Education should play an active role in assessing the suitability and functionality of such centres.

Mosa, a 20-year-old lady with a physical impairment, is a wheelchair user. She was raised by her parents in one of the high-density suburbs in Harare. Mosa narrates her personal experiences:

> I was 6 years old and living in Glen-Norah. There was a crèche nearby, which was run by the church; so we were not paying anything. I was going for free. There were swings and slides and I enjoyed the play. We were told to bring our own food from home, but at times there was no bread in our house. So I could not bring any. I liked the school, but it was hard at break time when others were eating and I was not, I would start feeling hungry and my friend would give me a little piece of his bread, until his mother told him not to give me.

A health and nutrition study carried out in Zimbabwe, revealed that many ECD centres in mainstream primary schools do not provide food as children are expected to bring their own food and drink from home (Makokoro, 2012). The study also revealed that some children in ECD programmes are infected with ringworms and bilharzia, which affects their development. The economic decline in the country has resulted in some children not being able to bring any food from home and they are forced to watch while others eat. To complement government efforts, Nhaka Foundation is working with nurses from local clinics who visit the schools to check on the health of children in an effort to contain ringworms and to ensure that health problems do not spread to other children. Families are educated on the importance of early education, balanced diets and good health for children, through community engagement, lobbying and activism.

Concluding insights and way forward

Considering challenges that surround early childhood learning for children with disabilities, there is evidence that some families can find themselves in limbo, unable to find appropriate ECE centres in their communities. Consequently, they live with the guilt of keeping their children with disabilities at home or delaying such enrolment until the children are of primary school age or beyond. Yet, children's learning is cumulative and ECE determines the outcome of later learning, in a scenario where the skills that are developed earlier in life, contribute greatly to a chain of outcomes. The result can be a strengthening of earlier skills and behavioural characteristics, or the worsening of initial difficulties, or new challenges may emerge (Moore, 2012).

In the context of the study informing this chapter, there is a possibility that the ECE sector can be infiltrated by opportunists, who set up sub-standard centres, in order to cash in on desperate parents trying to afford their children with disabilities early childhood learning. There is need for the Ministry of Primary and Secondary Education to establish machinery that conducts periodic checks on the status of all ECE centres (private and public). Also, the delivery of the curriculum, staff and well-being of the children should be supervised. Teachers capable of catering for children with and without disabilities should be appointed if there are to be chances of realising positive learning outcomes and child development.

The Ministry of Primary and Secondary Education needs to re-examine the broader aspects of inclusion in ECE and pay more attention to key aspects such as support, access and participation. As stated by Moore *et al.* (2013), educational policy and practice should stretch beyond professional development, to include appropriate implementation of inclusive practices that support children with disabilities. There is need to consciously create support platforms, upon which opportunities for collaboration and communication between families and educational staff can take place to ensure high-quality ECE. Access can be achieved by offering a diversity of environments and activities, which cater for the needs of all children including disabled children. Both physical and attitudinal barriers ought to be dealt with, within contexts that offer different and multiple ways of promoting early childhood learning and development, so as to ensure effective participation.

Enrolling deaf children who lack pre-primary education in mainstream schools that do not cater for their needs, and allowing such children to spend days without participating in class activities due to communication barriers, is a serious violation of their human rights. To enhance participation, there is need for the creation and sustenance of ECE programmes that use different mediums of instruction, so as to promote engagement of children with disabilities in appropriate learning and playing activities alongside others. Considering that Moore *et al.* (2013) assert that participation is the engine of development, efforts should be made to create a sense of belonging for all children, including children with disabilities.

Implementing policy on ECE does not on its own yield much, if the initiative is not accompanied by a rigorous awareness-raising campaign. The Ministry of Primary and Secondary Education, civil society and disabled people's organisations need to raise awareness about the value of ECE to all children, including disabled children. Such awareness will enable families and communities in both rural and urban areas to realise the need for including children in ECE programmes and demonstrates the negative impact of a lack of such education. Involving teenage or adult persons with disabilities in such awareness-raising campaigns, could go a long way in demonstrating the advantages of gaining access to ECE and the disadvantages of a lack thereof, to families and communities.

The involvement of families and communities is an acknowledgement that children do not live in isolation; the well-being of the children's families is likely to enhance the success of the children's learning experience, which is evidently linked to the home environment. Families need to realise that having any form of impairment does not mean that a child should start school later than his or her non-disabled peers. In any case, the government has directed two years of ECE plus an additional two years that are embedded in Grades 1 and 2 (the four years that are known as infant school). A diverse range of activities that assist young people to develop various skills, including language and social skills that are critical in their current and future well-being, are therefore required (UNESCO, 2006). Such an approach tends to promote holistic development of children and allow them to be ready for formal education.

Children who are enrolled at ECE centres could be assessed, perhaps at the beginning of the year, by a multidisciplinary team of practitioners, who include educationists with inclusive education background, health professionals and parents. A detailed assessment report could then be used to determine the needs of the child, including their unique educational needs. Considering that UNESCO (2006) recommends a holistic approach, which integrates educational activities with additional services such as nutrition, health and social services, the involvement of multidisciplinary teams would go a long way in offering a wholesome ECE programme, which eases the transition into primary school. In any case, early development of a child begins from birth to school-entering age. Therefore, a full package with more benefit for ECE programmes would yield more results (Carlis, 2011).

In resonance with the above assertion, Carlis (2011) states that the multidimensional nature of early childhood learning calls for the removal of barriers among separate domains if the comprehensive nature of child development is to be effectively attended to. The Ministry of Primary and Secondary Education should consider the establishment of a holistic policy, which directs synergy of education, nutrition, health and social welfare so as to provide a wholesome supportive and rich experience for all children, including children with disabilities. However, while there is growing international interest in the early learning of children, the topic of ECE for children with disabilities is under-researched within the global South. I therefore call upon interdisciplinary scholars to undertake further research on this valuable topic, particularly within African contexts.

References

Allan, G. & Skinner, C. (1991). *Handbook for Research Students in the Social Sciences.* London: The Farmer Press.

Carlis, L. J. (2011). *Evaluating which Classroom and Student Variables in an Early Childhood Program Best Predict Student Language and Literacy Achievement* (Order No. 3461500). Available from Education Database; ProQuest Dissertations & Theses A&I. (880396481). Retrieved from https://search.proquest.com/doc view/880396481?accountid=14500 on 14 April 2017.

Chataika, T. (2013). *Gender and Disability Mainstreaming Training Manual: Prepared for Disabled Women in Africa.* Germany: GMZ and GIZ, pp. 1–75. Retrieved from www.diwa.ws/index.php?option=com_ phocadownload on 19 April 2017.

Government of Zimbabwe (2011). *Education Medium Term Plan (2011–2015) Ministry of Education, Sports, Arts and Culture.* Retrieved from www.google.co.za/search?q=education+medium+term+plan+zimb abwe&rlz=1C1CHBF_enZW746ZW746&oq=EDUCATION+MEDIUM+TERM+PLAN+&aqs= chrome.1.69i57j0l4.14233j0j7&sourceid=chrome&ie=UTF-8 on 17 April 2017.

Gray, D. E. (2009). *Doing Research in the Real World.* London: Sage Publications Limited.

Hakim, C. (2015). The male sex deficit. *International Sociology* **19**(4), 314–335.

International Labour Organisation (n.d.). *What Is Child Labour?* Retrieved from www.ilo.org/ipec/facts/ lang--en/index.htm on 17 April 2017.

Makokoro, P. (2012). *Why ECD in Zimbabwe?* Retrieved from http://nhakafoundation.blogspot. com/2012/03/why-ecd-in-zimbabwe.html on 20 June 2017.

Makokoro, P. (2017). *The Status of Education and Early Childhood Development (ECD) in Zimbabwe.* Retrieved from www.nhakafoundation.org/the-status-of-education-and-early-childhood development-ecd-in-zimbabwe/ on 9 April 2017.

Ministry of Education, Sport, Arts & Culture (2005). Director's Circular Minute No. 12 of 2005. Implementing Early Childhood Development Education Development Education Programme in Schools and Centres. Harare: MoESAC.

Moore, T. G. (2012). Rethinking early childhood intervention services: implications for policy and practice. Pauline McGregor Memorial Address to the *10th Biennial National Early Childhood Intervention Australia (ECIA) Conference and 1st Asia-Pacific Early Childhood Intervention Conference 2012,* 9 August, Perth, Western Australia. Retrieved from www.rch.org.au/uploadedFiles/Main/Content/ccch/ profdev/ECIA_National_Conference_2012.pdf on 13 July 2017.

Moore, T. G., Symes, L. & Bull, K. (2013). *Strengthening Inclusive Practices in Early Childhood Intervention Services: Background Paper.* Centre for Community Child Health, Murdoch Children's Research Institute, The Royal Children's Hospital, Melbourne.

Obama, B. (2013). *Obama's 2013 State of the Union Speech: Full Text.* Retrieved from www.theatlantic.com/politics/archive/2013/02/obamas-2013-state-of-the-union-speech-full-text/273089/ on 13 June 2017.

Palmer, V. (2015). *The 13 Key Benefits of Early Childhood Education. A Teacher's Perspective.* Retrieved from www.huffingtonpost.com/vicki-palmer/the-13-key-benefits-of-ea_b_7943348.html on 13 June 2017.

Peta, C. (2017). Gender based violence: a 'thorn' in the experiences of sexuality of women with disability in Zimbabwe. *Sexuality and Disability* **35**(3), 371–386.

Philpott, S. & McLaren, P. (2011). *Hearing the Voices of Children and Caregivers: Children with Disabilities in South Africa: A Situation Analysis, 2001–2011.* Department of Social Development, Republic of South Africa/UNICEF: Pretoria.

Spice, W. (2007). Management of sex workers and other high-risk groups. *Occupational Medicine* **57**(5), 322–328.

UNESCO (2006). *Strong Foundations: Early Childhood Care and Education.* Paris: UNESCO.

UNESCO (2013). *Out-of-School Children and Adolescents in Asia and the Pacific: Left Behind on the Road to Learning Opportunities for All.* Bangkok: UNESCO. Retrieved from http://uis.unesco.org/sites/default/files/documents/out-of-school-children-and-adolescents-in-asia-and-pacific-left-behind-on-the-road-to-learning-opportunities-for-all-2015-en.pdf on 4 April 2017.

UNICEF (2014). *Research Study on Children with Disabilities Living in Uganda: Situational Analysis on the Rights of Children with Disabilities in Uganda.* Paris: UNICEF. Retrieved from www.unicef.org/uganda/UNICEF_CwD_situational_analysis_FINAL.pdf on 15 August 2017.

United Nations (2006). *Convention on the Rights of Persons with Disabilities (CRPD).* Retrieved from http://www.un.org/disabilities/convention/conventionfull.shtml on 15 July 2017.

William, R., Henninger, I. V. & Sarika, S. G. (2014). How do children benefit from inclusion? In S. G. Sarika, R. William, I. V. Henninger & E. V. Megan (eds) *First Steps to Pre-school Inclusion* (pp. 33–57). Baltimore, MD: Brookes Publishing.

8

EDUCATING DEAF CHILDREN IN MAINSTREAM AND SPECIAL SECONDARY SCHOOL SETTINGS

Inclusive mirage or reality?

Martin Musengi and Barbra Nyangairi

Introduction

In this chapter, we examine the inclusive education of deaf children by exploring the extent to which normative pedagogies allow them to participate in mainstream and special school settings. We understand inclusive education as participation in acquiring knowledge and we discuss the circumstances under which this is attainable for deaf children when teaching approaches are derived from the usually hearing peers. We trace inclusive education from primary socialisation in homes where parents might be deaf or hearing so that the different language development paths of deaf children are compared. The different language development patterns are used to understand the extent to which deaf children are able to participate in mainstream and special secondary school settings. Thus, we conceptualise inclusion in these secondary schools as the extent to which deaf children are able to participate in acquiring the norms, values, beliefs and knowledge in these settings. In order to put this into context, we discuss international charters that inform inclusive education, starting from the UNESCO (1994) Salamanca Statement up to Article 24 of the Convention on the Rights of Persons with Disabilities (CRPD; United Nations, 2006). We then use empirical evidence to explore Zimbabwean deaf school-leavers' reflections of their experiences when they were in school.

Inclusive education: different understandings

Inclusive education started as an attempt to create equity for children with disabilities so that they become integrated into the school community (Pantic & Florian, 2015; Ballard, 2012). Voss and Bufkin (2011) and Forbes (2007) explain that inclusive education has evolved into a much wider process of eliminating all forms of exclusion and marginalisation for all learners whose diverse needs and abilities might otherwise make them vulnerable to discrimination. Previously, schools tried to create equity for children with disabilities by offering remedial activities that would help 'fix' the children's deficits so that they could join non-disabled peers in mainstream school activities. It was understood that being placed in a mainstream school would remove restrictions to social interaction with non-disabled peers and help to provide an education that was of similar quality.

Placement in mainstream schools was considered less restrictive than placement in a hospital-based school or special school. This is because in the latter, there were fewer chances of interacting with non-disabled peers as models as illustrated in Deno's (1970) seminal cascade model. The model highlights a continuum of service provision for learners with diverse needs in which hospital-based schools and special schools are on the most restrictive end while mainstream schools embrace diversity. This general understanding of inclusive education as placing children with disabilities in mainstream education is partially supported by the Salamanca Statement (UNESCO, 1994), which is widely considered to be the founding international charter on inclusive education. The Salamanca Statement, however, does have a caveat in which it gives the specific examples of deaf-blind or deaf children. The Salamanca Statement states that in special schools where there is use of Sign Language, deaf children learn better.

The deficit-oriented stance, in which children with disabilities are supposed to be fixed first in order to fit into schools, is grounded in a medical model of disability. School practices that focus on remediating children to enable them to become better learners are considered as part of an 'incrementalist' perspective of inclusive education (Stubbs, 2008). Inclusive education has evolved from this medical model of wanting to increasingly change individuals so that they fit into schools, to a socio-cultural reconceptualisation of striving to change schools so that all children can participate fully in acquiring knowledge (ibid.).

Incrementalist and reconceptualist perspectives result in widely different practices, which all claim to be inclusive education. Some of these practices might, however, actually deny children with disabilities equitable access to knowledge in the schools. As a result of their unique mode of communication, the case of deaf children in schools magnifies this argument. The heterogeneous group of deaf children experiences incrementalist and reconceptualist education. Their varying experiences in different settings need to be explored in light of the right to inclusive education as enshrined in Article 24 of the CRPD (United Nations, 2006).

Article 24 of the CRPD exhorts governments not to exclude children with disabilities from the mainstream education system on the basis of having impairments (United Nations, 2006). It also urges governments to provide reasonable accommodation and support, such as facilitating the learning of Sign Language and ensuring that education is delivered in the most appropriate language that maximises academic and social development. In the reconceptualist spirit of endeavouring to change schools rather than changing deaf children, Article 24 advocates for the employment of teachers who are qualified in Sign Language, including deaf teachers. There is a need to analyse the extent to which the education system embraces deaf children as a group with a different language rather than as a group of children with a disability needing remediation. These two different understandings of deaf children are discussed in the next section.

Deaf or hearing impaired: different understandings

In the deficit perspective, deafness is understood in relation to the characteristics or goals of children with normal hearing, placing value on speaking and listening while viewing a deaf life as silent and segregated from mainstream society. In this pathologic view, policy would strive for the remediation of the deficiencies of deaf children so that they can be assimilated into the hearing society (Power & Leigh, 2011). In Zimbabwe, deaf people are referred to as 'hearing impaired' in official educational policy documents. This conception of the condition as a deficit is inconsistent with the CRPD's intention to promote linguistic identity as enunciated in Article 24 (United Nations, 2006). The term 'hearing impaired' suggests that hearing and speaking are normal and desirable, hence 'impaired'. This might cause the education system to view the condition as requiring remediation that focuses on learning to hear and speak. According to Power and Leigh (2011), how deafness is defined and valued, and perceptions of what a deaf life means, will determine aspects of the curriculum for deaf children.

The alternative is to view deaf children as having a cultural difference and valuing their linguistic difference so that their lives can be perceived as complete and wholesome as they are. This view concurs with deaf people's argument that they are a cultural and linguistic community, rather than a grouping of people with disabilities (Parasnis, 1998; Ladd, 2003). In support, Baker (2008) believes that being deaf is a difference, a characteristic that distinguishes deaf people from hearing people. This idea is the key tenet in the socio-cultural model of deafness where deaf people are viewed as a linguistic minority using Sign Language. This is supported by the CRPD Article 24's intention of promoting linguistic identity. Hence, the need to analyse the inclusion of deaf children attending various educational settings in a policy environment in which they are referred to as 'hearing impaired'. The education of such children has many issues, challenges and concerns as discussed in the next section.

Challenges and concerns in the education of deaf learners

In light of the differing perceptions about inclusive education and deafness, the educational experiences of deaf learners in Zimbabwe become intriguing. This is because education policy-makers and implementers are mostly socialised into Zimbabwean Shona or Ndebele culture, are all hearing and therefore not necessarily members of what Ladd (2003) calls the Deaf community. The intrigue has the backdrop of deaf children's educational outcomes, which are a long-term challenge not only in Zimbabwe, but globally. Literature is replete with research studies recording how most deaf high school-leavers barely manage to achieve a fourth grade reading level (Brueggemann, 2004; Wauters *et al.*, 2006) and how their mathematics attainments are lower than those of their hearing peers (Nunes & Moreno, 2002; Zarfaty *et al.*, 2004; Bull *et al.*, 2005). These global low levels of academic achievement are also evident in the education of deaf children in Zimbabwe (Musengi, 1999, 2014; Hlatywayo *et al.*, 2014). This is in contrast to the country having the highest literacy rate of 92% in Africa (United Nations Development Plan, 2010). In Zimbabwe, deaf children are mostly placed in boarding institutions where they undergo elementary education, after which most of them are then taught practical skills such as basketry, woodwork, leatherwork, sewing and cookery (Chitiyo & Wheeler, 2004). Peresuh and Barcham (1998) reported that, traditionally, teaching children with disabilities was considered more of a moral and religious obligation than a right in Zimbabwe. Since deaf children were also considered as disabled by humanitarian organisations, they also received education as a moral and religious obligation rather than a right.

In the pre-independence era, elementary special schools were established by churches and humanitarian organisations to cater for the needs of children with disabilities in Zimbabwe. Among these were special elementary schools for deaf children. These schools offered an academic and technical-vocational curriculum up to seventh grade, which is the end of the primary school cycle in Zimbabwe. After primary school, deaf children focused solely on vocational training in two- to three-year programmes, which were certified locally by the teachers at the schools. Prior to Zimbabwe's independence (1990), there was no secondary school education specifically meant for deaf children in Zimbabwe (Musengi, 1999).

After independence, the Zimbabwean government began to coordinate and regulate the education of children with disabilities (Peresuh & Barcham, 1998; Mpofu *et al.*, 2007). Education of such children was extended to mainstream schools. Much research has been carried out in Zimbabwe on the education of children with disabilities in general who attend mainstream schools (e.g. Mpofu *et al.*, 2007; Barnatt & Kabzems, 1992). Studies have also been carried out on the education of pupils with specific impairments (e.g. Ncube, 2015; Nyandoro, 2015; Svubure, 2015). Few studies have focused on policy implementation issues for these pupils (e.g. Mnkandla & Mataruse, 2002). The few studies that exist on the implementation of inclusive policies for deaf children, are based on Deno's (1970) popularised notion of mainstream schools as necessarily inclusive (e.g. Musengi & Chireshe, 2012). To our knowledge, there are no local studies on how inclusion might work for deaf children in special schools. The education of deaf children in mainstream schools is particularly interesting in light of the cultural ambivalence on whether they are disabled or non-disabled; as well as their low levels of academic achievement as compared to those with visual impairment, which involves challenges in seeing.

The interface between localised cultural conceptions of deafness and inclusive education of deaf children remains an under-researched area. It is imperative to analyse the mediation of local conceptions of deafness and how this influences their inclusion in mainstream education. This is particularly important in light of Hargreaves' (2009) observation that the vital work of ensuring children's intellectual growth and preparing them to meet the challenges of the future is carried out by hearing adults working with deaf children whose culture might be different. Yet, Deaf culture is somehow different from the hearing culture (Padden & Humphries, 2005). A basic premise of this chapter is that systematic information should be collected about the inclusive education of deaf children. Such information would improve the understanding of practices and inform what might need to be done to ensure the inclusion of such children in learning. The next section outlines this problem in greater detail.

Unpacking the problem

Many deaf children in Zimbabwe are identified rather late (Director, 2006) and arrive at school without any acquired language, spoken or signed (Musengi *et al.*, 2013) thereby complicating decisions about predisposition toward a first language. The educational experiences of such deaf people who attended various school settings can therefore be used to ascertain the extent to which deaf children participate in learning and, by implication, their inclusion in or exclusion from education. A research study was therefore carried out to address the question: To what extent do deaf children experience education as inclusive in mainstream and special school settings? The manner in which the study was carried out is described in the following sections.

Methodology

A qualitative approach was seen to be appropriate for this study, given that it is interpretative and focuses on the complex creation and maintenance of meaning (Liamputong & Ezzy, 2005). Key informant interviews were used as data collection methods that assisted in understanding educational experiences of deaf school-leavers. Key informant interviews were conducted with 18 deaf adults who had either been to mainstream or special school up to Ordinary level in Zimbabwe. Qualitative techniques allowed for contextualised experience and action, which led to a thick description of the experiences of deaf adults during their years in school (Liamputong & Ezzy, 2005). Key informant interviews were useful for gathering information on the inclusion of deaf children from a limited number of deaf adults. The method allowed us to get an in-depth understanding of the reflections of deaf school-leavers. Thus, participants were drawn from deaf school-leavers who were above the age of 18, who either attended resource units in mainstream schools or special schools. This proved significant as it ensured varied experiences by people who had been to different schools throughout the country. A total of 18 participants from the deaf community were identified through snowball sampling. The targeted age groups were above the age of 18. Three groups of 18–30 years, 31–40 years and 40–50 years were identified. Key informants were therefore mature people with first-hand experiences of the issue under investigation and, as school-leavers, were sufficiently detached from the schools to be objective and reflective.

A key informant interview guide was used to collect data from participants over a period of six weeks in all ten provinces of Zimbabwe. The interviewers were trained in collecting data from key informant interviews. Consent to the interview and to recording was established at the beginning of the interview. During the interviews, deaf participants gave brief narratives of their lives and experiences of their education, which were captured through audio-recording and field notes. Interviews were transcribed verbatim at the end of the data collection session.

We utilised thematic content analysis (Anderson, 2007) to make sense of the gathered data. After preparing all data, we developed codes or categories based on the words used by the participants more frequently and the themes that seemed to come out during these conversations. For every code we made, we placed all the excerpts from the data that fell into that category.

In drawing out the themes, we conducted an analysis of the language and noticed that some words were used more than others by the participants. Focus was on the language used by the participants as it provided a system of meanings and practices that construct reality. Creswell (2003) argues that words that occur frequently show their salience in the minds of research participants. In this research, words such as marginalised, discriminated, unloved, unwanted were used quite often.

In order to analyse the data provided by the deaf participants, we also utilised narrative analysis. Narrative analysis is an important tradition dealing with communication through which we enact important aspects of our identities and relations with others (Labov, 1972). Data from the participants were analysed for linguistic identity and relations with hearing and other deaf peers. As Liamputong and Ezzy (2005) observe, narrative analysis has explicit moral and political dimensions. Analysis therefore aimed at making explicit how deaf school-leavers had experienced inclusion or exclusion during learning.

Ethical considerations relating to confidentiality dictated that the findings be reported anonymously. Participants are therefore coded using single letters of the alphabet randomly selected from A to X. Two participants, D and F, had deaf parents while the rest had hearing parents. Seven participants had attended mainstream schools while 11 had attended special schools. Where participants state the names of institutions they attended in the interviews, this is coded using double letters of the alphabet, for example XX and ZZ for special schools and YY for resource unit. This was done to hide identities and maintain the integrity of the institutions.

Emerging findings

Data analysis resulted in five themes emerging from the participants' views: The home as a learning place; inability to understand English; lack of Sign Language in the instruction of deaf learners; Sign Language not recognised or used for instruction; and the teacher as the critical but missing link in deaf education.

The home as learning place

Participants reported that due to communication problems with their parents and guardians, they were not able to learn much at home. Participant C who has hearing parents and attended a special school had this to say:

When a mother is breast feeding her child, she will be talking to the baby and the baby learns things; while a mother is feeding a deaf child, she will be talking, but no communication is taking place. So no learning of new words takes place.

It is evident in the above statement that failure to communicate in the home hindered the foundation learning that is supposed to take place at home. Participants reported that at times, hearing parents of deaf children are a problem because they have bad attitudes toward their children and do not include them in the events that happen in their homes. Participant G who has hearing parents and attended a resource unit in a mainstream school reported that 'some parents do not love their deaf children and become impatient when the child asks questions'. This implies that regardless of whether participants had attended mainstream or special schools, they had initially experienced their homes as not providing as good a learning environment as it does for their hearing siblings. This was said especially in situations where the parents were hearing. Although some hearing parents might not accept their deaf children unconditionally, it is possible that the parents' impatience resulting from poor communication with deaf children might easily be misconstrued as lack of love. What seems to be more certain is that poor communication is a hindrance to early learning for deaf children in the home. Hindrances on early learning in the home are said to have had effects on later learning in schools. This view was expressed by participant B who attended a special school: 'Mathematics was difficult for me because I did not understand the words and also my parents did not teach me because they focused more on the hearing children'.

Thus, the lack of adequate communication and language development was reported to have hindered development of other academic disciplines which require an understanding of language. Learning mathematics using the English language was found to be difficult because a primary language (Sign Language) had not been developed.

Inability to understand English

English is the formal language of instruction in Zimbabwe and yet all participants indicated that it is problematic for them. The lack of primary language development makes learning and understanding a second language such as English more difficult. Participant D who attended a resource unit in a mainstream school said: 'English was the most difficult subject for me because the teacher used oral English and would not use Sign Language. When reading stories in the book he did not sign for me.' Although specific reference is made to Sign Language not being used, this participant's highlighting of the use of oral English suggests that a more visual rather than auditory form of English might have helped him. This becomes more explicit when the participant said that the stories in the books were not signed, which might suggest that he thought that Signed English might have helped him to understand much better.

Participant F who attended a special school said:

I did not like English. The teacher would hit me for writing wrong English. For instance, I would write 'Me go' instead of writing 'I want to go'. If you look at a grade 3 English book, a deaf adult who is 30 years old cannot read it but a 10-year-old hearing child can read. My daughter is 10 years old but she can read English better than me. I am not even able to help her because she is far much better than me.

Evidently, the teacher's use of corporal punishment for deaf children writing English using the correct grammar of Sign Language resulted in the children hating the subject and, eventually, failing to master it.

Lack of Sign Language in the instruction of deaf pupils

Most of the participants indicated that Sign Language was not used as a language of instruction. Participant T who attended a special school said: 'I went to (XX Special School) and I was taught in English but it was difficult for me to understand.' Participant W who went to a mainstream school commented: 'I went to (YY Resource Unit in Mainstream School) and my teacher used Shona. I knew some of the words because I played with hearing children.'

Shona is one of the main local languages in Zimbabwe. It is clear that whether the deaf children were in special or mainstream schools, spoken rather than signed languages were used. Instead of using Sign Language, most teachers are reported to have used spoken languages and can, therefore, be presumed to have employed the oral method of teaching. Participants indicated that while the teachers spoke and used the oral method, they themselves preferred Sign Language as this would ensure more effective learning. The participant who attended a mainstream school reported a slight advantage over those from special schools because he had acquired from hearing peers some of the Shona words that were being used in class. Such an advantage would, however, be minimal as the spoken language of teaching and learning for most secondary school subjects is English rather than Shona.

Sign Language not used as a language of instruction and learning

Deaf participants reported that Sign Language was not recognised as a language of similar weighting with other languages. Participant E from a mainstream school argued:

> Why is it that the government wants 5 'O' level passes including English subject yet that is not our language, our language is Sign Language. They expect us to have English whilst the deaf people are not taught in Sign Language which is their first language. Then why does the government expect the deaf people to have 5 subjects when they are being taught in a language that we don't understand.

The participant was not happy with the requirement that a school-leaving certificate was only considered as complete if it had five Ordinary level passes, one of which must be English language. Her argument was that it is unfair to insist that deaf people must pass a language that they have not mastered while ignoring the Sign Language. Participant H who attended a special school said:

> There should be teachers who are specialised in Sign Language. If a word is correct in Sign Language, to us, it is correct. Then why does the government want the deaf people to use proper grammar when it is difficult for us?

Underlying this participant's view is the argument that if Sign Language is accepted as a real language, then there is a need for it to be taught by teachers who are properly trained in the language. She is arguing that Sign Language is legitimate as it has its own structures that do not have to follow the structures of any other language. Instead of prioritising English, Shona and other spoken languages in the education system, Sign Language should be recognised as a language capable of being used for teaching, learning and examination.

The teacher as the critical but missing link in deaf education

Most participants felt that their teachers had let them down during their school years. The inability of teachers to communicate in Sign Language was said to be a major barrier to learning. Participant L who attended a special school had this to say:

> I think (hearing) teachers should be trained by deaf teachers to teach deaf children because most of them are not proficient in Sign Language. For example if a new teacher comes to a school for the deaf; it is wise for the deaf to teach the teacher Sign Language so that he/she will be able to teach the children in the language that they understand.

The observation is that since most hearing teachers who are already in service either in special or mainstream schools are not proficient in Sign Language, there is a need for them to be given in-service training in the language from deaf adults. Such training could be done through workshops led by deaf adults. Participant X who attended a mainstream school explained:

> We want specialised Sign Language teachers from primary, secondary to tertiary level. Just like in the mainstream schools, they do have teachers for primary who are specialised in that; they also have teachers who teach specifically secondary and those who teach tertiary education. Thus, it should be the same for deaf people; they need teachers in all those levels.

The position that specialised Sign Language teachers are necessary at all levels of education is consistent with the argument that this would properly recognise it as a real language. This would also recognise Deaf people as a linguistic minority rather than as a group of people with disabilities. In addition to teachers' lack of proficiency in Sign Language, participants who had attended mainstream schools indicated that they faced discrimination from their teachers. Participant S who attended a special school said: 'Some teachers have no heart for deaf children. They do not support deaf children. It also does have changes in our learning.'

It is possible that some teachers might have negative attitudes toward pupils with additional educational needs but it is more likely that the teachers did not give their deaf pupils adequate time and attention since there were many competing demands in the mainstream classes. Paying inadequate attention to these pupils would then be viewed as failing to support their learning. This was made explicit by participant A, who attended a special school PP which practises reverse inclusion. This is where learners without disabilities are placed in special school: 'Teachers give much attention to hearing students and neglect deaf children. If you have an inclusive class for hearing and deaf children, the teacher will be lazy to teach deaf students and focus on hearing children.'

Participant J who attended a mainstream school explained: 'We were marginalised in class and they put the deaf on one side and the hearing on one side.' Participants in both mainstream and special school settings where there were hearing peers felt neglected by their hearing teachers who can be presumed to have better communication with hearing children than with deaf children.

Discussion

The study established that a home environment in which a deaf child's language does not develop spontaneously contributes to them not being able to fully participate in later mainstream and special school education. The lack of spontaneous language development at home is often compounded by hearing parents' negative attitudes toward their deaf children as many might still be grieving for the loss of a hearing child (Musengi, 2014). Many deaf children, therefore, might not be included in the events that happen in their homes as many parents are unable to use Sign Language and some might have negative attitudes. The lack of a strong foundation in Sign Language at an early age affects future learning outcomes as the negative effects of missing the window of opportunity for language development are well documented (Fox *et al.*, 2013). As Caselli (2014) and Herman (2014) observed, many deaf children had a deficit in language development prior to entering school.

Once these linguistically deprived deaf children get into the formal education environment, the exclusion continues as most participants indicated that they were unable to understand English and that there was lack of Sign Language instruction. Kiyaga and Moores (2009) found that most teachers of deaf children in sub-Saharan Africa cannot sign and do not believe Sign Language to be a real language. Not using the Sign Language of deaf people results in a barrier to learning, as well as to inclusion, as the deaf children are not well versed in any spoken language. This is regardless of whether deaf pupils are enrolled in mainstream or special schools. The implication is that it is not the placement that determines whether the deaf pupils are included or excluded. Rather it is the ability to access a language that ensures inclusion in whatever educational setting. This is supported by Powers (1996) who argued that inclusion is not a place, but an attitude that allows participation in learning. Participants indicated their preference for Sign Language to learn as this would ensure effective learning and therefore inclusion. This might indicate the need to develop Sign Language into an examinable language. This is particularly important since Sign Language is now recognised as one of the 16 official languages in Zimbabwe's revised national Constitution (Government of Zimbabwe, 2013).

There was agreement among deaf participants that forcing them to talk is not desirable as they are not willing to learn to talk. Teachers' insistence on teaching articulation skills is premised on what Knoors and Marschark (2012) call the social desire for deaf children to eventually integrate fully into the larger society. The deaf participants' objections to being forced to talk are, however, understandable in light of the finding that most are identified late, with intervention beginning upon entry into school at 6 or 7 years of age (Musengi *et al.*, 2013). Such late intervention cannot achieve optimal results as it misses what Fox *et al.* (2013) call the sensitive period of language acquisition. This situation is compounded by the observation that in Zimbabwe the teaching of articulation is done by teachers who are not professional speech therapists. In this context, being preoccupied with making deaf pupils speak would be a practice that Baumann (2004) calls 'audism', which is discrimination on the basis of preference for sound-based, spoken language; thus, excluding the three-dimensional, kinaesthetic Sign Language of deaf people. Such discrimination was also perceived when teachers failed to give deaf pupils adequate time and attention in classrooms practising reverse inclusion. The focus on hearing pupils was perceived as discriminatory as it affected deaf pupils' educational outcomes.

Conclusions and recommendations

The purpose of this chapter is to analyse the extent to which deaf children view mainstream and special schools as inclusive. The initial understanding of inclusion based on deficiency views of allowing deaf pupils to learn alongside hearing peers was found to be perpetuating exclusion rather than inclusion. Similarly, emphasising the teaching of speech to deaf learners also has exclusionary implications. A more evolved understanding of inclusion focuses on whether deaf pupils can participate in acquiring knowledge in the schools. Emphasis would then be on using the language that is most accessible and therefore usable by these pupils for the purpose of learning. Such access to language would ideally begin at home before the child comes to school. This would allow continuity into the school system. The least restrictive environment is therefore one in which deaf pupils can acquire knowledge using an accessible language they prefer. Since many deaf school-leavers preferred their visual Sign Language, this may then be used in order to practise inclusive education regardless of location. Such an approach has several implications for teacher preparation as outlined in the following recommendations.

It is clear from this chapter that resource units for deaf pupils that were created in mainstream schools did not meet the criteria of 'schools for all' as there is inadequate training of teachers in Sign Language, and a shortage of Sign Language materials and financial resources. All these inadequacies apply to special schools for the deaf as well. These inadequacies therefore need to be addressed by government in order to create school environments suitable for the education of deaf children in both mainstream and special schools.

It also emerged that deaf school-leavers from both mainstream and special school settings were dissatisfied by their educational experiences. This implies that the educational setting itself does not make education inclusive or discriminatory. What makes education inclusive are practices that make academic content accessible. Educators and parents of deaf learners should, therefore, use effective participation in learning as the only yardstick for judging whether such learners are included or excluded. This means that practices such as reverse inclusion in special schools for deaf pupils should be judged to be inclusive only if there is optimal learning by both hearing and deaf pupils. The education of deaf children is likely to become inclusive if these key recommendations are addressed; otherwise it remains an elusive mirage.

Reflective questions

1   Using insights from this chapter, develop your own definition of inclusive education.
2   Reflect on incremental and reconceptualist perspectives of inclusive education.
3   How can you apply the concept of the least restrictive environment to the education of deaf children?
4   Discuss Article 24 of the CRPD of 2006 in light of the provision of inclusive education for deaf children.

References

Anderson, R. (2007). *Thematic Content Analysis (TCA): Descriptive Presentation of Qualitative Data.* Course material for Institute of Transpersonal Psychology, Palo Alto, CA.

Baker, C. (2008). *Foundations of Bilingual Education and Bilingualism,* 2nd edn. Bristol: Multilingual Matters.

Ballard, K. (2012). Inclusion and social justice: teachers as agents of change. In S. Carrington & J. Macarthur (eds) *Teaching in Inclusive School Communities* (pp. 65–87). Sidney: John Wiley and Sons.

Barnatt, S. N. & Kabzems, V. (1992). Zimbabwean teachers' attitudes towards integration of pupils with disabilities into regular classrooms. *International Journal of Disability, Development and Education* **39**(2), 135–146.

Baumann, H. D. L. (2004). Audism: exploring the metaphysics of oppression. *Journal of Deaf Studies and Deaf Education* **9**, 239–246.

Brueggemann, B. J. (2004). *Literacy and Deaf People,* 2nd edn. Washington, DC: Gallaudet University Press.

Bull, R., Marschark, M. & Blatto-Vallee, G. (2005). Examining number representation in deaf students. *Learning and Individual Differences* **15**, 223–236.

Caselli, C. M. (2014). *Language Development of Deaf Children in the Era of Cochlear Implantation: Implications for Teaching E-learning Through Visual Environments.* Paper presented at the 1st International Conference on Teaching Deaf Students. Amsterdam, the Netherlands.

Chitiyo, M. & Wheeler, J. (2004). The development of special education services in Zimbabwe. *International Journal of Special Education* **19**, 46–52.

Creswell, J. W. (2003). *Research Design*, 3rd edn. Thousand Oaks, CA: Sage Publications.

Deno, E. (1970). Special education as developmental capital. *Exceptional Children* **37**, 229–237.

Director (2006). *Guidelines on Over-aged Learners in Special Education*. Ministry of Education Director's Policy Circular. Harare: Ministry of Education.

Forbes, F. (2007). Towards inclusion: an Australian perspective. *Support for Learning* **22**(2), 66–71.

Fox, N. A., Nelson, C. A. & Zeanah, C. H. (2013). The effects of early severe psychosocial deprivation on children's cognitive and social development: lessons from the Bucharest Early Intervention Project. In N. S. Landale, S. M. McHale & A. Booth (eds) *Families and Child Health* (pp. 147–182). New York: Springer.

Government of Zimbawe (2013) *The Revised National Constitution*. Harare: Government Printers.

Hargreaves, L. (2009). The status and prestige of teachers and teaching. In L. J. Saha & A. G. Dworkin (eds) *International Handbook of Research on Teachers and Teaching* (pp. 217–229). New York: Springer Science.

Herman, R. (2014). *Language Assessment in Deaf Learners*. Paper presented at the 1st International Conference on Teaching Deaf Students. Amsterdam, the Netherlands.

Hlatywayo, L., Ncube, A. C. & Mwale, F. (2014). Examination question paper development and administration for deaf learners at grade 7 level: reflections of the Zimbabwe school examinations council (ZIMSEC). *IOSR Journal of Humanities and Social Science* **19**(11), 96–107.

Kiyaga, N. B. & Moores, D. F. (2009). Deafness in sub-Saharan Africa. In D. F. Moores & M. S. Miller (eds) *Deaf People around the World* (pp. 333–352). Washington, DC: Gallaudet University Press.

Knoors, H. & Marschark, M. (2012). Language planning for the 21st century: revisiting bilingual language policy for deaf children. *Journal of Deaf Studies and Deaf Education* **17**(3), 291–305.

Labov, W. (1972). The transformation of experience in narrative syntax. In W. Labov (ed.) *Language in the Inner City* (pp. 352–396). Philadelphia, PA: University of Pennsylvania.

Ladd, P. (2003). *Understanding Deaf Culture: In Search of Deafhood*. Clevedon: Multilingual Matters.

Liamputtong, P. & Ezzy, D. (2005). *Qualitative Research Methods*. Oxford: Oxford University Press.

Mnkandla, M. & Mataruse, K. (2002). The impact of inclusion policy on school psychology in Zimbabwe. *Educational and Child Psychology* **19**, 12–23.

Mpofu, E., Kasayira, J. M., Mhaka, M. M., Chireshe, R. & Maunganidze, L. (2007). Inclusive education in Zimbabwe. In P. Engelbrecht & L. Green (eds) *Responding to Challenges of Inclusive Education in Southern Africa* (pp. 66–79). Pretoria: Van Schaik.

Musengi, M. (1999). *The Impact of Hearing Aid Fitting Practices on Ways of Teaching Hearing Impaired Pupils in Zimbabwe's Special Schools*. Unpublished Bachelor's Dissertation, Educational Foundations Department, Faculty of Education, University of Zimbabwe, Harare, Zimbabwe.

Musengi, M. (2014). *The Experience of Teaching in Residential Schools for the Deaf in Zimbabwe*. Unpublished PhD Thesis, Wits Centre for Deaf Studies, School of Education, University of the Witwatersrand, Johannesburg, South Africa.

Musengi, M. & Chireshe, R. (2012). Inclusion of deaf students in mainstream rural primary schools in Zimbabwe: challenges and opportunities. *Studies of Tribes and Tribals* **10**(2), 107–116.

Musengi, M., Ndofirepi, A. & Shumba, A. (2013). Rethinking education of deaf children in Zimbabwe: challenges and opportunities for teacher education. *Journal of Deaf Studies and Deaf Education* **18**(1), 62–74.

Ncube, E. (2015). *Barriers Faced by Learners with Severe Learning Disabilities in an Inclusive Setting in Beitbridge West*. Unpublished Bachelor's Dissertation, Jairos Jiri Centre for Special Needs Education, Robert Mugabe School of Education, Great Zimbabwe University, Masvingo, Zimbabwe.

Nunes, T. & Moreno, C. (2002). An intervention program for promoting deaf pupils' achievement in mathematics. *Journal of Deaf Studies and Deaf Education* **7**(2), 120–133.

Nyandoro, P. (2015). *Challenges Faced by Children with Physical and Motor Impairments at a Regular School in Zaka*. Unpublished Bachelor's Dissertation, Jairos Jiri Centre for Special Needs Education, Robert Mugabe School of Education, Great Zimbabwe University, Masvingo, Zimbabwe.

Padden, C. & Humphries, T. (2005). *Inside Deaf Culture*. Cambridge, MA: Harvard University Press.

Pantic, N. & Florian, L. (2015). Developing teachers as agents of inclusion and social justice. *Education Inquiry* **6**(3), 331–351.

Parasnis, I. (1998). *Cultural and Language Diversity and the Deaf Experience*. Cambridge: Cambridge University Press.

Peresuh, M. & Barcham, L. (1998). Special education provision in Zimbabwe. *British Journal of Special Education* **25**(2), 75–80.

Power, D. & Leigh, G. (2011). Curriculum: cultural and communicative contexts. In M. Marshark & P. Spencer (eds) *The Oxford Handbook of Deaf Studies, Language and Education*, Vol 1. (pp. 174–212). Oxford: Oxford University University Press.

Powers, S. (1996). Inclusion is an attitude not a place Part 1. *British Association of Teachers of the Deaf* **20**(2), 35–41.

Stubbs, S. (2008). *Inclusive Education Where There Are Few Resources*. Oslo: The Atlas Alliance.

Svubure, M. (2015). *Interrogating the Attitudes of Teachers towards Students with Epilepsy in Primary Schools in Gutu District*. Unpublished Bachelor's Dissertation, Jairos Jiri Centre for Special Needs Education, Robert Mugabe School of Education, Great Zimbabwe University, Masvingo, Zimbabwe.

UNESCO (1994). *The Salamanca Statement and Framework for Action on Special Needs Education*. Paris: UNESCO.

United Nations (2006). *Convention on the Rights of Persons with Disabilities and Optional Protocol*. New York: United Nations.

United Nations Development Plan (UNDP) (2010). *Human Development Report 2010*. Basingstoke and Switzerland: UNDP.

Voss, J. & Bufkin, L. (2011). Teaching all children: preparing early childhood pre-service teachers in inclusive settings. *Journal of Early Childhood Teacher Education* **32**(4), 338–354.

Wauters, L. N., van Bon, W. H. J. & Tellings, A. E. J. M. (2006). Reading comprehension of Dutch deaf children. *Reading and Writing: An Interdisciplinary Journal* **19**, 49–76.

Zarfaty, Y., Nunes, T. & Bryant, P. (2004). The performance of young deaf children in spatial and temporal number tasks. *Journal of Deaf Studies and Deaf Education* **9**(3), 315–326.

9

USING THE INTERNATIONAL CLASSIFICATION OF FUNCTIONING, DISABILITY AND HEALTH MODEL IN CHANGING THE DISCOURSE OF DISABILITY TO PROMOTE INCLUSIVE EDUCATION IN ZAMBIA

Gloria Azalde, Jacob R. S. Malungo, Nchimunya Nkombo,
Sarah Banda, Ravi Paul, Chibesa Musamba
and Arne H. Eide

Introduction

The fourth goal of the Sustainable Development Goals (SDGs) reflects the international commitment to achieving education for all. In order to achieve this goal, quality education has to be available for everyone, including disabled people who are among the populations that are routinely denied their right to education (United Nations, 2015; World Bank, 2015; UNESCO, 2016). The right of disabled children to education is enshrined broadly in the United Nations Convention on the Rights of the Child, and more explicitly in Article 24 of the United Nations Convention on the Rights of Persons with Disabilities (CRPD) (United Nations, 2006). Thus, the CRPD is the first legally binding instrument to proclaim the right of disabled children to inclusive education (United Nations Committee on the Rights of Persons with Disabilities, 2016). However, disabled children face many barriers, both societal and structural, which need to be addressed in order for them to enjoy high-quality education. The International Classification of Functioning, Disability and Health (ICF), which includes both a functional and a social perspective of disability, could be a useful tool to change the perspective of provision of education of disabled children from segregation to inclusion. This could be done by shifting the locus of limitation from the child to the environment (WHO, 2001). In this chapter, we look at how this would apply to inclusive education in Zambia.

Understanding inclusive education

Inclusive education is a process of enabling all children to learn and participate effectively within mainstream school systems. It does not segregate children according to abilities or needs. It is child-centred, flexible and allows children to develop to their own potential (Rieser, 2012). In order to achieve this, it requires a whole systems approach where all elements within the educational system are working interactively to ensure that education is available, accessible, acceptable and adaptable to all children regardless of vulnerability. Availability secures provision, both quantity and quality. Accessibility attends to removing obstacles in the built environment, curricula, education materials, pedagogical methods, support services, and more. Acceptability means providing quality and equitable education, one that is appropriate and respects the dignity and autonomy of the child. Adaptability also means creating adaptable learning environments where instead of providing 'one-size fits-all' curricula, one provides multiple options for children to perceive information, express knowledge and engage in learning as illustrated in Figure 9.1 (Stubbs, 2008). Thus, inclusive education does not include asking the child to fit into the system. Rather, it adapts the system to include the child, and acknowledges that all children are different and have the capacity to learn (UDL Center, no date; United Nations Committee on the Rights of Persons with Disabilities, 2016).

The ICF, endorsed by the World Health Assembly in 2001, is the result of more than 20 years of work in developing a new concept, which went beyond diagnosing disease and capturing the consequences of disease on the lives of people (Ingstad & Eide, 2011). The forerunner to the ICF, the International Classification of Impairments, Disability and Handicap (ICIDH) (WHO, 1980) was based on the biopsychosocial disease model and described consequences of disease in three dimensions: structural and functional body impairments, restrictions of activities of daily living, and handicaps (*sic*) or participation limitations in social integration. ICIDH was heavily criticised by the disability movement and was challenged by the emergence of a social model of disability for ignoring the environment and for lack of conceptual clarity (Fougeroyrollas & Beauregard, 2001). A revision of ICIDH was initiated in the early 1990s, and resulted in ICIDH-2 and later ICF. The strength of the ICF concept is in offering a common language to study the dynamic interaction between health condition, environmental factors and personal factors and therefore enabling to define what can improve the life situation of disabled people (Hollenweger, 2014).

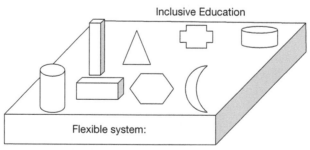

Figure 9.1 Differences between special, integrated and inclusive education
Source: Stubbs (2008).

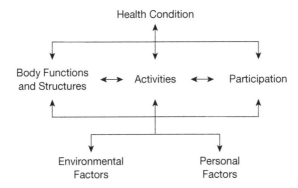

Figure 9.2   The ICF model: interaction between ICF components
Source: WHO (2001, p. 18, Figure 1).

The ICF, and its Child and Youth Version, the ICF-CY, has a broad scope, which can describe the impact of the environment on activity and participation and thus social inclusion of people and disabled children as illustrated in Figure 9.2 (WHO, 2001).

The ICF can highlight discrimination and environmental barriers within human-rights issues such as exclusion in education systems. Though research in education has primarily used ICF as a tool for educational assessment of children with disabilities, since it defines components of functioning and disability, ICF itself does not establish who is 'disabled' or who is 'not disabled' (Hollenweger, 2014; Sanches-Ferreira *et al.*, 2014). This biopsychosocial model is interested in the interactions that exist between the biological, psychological and social factors. It is, therefore, an effective tool that can be used to include all vulnerable groups, as well as children, who would not currently be categorised as having impairments, or other children who are at risk of underachieving or falling out of the educational system early. The advantage of the ICF model is that it views functioning as continuous, and in interaction with its surroundings. Participation then becomes very important from an ICF model perspective and its use about creating opportunities and enabling environments in schools and other settings to ensure that all children learn to their potential (Hollenweger, 2014).

Since outcomes in education can be linked to participation, there is a potential in the use of the tool beyond its current use. That is, to enable the inclusion not only of disabled children, but also of all children who need additional support to obtain individualised academic achievement. Just by applying a broader definition of what is defined as 'special needs', a study in Belgium found that an additional 15% of primary school age children had additional educational needs (Lebeer *et al.*, 2012).

So far, research on conceptual systems used in inclusive assessment, including the ICF model, have been based in high-income country contexts (Sanches-Ferreira *et al.*, 2015). In addition, the ICF model has only been used to assess the eligibility and interventions of students in need of specialised support, or as a tool for collaboration among various professionals in the field of education for disabled children (Sanches-Ferreira *et al.*, 2014). There is no evidence of its use in low-income contexts, or of its use in including vulnerable children in general. Since most tools are based on the reality of high-income countries, they are complex and require the involvement of an army of professionals to work together to include disabled children. The reality of low-income contexts is that there are very few resources, though this does not mean that inclusion cannot be realised. This chapter, therefore, highlights the barriers disabled children face in Zambia with respect to education and how the ICF model could be used as a tool to uncover barriers in Zambia and to change the discourse of disability in order to achieve inclusive education.

Disability and education in Zambia

Zambia ratified the CRPD in 2008. However, Zambia has included disabled people in different policies and laws since the amended Constitution of 1996 (Republic of Zambia, 1996a). Currently, there are several laws and policies in place that include disabled people, and some specifically within the area of education, including the National Policy on Education (Ministry of Education, 1996), the Education Act (Republic of Zambia, 2011) and the Technical Education, Vocational and Entrepreneurship Training (TEVET) Act (Republic of Zambia, 1996b). Nevertheless, the most important act pertaining to disabled people and influencing education is the Persons with Disabilities Act (Republic of Zambia, 2012).

The 2012 Disability Act provides for free primary education, access to secondary and higher education in the communities in which disabled children live, vocational training on the basis of impairment and for special schools for persons who cannot be enrolled in inclusive educational schools. It also ensures physical access to educational institutions, support and access to alternative forms of communication as well as allowances to cover extra costs attributed to learning. However, these measures are far from being implemented (Republic of Zambia, 2012).

Currently, the welfare of disabled people is the responsibility of the Ministry of Community Development and Social Welfare (MCDSW). The ministry has several departments working in one way or the other to provide support for disabled people. For instance, while the Department of Community Development works to empower vulnerable people in the community, the Social Welfare Department deals with disabled people needing welfare support, such as cash transfers. This ministry is also responsible for the Zambia Agency for Persons with Disabilities (ZAPD). Briefly described, ZAPD has the responsibility to implement the Disabilities Act of 2012 and any policy or national strategy on disability. This agency, under the MCDSW was established under the Persons with Disabilities Act of 1996 and continued under the Act of 2012.

In 2002, free education for all children in the first six years of primary school was introduced. This had a direct effect of increasing the net enrolment rate from 68% in 2000 to 96% in 2006 (Miles, 2011). However, the same trend was not observed among disabled children. A 2006 survey of living conditions among disabled people in Zambia reported that around 25% of disabled individuals, though eligible, did not attend primary school (Eide & Loeb, 2006). However, given the opportunity to attend school, disabled people matched the achievements of non-disabled people. The current study has provided the MCDSW not only with more general knowledge about disabled people in Zambia, but also provided insight into factors relevant for inclusion of disabled people in education in Zambia.

Methodology

The Zambia National Disability Study (ZNDS), financed by UNICEF Zambia was carried out in 2015. The study was conducted in collaboration with the Central Statistical Office of Zambia (CSO), the University of Zambia (UNZA) and SINTEF Technology and Society in Norway. The ZNDS was designed to determine impairment prevalence among adults and children in Zambia; to analyse the socio-economic and demographic characteristics of disabled people, including children; and to assess the main issues that affect their quality of life in terms of participation and use of basic social services. The results of the study will be used by the MCDSW in Zambia for policy formulation and programming in order to promote the inclusion of disabled people (including children), and to contribute to the effective implementation of the Persons with Disabilities Act of 2012. It will also be used to inform national agendas and various policies and programmes.

A national, representative household survey was carried out in all ten provinces in Zambia. A cross-sectional study design was used. Households were recruited using a two-stage stratified cluster sampling method. The sample consisted of 3,685 households, which was adequate to give reliable estimates at national and provincial level. All individuals in the selected households were screened to determine whether the household would be classified as a disabled or non-disabled household. A census of the entire household was undertaken by administering a questionnaire to the head of each selected household. The survey was conducted by 38 teams. Each team consisted of a supervisor, three to four interviewers and a driver. Analysis was conducted at both the individual and household levels, with comparisons done between persons with and without disabilities as well as between households with and without at least one person with disability.

The questionnaires used included a Child Module questionnaire developed by UNICEF and the Washington Group on Disability Statistics. This was applied to a sample of 3,882 children aged between two and 17 years, of which 954 were children with disabilities and 2,908 non-disabled children. The advantage with a specific child module is that it provides a much more detailed and age-relevant picture of functional problems among children in Zambia.

The ZNDS also comprised a qualitative component, an in-depth study of the barriers and facilitators for life-long learning and skills development for disabled children and young people in Zambia. Four study sites were selected: two urban sites, one in Lusaka and one in Copperbelt, and two rural sites, one in Western Province and one in Eastern Province. The informants were identified through pre-visits to the four study sites and community mapping of key informants as well as through snowballing. A combination of focus group discussions (FGDs) and individual in-depth interviews were carried out among service providers, disabled children and young people, as well as their family members. Some of the in-depth interviews formed part of case studies used in the research. In total, 41 FDGs and 70 individual in-depth interviews were carried out in the four sites, comprising 94 disabled young people, 104 service providers and 83 family members. The following types of impairments were represented in the interviews with disabled children and their family members: sensory, developmental and psychosocial impairments, including those with epilepsy. A team of four experienced qualitative researchers from the University of Zambia and 12 research assistants carried out the qualitative fieldwork. The qualitative data from all four sites were analysed using thematic analysis.

Quantitative findings

The study showed that on key indicators on level of living, disabled individuals are worse off compared to those without disabilities. The analyses also showed that these differences increased with severity of impairment. Looking specifically at education, the study found that though the large majority of people in Zambia had accessed formal education, disabled individuals, rural participants and females reported lower levels of access and lower levels of education.

The study also provided a profile of child disability in Zambia. The survey found that disabled children reported more environmental barriers than those without disability. Between 20% of disabled children reported being affected by transport problems, negative attitudes and discrimination, with approximately 10% being affected on a daily basis. In addition, disabled children were more exposed to abuse compared to children without disabilities, both within the family and in their daily environment. Disabled children also experienced several service gaps. Few disabled children received counselling and any form of assistive technology. Thus, only half of the disabled children who required educational services (e.g. remedial therapist/tutor, special school, early childhood stimulation and educational psychologist), accessed them. In services where the need gap was smaller in the population in general, as in health information services and general health services, there was a greater gap for disabled children.

Looking specifically at formal education, many more children have recently accessed formal education. However, findings among disabled children aged 12–17 years, mirrored in part those of the adult population. Schools were either not accessible or not available for 30% of disabled children, though few disabled children reported that they had been refused entry to formal education. However, many did report that their families did not register them in schools. Nevertheless, 86.8% of disabled children have managed to access formal education compared to 95% of non-disabled children. There were also fewer children with disabilities who were able to read (33.3% vs. 18.3%). In addition, fewer disabled children studied as far as they had planned, and fewer were still studying. Finally, only 4.1% of the total population of children surveyed confirmed that they had a skill, of which only 1.3% had received these skills at a formal learning institution.

Qualitative findings

The qualitative findings uncovered several environmental factors limiting social participation in educational services for disabled children.

Barriers in societal knowledge and attitudes

Most informants had good general knowledge on disability. They were able to give examples of different types of impairments, and most cited infectious diseases, accidents and congenital causes as reasons for being disabled. However, most informants saw the barriers experienced by disabled people as an inherent part of the impairment itself. Nevertheless, others attributed the barriers of disabled people to the stigma in the community and its inability to see beyond the impairment. Discriminating attitudes were also present within the educational system. Special education teachers described having to defend their career choices: 'Sometimes they even ask you saying "why did you choose to teach *'imingulu'* [senseless children] of all the things; why did you choose to teach these children?"' (Special school teacher, Copperbelt Province).

Others experienced being excluded from promotion for the same reason:

> it not only that we are offering service without papers, we just have same papers like those teaching at the mainstream schools. We are going to the same university, getting the same degree, and they are saying 'those in special education, they are not going to be upgraded.' And those our colleagues once they have finish, they get their degrees, they are upgraded.
>
> *(Special education teacher, Lusaka Province)*

Societal structure barriers

Local mainstream schools are generally not accessible for disabled children. Several informants also pointed out that there are few special schools and vocational schools for disabled children. Special schools tend to be located in urban areas, have many students per teacher, provide few enrolment and boarding spaces and lack assistive technology. An additional barrier is poverty. Even though there are no primary school fees, there are still added costs to school, like food allowance and uniforms. Parents of disabled children have additional costs such as transport costs due to long distances to schools, and the cost of assistive technology.

> For example in my area, . . . there is no special school . . . so when you approach parents about their children starting school, they say I will not manage because the bus cannot go round picking minus fuel, so every month they do make a contribution of K50 . . . (but) K50 is very difficult to find by some parents.
>
> *(Special education teacher, Copperbelt Province)*

Another teacher describes the interaction between limited resources, lack of assistive technology:

> It is difficult. It is not easy, say for children . . . unable to walk. For them to come is a burden, already we have one who is just being carried on the back to come here, so we asked them to maybe find a wheelchair for that child because how will that child be sitting in class, but since the parents left up to now, they have not come back. It is not easy for them to come here due to distances.
>
> *(Primary school teacher, Eastern Province)*

Discriminatory practices surrounding the availability of stipends for disabled children in schools, boarding schools, trade schools and higher education only make it less likely that disabled children will be able to attend any kind of schooling. For those who have assistive technology and can independently come to school, their school routes are often not safe, due to lack of sidewalks, heavy traffic and wide and dangerous roads to cross.

Barriers in learning environment

Inaccessible educational building structures were mentioned by almost all informants. Stairs, lack of ramps, distances between facilities such as dormitories and classrooms, uncleared bushes, lack of lighting, all contribute to making the physical environment inaccessible to disabled children. Lack of accessible toilets is one of the major deterrents. Since wheelchairs usually do not fit in the space allowed for the toilet, children with physical impairments find themselves crawling on dirty floors in order to use the toilets: 'you try to crawl on the ground but on the floor of the toilets there is a lot of liquids and you don't have protective equipment, so you just suffer inwardly' (Young man with physical impairment, Eastern Province).

Lack of resources, such as books and computers, is a general problem in schools, but it disproportionately affects disabled students in all types of schools. Even in special schools, there is a lack of computers and adaptive learning materials. People with visual impairment lack textbooks and books in braille, as well as braille paper. Equipment for hearing-impaired learners is also scarce. In addition, special schools are often dependent on support from NGOs for these types of resources.

In mainstream schools, teachers complain that disabled students are enrolled without increased financial resources, support staff or in-service training of teachers. It is also common for special education teachers to work with either old, unrevised curricula or curricula for mainstream students and mainstream books, which they need to adapt.

Another problem expressed by teachers is that disabled children do not undergo clinical or pedagogical assessment before they begin school. However, an informant stated that disabled children are required to be clinically assessed before starting school, though this is not standard-ised. This results in children with varying degrees of impairments, knowledge and abilities being randomly assigned to a class, instead of optimally assigned according to intellectual potential, availability of assistive technology, flexibility of teacher and environmental adaptation.

> I think that the system has not followed the principal of placement because they haven't been assessing these children . . . you find one has an extreme disability and another has a moderate or mild, yet they are put together. You will find that that will affect the teacher to ensure that the child acquires knowledge that is supposed to be given to each and every child in the class and then the child also will be derailed.
>
> *(Teacher in school with inclusive education, Lusaka Province)*

There is also no coordinated effort or systems in place to ensure life-long learning of disabled children. They might be able to progress with schooling up to a certain grade level, but there are no plans or policies in place to ensure further success. Many find that they are unable to sit for qualifying examinations because institutions are not physically accessible to them due to distances. Another challenge is that examinations are not designed to meet their individual impairment-specific needs. Lack of accommodation in exams and lack of opportunities for disabled children following education make them feel that, though important, their education is irrelevant since they just return to the same life they led before they started school.

> My mother has no problem but dad still call(s) me names especially when he is drunk. This problem of the results missing, he says it is not the results, he feels that I did not just pass and he says it was time wasted being in school for all those years.
>
> *(Girl with visual impairment, Western Province)*

Barriers mentioned above are having a significant impact on the quality of education that disabled children receive. Despite these barriers, there are disabled children who do well in mainstream schools. However, their opportunity for secondary education and higher education is often cut short due to additional systemic barriers, e.g. lack of stipends and lack of individual education plans.

Following are the stories of two young people who have attained some measure of success in the educational or skills training opportunities they have been allowed to access despite the many barriers they have had to overcome. These two cases arise from key informant interviews conducted in 2015 in the Copperbelt region in Zambia. They involve children with very different impairments and activity limitation profiles. However, these two cases emphasise the importance of having an ICF perspective in inclusive education, especially for disabled children.

Susan: making the most of her skills training

Susan receives vocational training at an all-female special school. At this school, students acquire practical skills like sewing, cooking and baking. The aim is to give students skills they can use to generate income. Susan believes her impairment is a result of witchcraft. She explains: 'Someone got my *chitenge* (material) tied some charms and I stopped walking. From there, I found my leg and hand bent.' She says she also has epilepsy. Her mother, however, recalls that Susan's impairment was due to contracting malaria at the age of six months, and their inability to reach a hospital early enough. Though she started having seizures at this age, her family was never counselled about how to deal with them or how the seizures would affect Susan's future.

Though Susan says she has accepted her impairment, it pains her to be laughed at by other people in the community. Even her siblings yell at her using derogatory terms such as 'cripple'. 'You are bewitched and have a crippled hand.' However, she is praised by her parents for being a hard worker. Despite the impairment, she sweeps the house, makes her bed and washes clothes. She is also able to bathe and dress herself and take care of most of her personal hygiene. She also collects her own medicines when needed. She is very independent in many ways. However, her impairment does not allow her to lift heavy things or carry delicate objects. She also does not cook for fear of being burnt during a seizure. Susan gets about four to five seizures a day.

Susan's parents are self-sufficient farmers who supplement their income by selling their own farm products. Her father was previously a soldier, but now he raises chickens. When Susan was little, she attended a preschool together with non-disabled children. However, she says she was not allowed to continue in mainstream schools. Her mother recalls that Susan started in a main-stream school, but a doctor came to assess her and determined that 'she (was) fine, but a bit slow' and that she could not learn in that school. Her mother continues, 'They recommended she goes to the special school and I accepted'. She was then transferred to a mixed gender rehabilitation centre, which was eventually closed. She now attends a vocational school, where she has learned to make doormats and bake. She hopes her education will enable her to learn to read, do mathematics and sew clothes, so that she will be able to make her own clothes and enable her to buy her parents' clothes. At school, besides solving mathematical questions, something she finds 'easy', she cleans the classroom, windows and blackboard. She finds reading difficult, especially holding books. She is also aware that the education she is receiving at the special school is different from the education her siblings are receiving. Though she is older, her siblings can already read and are taking subjects like mathematics, English and Bemba. She also knows that her siblings' education will allow them to sit for Grade 9 examinations, which is needed if they wish to continue study-ing, whereas in her school, they do not sit for these examinations, since 'after completing, (they) get a certificate and go home'. However, Susan's mother seems appreciative of her education:

> It's very different in there are many people who are like Susan . . . but she doesn't beg because you find that most of those who are like her are beggars and pick things in the streets, but she is not like that, so they ask me like how did you educate her and I say I took her to school.

In her interview, Susan comes off as a very enterprising individual. Susan currently uses the skills she has learned at the special school to make an income. She sells doormats and scones. At the time of the interview, she sold the doormats she made by the side of the road for 20.00 Zambian Kwachas (ZMK) each. She is also instrumental in having provided her family with a new source of income; that is, selling of scones. Though she does not put the scones in the oven herself, she introduced the knowledge of baking scones to her family from what she learned at school. Susan and her family make from 40.00 to 100.00 ZMK per day from selling scones. Her family has been so successful that according to her teacher when they first started 'they just bought her one kilogram of flour at the market; but this time they have gone into a 50 kg bag'. When asked what Susan does with the money she earns from both the mats and scones, she replied:

> I buy my clothes; supplement some food stuffs at home and my cosmetics. All my family members benefit from (the) money I realise from scones and doormats. When I come to school my sisters bake scones and sell together with my mother who also sells sweet potatoes and wild fruits . . . I use them for any group contributions at school and church, sometimes I pay my school fees and buy groceries at home.

Susan's mother describes her daughter as both hard working and intelligent. She might not think much about Susan's ability to write 'but whatever else she learns, she comes back to teach us'. She describes Susan as tough, ambitious, driven and not easily dissuaded and having an instinct for business. She says that it is easy to teach Susan new things: 'That's what I was saying she doesn't delay in learning new things easily.' Her teacher at the special school is also impressed with Susan's abilities:

> Susan's story has given a very big story: no one, no one is not able: Everyone is able whether with disability or no disability . . . If Susan can do it, we believe even the other disabled students out there can make it in life.

Mutalo: academic success in the face of barriers

Mutalo was born with a congenital hearing loss. His parents said that he has 'holes on the neck, which form pus', and when this happens, he is only able to hear the sound of water and ringing in his ears, and nothing else. It is when these holes clear that he is able to hear again. Therefore, his hearing impairment is not constant. His parents have taken him to different doctors but he has never been referred to specialists. His parents feel that they are taken seriously by the medical profession.

Mutalo has only attended mainstream schools and therefore has not learned Sign Language, but he seems to be very good at lip reading. He is currently attending a boarding school together with his younger brother. An NGO is paying for their tuition, uniforms and books. Mutalo is in Grade 11. He should have finished school earlier, but since his teachers did not seem concerned whether he was hearing or learning, his parents decided to hold him back three years when he was young. They meant that in this manner 'your young brother will be explaining to you where you don't understand'.

Mutalo's classmates communicate with him by either shouting or pointing. In the classroom, Mutalo sits on the last bench of the middle row. Since his hearing is not stable, his participation in class is deeply affected by his ability to hear. He only participates when he is able to hear. One of his classmates has observed that he does not understand what teachers are saying most of the time, 'He just learns through guessing, especially when the teacher is not speaking loudly. He only studies notes on his own.' When he cannot hear, and no one can communicate with him, it makes it difficult for him to learn. As his friend points out, sometimes written communication is not enough to understand new concepts: 'There are some topics you can't understand (unless) it is explained.' He is very bright though, and does well in mathematics and chemistry. He is often first or second in his class.

His lack of hearing also affects his relationships with others. His family and friends think he is short-tempered and fear him. His best friend does not think that Mutalo is particularly moody, just that his hearing problem causes him to be like that. When he suddenly suffers hearing loss, he just wants to be alone and sleep. As for his future, Mutalo seems to have considered several types of careers as related by those who know him. Depending on whom one asks, Mutalo has said he wants to be a teacher, a pilot, a mechanic, a driver and a soldier. His father says that Mutalo has an interest in computers, and that this could be a skill he could acquire which could help him get work.

His teachers at both his present school and past school describe him as very competent and friendly. The teacher at his current school says that he excels in general science, chemistry and physics despite having no learning material adapted to his needs. Though Mutalo does not respond in class, his test results are very good. The teacher acknowledges that though the school policy warrants the inclusion of disabled children, it is unable to accomplish inclusion because the school lacks personnel trained for this. However, they do try to adapt for children with hearing impairment by having them sit closer to the blackboard. In this manner, students can see and read the teacher's lips. The teacher in his past school used the same approach to include children with hearing impairment, though he did not have a positive view on inclusive education:

> [W]hen teachers teaching those who are normal using speech, it was very difficult for Mutalo to get what the teacher was teaching hence, there was no special tool which was being used to the learning of Mutalo, that's why I am saying this inclusiveness is not good. It is better those children with Special Education Needs go to special schools so that they learn fully, unlike just being put together with normal children, only normal children benefit (then), (the others), they lag behind.

This teacher's explanation shows that inclusive education policy has been introduced in schools without implementation. Mutalo's educational path has been marred by systemic barriers and stigma. He has yet to be helped by health providers and his education has never been adapted to his disability. Most of his time in school, has been spent reading lips, and guessing what teachers and friends say to him. His impairment has greatly affected his participation in society because he often does not feel physically well and because he finds it easier not to be social. At the time of the interview, he had yet to receive counselling on what career options he had and how he could attain them. His future seems very unsure despite the fact that he is both intelligent and a hard worker. The fact that he is still in school attests more to his strong character and persistence than to implementation of inclusive education.

Similarly, Susan has yet to achieve her full potential. Fortunately, she is receiving care for her epilepsy, and has been able to learn skills at a vocational school, so, in many ways, she could be considered a success for the system and her family, but we do not know what else she could be able to learn and achieve. She has demonstrated that she is able to learn quickly and is clever in mathematics and business. However, reading is a skill she cannot do, or could adapted education provide her with this one skill she so dearly wants?

Discussion

Having an ICF model perspective in implementing inclusive education is important because it can change how people view disability. The model clearly shows that the activity of a person is limited not only by their health condition, but also by the individual's contextual factors (environmental and personal factors). Environmental factors are something that can be changed so that an individual's life can change from one of constant limitations to increased participation. If an individual is not participating, whether the individual has a health condition or not, one has to look at this individual's environment to see whether there are factors that can be changed for that person to participate.

In the ICF model, environmental factors comprise products and technology, natural and human-made changes to the environment, support and relationship, attitudes, and services, systems and policies. The findings of the study showed that there were many barriers with respect to attitudes as well as services, systems and implementation of policies.

Barriers in attitudes

An attitudinal barrier is perhaps one of the most important environmental barriers to work with, because it affects relationships, systems, policies and availability of quality services

(Chataika, 2013). The most important view to change is that participation is solely dependent on an individual's health condition. This view allows society to accept limitations as inevitable and encourages passivity instead of action for change and solutions. The study found that approximately 20% of children with disabilities had problems with people's attitudes, prejudice and discrimination, while one quarter experienced abuse from both family and their community. In interviews, description of experienced abuse and stigma, inability to see potential in disabled people, prejudice toward teachers working with disabled children, as well as descriptions of disabled people as not 'normal', are all a result of the limiting disease-based concept of disability where barriers are an inherent part of disability. Changing attitudes depend on provision of information, which in turn is dependent on quality of services in general. Disabled people's organisations are in a unique position to work in communities to provide information based on a new disability discourse and thus, change societal values (Chataika *et al.*, 2015).

Barriers in services

Most of the institutional barriers experienced by disabled children in education fall under what ICF calls services 'systems and policies'. Many policies are in place but implementation of these policies is lacking. The survey found that about 20% of children were having problems accessing transport services and many more were having problems accessing educational services. It also found a problem with physical access to public institutions, including educational institutions, and access to assistive devices. Where services were being provided, there were issues with the quality of these services, as illustrated by the low percentage of disabled children being able to read. The interviews pointed to a lack of assessments and plans, lack of services, lack of accessible environments and quality of education as important factors for inclusion into education.

Bio-medical and pedagogical assessments of children as well as environmental assessment are necessary in order to be able to provide quality education. An assessment based on the ICF perspective would enable local schools and teachers to adapt education to the gaps experienced by all children, including disabled children. This type of assessment would not only uncover the bio-medical needs of children but also the physical environmental needs, the technical needs, the financial needs and the services needs necessary to achieve the educational goals set for each child. The emphasis would not be on the impairment but on the gaps hindering children from achieving educational goals (Stubbs, 2008). Though schools could not be responsible for describing health states based on ICF or providing health services, they could uncover children who have fallen through the system and not received necessary health services, such as provision of medication or assistive technology needed to function in daily life. They could also uncover whether there were other services, which school children were entitled to but not receiving, such as cash transfers or other financial support needed for educational participation. This would require a whole systems approach as described in the CRPD (United Nations, 2006).

Once established, schools could concentrate on pedagogical assessments, individualised goals and individualised learning plans in order to ensure quality education. In order to do this, there is a need of professionalisation and additional training of teachers, not only of 'special education teachers', but also mainstream teachers. As the interviews uncovered, pedagogical training needs to focus on inclusive education. ICF and UDL training could be an integral part of the competency development of teachers. However, the interviews also uncovered that quality also depended on the amount of support being received by the teachers. They often felt overwhelmed by large classrooms, children with different pedagogical needs, as well as children needing care. Therefore, many teachers are not only in need of pedagogical support staff but also of care support staff. Using ICF as a tool could uncover these needs. It could also uncover physical environmental barriers present in schools, such as stairs, non-accessible bathrooms, lighting and resources (Eide & Loeb, 2006).

In addition to change in disability discourse, there is a need for provision of information about policies guaranteeing education or training for disabled people. This will empower communities and help develop their voice to demand better access to educational services. Again, this is something DPOs could actively work on. Together, these initiatives could perhaps change the willingness of the community to work together with school administration and teachers to help improve educational environments so that they become inclusive schools. The perception of quality in education could help increase school enrolment among disabled children and increased appreciation of the advantages of education, such as increased opportunities and independence (Hollenweger, 2014).

Finally, it is important to consider the findings presented here in light of the context. Some laws might be in place, but overall, large investment in education is needed. It is necessary to improve the quality of children's education and teacher training. It is also important to provide pedagogical assessment of children, inclusive educational curricula and plans, learning and human resources that promote inclusive education (Hollenweger, 2014). In addition, there is a need to provide career counsellors and to improve physical accessibility in schools; hence, providing quality education that is accessible, acceptable and adaptable (United Nations, 2006).

Article 24 of the CRPD requires a whole systems approach, with changes in legislation, policy, mechanisms for financing, administration, design, delivery and monitoring of education (United Nations, 2006). Though this might seem like a huge investment for a country with limited resources, it is more costly not to invest in education and not to take advantage of the years of latent productivity among disabled people. In addition, the CRPD is aware of the limitations of the context of some countries and does not expect inclusive education to be achieved within a short time; rather it expects that countries progressively accomplish their obligations under CRPD by providing reasonable accommodations for inclusion, and not allowing countries to use limitations in resources as excuse. What would this mean in terms of resources to achieve the right of disabled children to inclusive education in accordance to the ratified CRPD? Knowledge of ICF's contextualisation in accordance to the expected goals of the CRPD and its application in low-income contexts for use in inclusive education could be a next step for research.

References

Chataika, T. (2013). *Gender and Disability Mainstreaming Training Manual: Disabled Women in Africa*. GIZ Sector Initiative Persons with Disabilities on behalf of BMZ. Retrieved from www.diwa.ws/index.php?option=com_phoca on 6 September 2017.

Chataika, T., Berghs, M., Mateta, A. & Shava, K. (2015). From whose perspective anyway? The quest for African disability rights activism. In E. de Waal (ed.) *Advocacy in Conflict: Critical Perspectives on Transnational Activism* (pp. 187–211). London: Zed Books.

Eide, A. H. & Loeb, M. (2006). *Living Conditions among People with Activity Limitations in Zambia: A National Representative Study. SINTEF Report A262*, SINTEF, Oslo.

Fougeroyrollas, P. & Beauregard, L. (2001). An interactive person-environment social creation. In G. L. Albrecht, K. D. Seelman & M. Bury (eds) *Handbook of Disability Studies* (pp. 171–194). London: Sage Publications.

Hollenweger, J. (2014). *Definition and Classification of Disability, Webinar 2, Companion Technical Booklet*. United Nations Children's Fund (UNICEF). Retrieved from www.inclusive-education.org/sites/default/files/uploads/booklets/IE_Webinar_Booklet_2.pdf on 10 September 2016.

Ingstad, B. & Eide, A. H. (2011). Disability and poverty: a global challenge. In A. H. Eide & B. Ingstad (eds) *Disability and Poverty: A Global Challenge* (pp. 1–13). Bristol: The Policy Press.

Lebeer, J. *et al.* (2012). Re-assessing the current assessment practice of children with special education needs in Europe. *School Psychology International* **33**(1), 69–92.

Miles, S. (2011). Exploring understandings of inclusion in schools in Zambia and Tanzania using reflective writing and photography. *International Journal of Inclusive Education* **15**(10), 1087–1102.

Ministry of Education (1996). *Educating our Future. National Policy on Education.* Republic of Zambia.

Republic of Zambia (1996a). *The Constitution of Zambia Act.* Republic of Zambia.

Republic of Zambia (1996b). *The Technical Education, Vocational and Entrepreneurship Training (TEVET) Policy.* Republic of Zambia.

Republic of Zambia (2011). *The Education Act.* Republic of Zambia.

Republic of Zambia (2012). *The Persons with Disabilities Act.* Republic of Zambia.

Rieser, R. (2012). *Implementing Inclusive Education: A Commonwealth Guide to Implementing Article 24 of the UN Convention on the Rights of Persons with Disabilities.* Second. Commonwealth Secretariat, London.

Sanches-Ferreira, M., Silveira-Maia, M. & Alves, S. (2014). The use of the International Classification of Functioning, Disability and Health, version for Children and Youth (ICF-CY), in Portuguese special education assessment and eligibility procedures: the professionals' perceptions. *European Journal of Special Needs Education* **29**(3), 327–343.

Sanches-Ferreira, M. *et al.* (2015). Evaluating implementation of the International Classification of Functioning, Disability and Health in Portugal's special education law. *International Journal of Inclusive Education* **19**(5), 457–468.

Stubbs, S. (2008). *Inclusive Education: Where There Are Few Resources.* Oslo: The Atlas Alliance.

UDL Center (no date). *The Three Principles of UDL.* Retrieved from www.udlcenter.org on 3 June 2017.

UNESCO (2016). *Global Education Monitoring Report – Education for People and Planet: Creating Sustainable Futures for All.* Paris: UNESCO. Retrieved from http://unesdoc.unesco.org/images/0024/002457/245752e.pdf on 27 August 2016.

United Nations (2015). *Sustainable Development Goals.* United Nations. Retrieved from https://sustainable development.un.org/?menu= 1300 on 15 March 2017.

United Nations (2006). *Convention on the Rights of Persons with Disabilities and Optional Protocol.* New York: United Nations. Retrieved from www.un.org/disabilities/documents/convention/convoptprot-e.pdf on 7 September 2017.

United Nations Committee on the Rights of Persons with Disabilities (2016). *General Comment No. 4: Article 24: Right to Inclusive Education.* United Nations Convention on the Rights of Persons with Disabilities (CRPD). Retrieved from www.refworld.org/docid/57c977e34.html on 3 February 2017.

United Nations General Assembly (1989). *Convention on the Rights of the Child.* United Nations.

United Nations General Assembly (2007). *Convention on the Rights of Persons with Disabilities.* Retrieved from www.refworld.org/docid/45f973632.html on 15 September 2016

WHO (1980) *International Classification of Impairments, Disabilities, and Handicaps: A Manual of Classification Relating to the Consequences of Disease.* Geneva: World Health Organization.

WHO (2001). *International Classification of Functioning, Disability and Health (ICF).* Geneva: World Health Organization. Retrieved from www.who.int/classifications/drafticfpracticalmanual2.pdf?ua=1 on 15 September 2016.

World Bank (2015). *Incheon Declaration: Education 2030 – Towards Inclusive and Equitable Quality Education and Lifelong Learning for All.* Retrieved from http://documents.worldbank.org/curated/en/167341467987876458/Incheon-declaration-education-2030-towards-inclusive-and-equitable-quality-education-and-lifelong-learning-for-all on 26 September 2016.

10

EXAMINING THE EFFECTIVENESS OF THE SPECIAL CLASS MODEL IN ZIMBABWE

Sitshengisiwe Gweme and Tsitsi Chataika

Introduction

The special class model intends to assist learners with difficulties in improving in the areas where they face challenges in mathematics, reading and spelling. This chapter is based on a study that explored the effectiveness of the special class model on primary school children with specific learning difficulties (SpLDs) in Hwange urban, which is in Zimbabwe. We begin by providing the background literature and outline the methodology used. We then present the major findings and then interpret them, intercepting with relevant literature. Finally, we present conclusions.

Background

Children with SpLDs vary in nature and in the areas where they face challenges. There are various forms of SpLDs, however, this chapter focuses on dyslexia and dyscalculia as these are the ones that are considered for placement in the special class in Zimbabwe. These are challenges faced in mathematics, reading and spelling. Florian and Hegarty (2010) describe dyslexia as a specific difficulty in reading, spelling and written language. Difficulties in mathematics, on the other hand are referred to as dyscalculia (Price & Ansari, 2013).

Learners are identified as having learning difficulties when they excel in other areas of the curriculum but face challenges in a specific area. The regular classroom practitioners are mandated with the task of identifying these individuals for placement in special classes for the purpose of receiving individualised assistance from the specialist teacher.

Most teachers in the mainstream classes tend to identify and refer those learners they feel they cannot handle in their classrooms. This makes it difficult for the special class teacher to make noticeable progress in assisting these individuals as some, if not most of them, would be under-performers in all areas of the curriculum. According to Aro and Ahonen (2011), in deciding which learners to refer for possible placement in special classes, teachers consider their perceptions of the child's performance. Mitchell (2008) observes that teachers refer learners whom they perceive as difficult to teach and who have serious academic and behavioural problems.

It is against this background that most regular teachers do not want learners with SpLDs to return to their classes. According to Fletcher-Janzen and Reynolds (2008), many teachers are sceptical of proposals to return all children with learning difficulties to general education classrooms because they feel that coping with the difficulties these children present is a challenging task.

The study was primarily based on the concept of inclusion, which implies that all learners, including those with difficulties, should learn in mainstream classes alongside their peers without difficulties under the supervision of one teacher (Mitchell, 2008). The inclusion of children with diverse needs in mainstream schools is a national and international development. According to Jenjekwa, Rutoro and Runyowa (2013), education for learners with diverse educational needs should be provided in ordinary schools, hence the concept of inclusion. As part of promoting inclusion, Zimbabwe has introduced the special class model in most mainstream schools to cater for the unique needs of children with SpLDs.

The special class model

Zimbabwe has introduced the special classes in most regular schools to cater for children with SpLDs. Learners are tested and placed in these classes by the Schools Psychological Services and Special Needs Education (SPS & SNE) after having been diagnosed as having SpLDs (Jenjekwa *et al*, 2013).

The class size in the special class model is between 15 and 19 (National Council for Special Education, 2014). In agreement, Mnkandla and Mataruse (2002) state that the number is smaller than in the mainstream classes where each learner gets individual instruction to reach their goal. This facilitates more individual attention and small group instruction (Mitchell, 2008). Hence, this creates more chances for learners to re-join their mainstream peers.

Concepts in the special class are covered at a slower pace (Department of Education and Science, 2007). This enables learners to learn at their pace, as they may not be forced into grasping too much information at the same time. Kay and Yeo (2003) also emphasise that special class teachers should repeat concepts to ensure understanding in learners. That way, learners will have a better chance of mastering concepts.

Learners in the special class are not supposed to share learning aids as they are encouraged to manipulate objects and gain information and knowledge using most if not all their senses. This allows the learners to manipulate the material in any way possible to solicit for information. Jenjekwa *et al* (2013) observe that multisensory teaching links listening, speaking, reading and writing through the simultaneous and alternating use of visual, auditory, kinaesthetic and tactile modalities. It then becomes important to adopt this approach when teaching learners with SpLDs, as they need a more individualised approach to learning.

Learners in the special class model do not learn all the subjects of the curriculum in this class. They are only taught mathematics, reading and spelling. Content subjects are learned alongside their peers in the regular classrooms while being instructed by the ordinary teacher. This is done mainly for integration. Hocutt (1996, p. 8) states that 'these students spend an average of 70% of their time in general education settings'. In Zimbabwe, learners in the special class spend half of the day in the special class and the other half in the mainstream classes (Mpofu, 2001).

Learner eligibility

For learners to be placed into the special class, they should first be identified as having SpLDs and then be tested. It is stated by Ncube and Hlatshwayo (2014) that special class eligibility is based upon evidence that the student does not achieve adequately for his or her age in either written expression, basic reading skills, mathematical calculations or mathematics problem solving. To ensure adequate identification, the school personnel should, according to Fletcher, Lyon, Fuchs and Barnes (2007), ensure that the child has been provided with appropriate instruction in regular education settings.

According to the Saudi Arabian Ministry of Education (2011), if a child has been identified as having an SpLD, the school should ensure that they get the parents' consent before the testing can be done. This implies that parents are the ones who will decide whether the child should be referred for further testing by the SPS and SNE or not.

For the special class model testing, a number of pupils are identified and recommended (Lerner, 2003). Those eligible are then selected depending on their performance in the test. Rose (2009) reported that the results of the test will indicate if the child has a learning difficulty and the level at which he/she is operating. Learners identified are usually from grades four to six though in some schools they also select learners from grade three. The programme in Zimbabwe, according to Samkange (2013), originally targeted grade four learners, but later included learners from all the other grades except grades one, two and seven.

Attitudes toward the implementation of the special class model

Chakuchichi, Chiinze and Kaputa (2003) argue that negative attitudes toward differences result in discrimination and can lead to a serious barrier to learning. Learners placed in the special class can at times be stigmatised and labelled by peers and teachers. Such ridicule and labelling might lead to a self-fulfilling prophecy on these learners, thereby leading to failure to improve. Similarly, Mafa (2012) established that teachers have no desire to teach children with learning difficulties and that they have the most negative attitudes. This could be due to the fact that these learners need more time for their learning. According to Maunganidze and Kasayira (2002), mainstream teachers indicated that they already have too much workload and having to deal with children with SpLDs would be an extra burden. Mnkandla and Mataruse (2002) assert that teachers have negative attitudes because of lack of knowledge and incompetence in teaching children with SpLDs.

Teachers are supposed to play an important role and their willingness to make a positive contribution to all children supports the goal of education. Samkange (2013) argues that the special class model calls for respect of differences, and this helps to break down barriers in negative attitudes.

Parents of children with SpLDs have an important role to play in the education of their children. According to Ministry of Education (2011), research has shown that parents' attitudes affect the success in the education of their children. In addition, Somaily, Al-Zoubi and Rahman (2012) state that vague understanding of the purpose and the benefits of the education of children with SpLDs on the part of the parents can be a main reason for holding negative attitudes toward their children's education.

In line with policies on advocating for inclusive education, schooling of children with SpLDs in content subjects takes place in a mainstream setting. However, access to the mainstream class does not necessarily guarantee full participation, and students with SpLDs often have limited social relationships (Vignes, 2009). This could be due to a number of reasons. Horne (2011) observes that this restriction of social participation is brought about by both personal and environmental factors, including negative attitudes of peers. Numerous studies have explored attitudes toward peers with SpLDs and they have established that many primary school students with SpLDs feel rejected by their peers and are rarely chosen as friends (Vignes, 2009). This regrettably impacts on their personal, social and academic growth.

Peer acceptance constitutes an important determinant of successful inclusion, because social rejection can contribute to the development of various emotional and behavioural problems. In order to facilitate full inclusion of children with SpLDs, there is a need to improve the attitudes of other children toward them (Kourkoutas, 2012).

Methodology

In an attempt to establish the effectiveness of the special class model in improving the learning outcomes of primary school learners with SpLDs in Hwange urban in Zimbabwe, we randomly selected three primary schools that are implementing the special school model. Data were gathered between June and July 2016.

The study adopted a qualitative approach, which focuses on the different ways in which people look at things. This type of research was relevant as it focuses on experience and data that cannot be adequately expressed numerically (Thomas, 2010). This type of research could also lead to the development of new concepts as people's views were considered. We utilised interviews and focus group discussions (FGDs) with heads, teachers, learners in the special class model and parents.

Data from natural settings allowed us to gain a sense of whether what the interview and FGD participants reported about the special class model practice was actually happening, or whether participants were telling and retelling stories that were speculation, hearsay or even distorted perceptions. It also allowed us to see if information given by participants were valid realities as it is usually easy to determine if a person is giving you false information through a face-to-face conversation.

A standardised, open-ended interview for the heads of schools and the District Remedial Tutor (DRT) was used for data collection. Kessler (2013) states that interviews allow the researcher to probe further based on what respondents have said so as to gather more information about their experiences and feelings. Thus, interviews allowed us to understand the meanings that everyday activities hold for people, as well as allowing for immediate follow-up and clarification on information (Haslam, 2014). Interviews also allowed us to 'examine attitudes, interests, feelings, concerns and values' (Gay & Airasian, 2002, p. 209). As interviews involve personal interaction, cooperation was essential. We were aware that interviewing had limitations and weaknesses. To overcome these, instructions were clearly explained to participants and we ensured that ethical considerations were upheld.

In FGDs, an environment conducive for everyone was created and questions asked were clear so that discussion could take place allowing the participants to freely express their individual views and opinions. We were aware that in FGDs, a person's beliefs and attitudes are usually guided by other people's views and opinions (Coolican, 2014). The aim of utilising this method was to ensure that participants could freely and independently share their views and thoughts in a natural environment.

Furthermore, FGDs provided quick results and permitted more people to be interviewed at the same time. The use of FGDs was relevant to the study because it brought a group of people together to share ideas, therefore providing diverse views.

The interviews and FGDs carried out yielded a great amount of data that had to be transcribed, analysed and interpreted. The reason for analysing data collected was to enable the researcher to extract information that was relevant to the study. According to Bell and Waters (2014), the analysis might give an account of the data collected by summarising it and noting similar contributions as well as comparing and contrasting the given data. Interpretation, on the other hand, is the process of attaching meaning to the data, as Coolican (2014) states that interpretation of data is the way in which the researcher moves from a description of what is the case, to an explanation of why it is the case.

To ensure ethical considerations were met, clearance was sought from the University of Zimbabwe, Educational Foundations Department to conduct the study. All the participants who were selected for the interviews and FGDs were given informed consent forms to read and sign if they agreed with what was written. We made sure that participants had full knowledge of what was involved. Participants were also assured of confidentiality, privacy and anonymity.

Participants were informed of the reason for the study, the data collection procedure and what would be expected of them before starting with the interview and FGDs. Participants were also guaranteed that they were not going to be put in a situation where they would be harmed as a result of their participation, physically or psychologically. The participants all appeared to engage freely in the discussions and this indicated that the interview and the FGD process allowed the participants to share their views in a safe environment and without being judged.

Permission to record the interviews and the FGDs was also obtained from the participants. It was further explained to them that their information would remain confidential. The identity of the participants was not included in the research and a key was used for the participants. They were assured that they had a right to withdraw from the interviews or FGDs at any time if they felt uncomfortable without giving any explanations. It if from these methodological resources that we managed to generate the findings that we present in the next section.

Major findings

Several themes emerged from the study, however, for this chapter we decided to focus on three major themes, namely, the understanding of the special class model, learner eligibility, and the challenges in the implementation of the model.

Understanding the special class model

Several views emerged from the study pertaining to the understanding of the special class model. According to the DRT, a 'special class model is whereby teacher pupil ratio is 1 is to 19, which makes it easy for the teacher to attend to individual difficulties of students'. It implies that the DRT's understanding of the special class model was based on the class size as opposed to SpLDs to be addressed. This is worrying as this participant holds an influential position in the district when it comes to the education of children with disabilities.

The three school heads and the teachers had similar understanding of the special class models as indicated by school head 2:

> My understanding of this model is that the children with learning difficulties are helped mostly individually. The teacher will take time to have a look at an individual child. The pace that they use is not the same as the pace which is used by the main classes. I think that alone helps them a lot. They are taught at their own pace and a lot of individual attention is given.

One of the teachers in the FGD at school 3 indicated that a special class model is where students who would have been identified to be having SpLDs are withdrawn into their class so that their specific needs are catered for, separate from the mainstream class. It is clear that most participants had a general understanding of what the special class model is about.

Learner eligibility

The study revealed that schools had slightly different ways of choosing learners who were eligible for the special class model. However, they all agreed, along with the DRT that there are Ministry of Primary and Secondary Education (MoPSE) expected criteria. The DRT shared the expected criteria:

> There is a standardised test which is administered before children are graded into the special class. This comprises maths and English whereby children answer questions on given answer scripts and then those are marked and they are selected into the special class. Normally we test from grade three to six those who are thought to be lagging behind in their performance. The criteria used by schools starts from remedial class selection whereby the diagnostic tests are administered to pupils and those who prove to be weak in both maths and English are given another standardised test for selection into the special class.

The above criteria slightly differed from what one of the teachers in school 2 shared:

> In this school, we choose the grade fours and fives, the reason being, grade three is a transitional stage and there are a lot of concepts that are being introduced there. So at times it will be that a child doesn't have problems as such, but, yes, some will be failing to cope and all. And then at grade four and five that is when you can realise that this child has a problem. Then grade six, we are looking at the fact that they have to complete the grade seven syllabi, so when the child is in grade six we cannot disturb that child because the remedy at times won't be effective because the child will have missed a lot of things. In grade seven the teacher helps the child.

The teacher indicated that they were not aware of the district's expectations. It then meant that they applied whatever method they thought was most suitable for them. However, another teacher at the same school 2 had a contradicting view:

> Actually at grade four level, we expect that almost all children should be able to read, make simple operations like simple addition and subtraction. Then from there that's when we discover that some pupils cannot read, add, they cannot even identify a figure or a letter, so those are the children that we choose; then they are tested before they can be admitted into the special class.

These different views from participants in the same school implied that teachers were not clearly conversant with the selection criteria of learners eligible for the model. If this is the case, then the success of the model in that school is hampered by contradictory implementation challenges.

Challenges in the implementation of the special class model

Several challenges were noted by participants. These included attitudes from teachers, peers and parents as well as the identification procedures.

TEACHERS' ATTITUDES

Participants indicated that some teachers held negative attitudes toward learners with SpLDs. Such attitudes pose a challenge in the successful implementation of the special class model. The DRT, school heads and the teachers held similar views to this regard. These views are well-articulated by the DRT:

In schools, the major challenge is that one of integrating these children into the mainstream classes in other subjects because normally the special class model concentrates mainly on mathematics and English which are the basics of all learning but then there are challenges such as negative attitudes from the regular class teachers in handling those children because they claim they are having an extra load.

Also, school heads indicated that teachers usually complain about numbers of learners, especially when the teacher–pupil ratio goes beyond 40. Hence, teachers felt that if learners eligible for the special class are excluded in the mainstream, this relieves them from having bigger class sizes. However, they still felt that when children come back into class for other subjects other than mathematics and English, they increase the burden again. Again, school heads noted that mainstream teachers felt that special class teachers have few children, meaning that they do not have much work to do, especially when it comes to marking of children's books. As a result, school head 2 was concerned about the attitudes of mainstream teachers:

> The challenges that I have noticed are that when these children (special class children) leave for the other subjects, I don't see them benefiting much in the mainstream classes. This is because there is a tendency that the teacher may not really like those children because they feel that they underperform. Also, they feel that they are doing the job of the special class teacher who does not have many children. That is a serious challenge that I have observed.

Similarly, some learners with SpLDs felt that some mainstream teachers label them. One learner noted that, 'When we are just seated quietly and others in our group make noise, our teacher says "you from the special class you are making noise"'. Such negative attitudes have adverse impact on the learning outcomes of learners with SpLDs as they might find it difficult to be part of the mainstream class. It, however, emerged that some teachers held positive attitudes toward these learners. This is applauded, as such attitudes have positive implications on learning outcomes and child development of children with SpLDs.

PEER ATTITUDES

It also emerged that some peers in the mainstream held negative attitudes toward children with SpLDs. School heads as well as the teachers shared similar views on the attitudes of peers. These attitudes affect the learning of the children with SpLDs in that they might feel stigmatised by peers and looked down upon. This implies that mainstream learners have limited understanding of what this special class model is all about. Also, appreciation of learner diversity seems to be missing from other learners, making it difficult for those with SpLDs to be readily accepted in the mainstream classes. However, some of the peer attitudes toward the learners with SpLDs were positive as they acknowledged that some of them treat them like any other learner. They also indicated that some learners share their belongings with them and they do not label them. Such positive attitudes are a positive catalyst to inclusion, an aspect that has implications on learning outcomes.

PARENTAL ATTITUDES

It emerged that some parents of children with SpLDs held negative attitudes toward the special class model, which unfortunately had a negative impact on the learning achievements of these learners. School head 3 was concerned that some parents seem not to understand the special class model as they believe that their children have been labelled and relegated into a non-learning class, yet the school will be trying to address the SpLDs before their children re-join their peers. The school head felt that such parents are not supportive of their children's learning. Also, one teacher from school 3 was concerned about the attitudes of parents:

> We also have parents who are negative towards this programme. If the child is identified, the parent refuses. It's due to ignorance. I had a certain parent who cried when they were told that their child was going to the special class. We discussed what is going to happen in the special class and they ended up agreeing. At the end of the year, they were very happy because their child had improved. So it's due to ignorance. I think if they are aware of what is happening then it would be better.

What is emerging from parents is that most of them are against the idea of the special class model. Such attitudes could be due to ignorance and lack of understanding of what the special class model entails. This might imply that the school is not providing enough information to parents about the special class model until their children are identified as learners with SpLDs, who require such services.

IDENTIFICATION PROCEDURE

Schools used various procedures in identifying children eligible for the special class. Some were the procedures highlighted by the DRT. Some, however, were crafted by teachers who seem to hold negative attitudes. Participants indicated that some of the procedures used posed a challenge in the implementation of this model as indicated by a teacher from school 1:

> The first challenge that we have is the testing instrument that is being used to test this class. We are using WRAT [Wide Range Achievement Test], which is not ecologically valid. Words that are in the WRAT test are not from our country. They are from those countries down there. Those people are well versed; those are the things they use here and there. The words are difficult. So you cannot effectively test using the WRAT; even an adult can fail the WRAT test. Then we use it as a testing instrument so that we place a child in the special class; that is not fair.

Another teacher from school 3 commented:

> There are some children who are recommended for the special class but those children might need more time with their teachers in the mainstream. They might be grasping concepts slowly and the class teacher can simply come up with a programme for the children. I am not subtracting anything from the special class, but there are children who are taken to the special class who might not even improve or do better because it might even kill them. The fact that the child has been seconded to the special class, it can even destroy that child at times because the special class is associated with slow learners. So some children will do better with their teacher in the mainstream than going to the special class. We have those rare cases where some children might not even progress because they are in the special class.

It emerged that the identification procedures used by some schools posed a challenge in the success of the special class model. School heads and teachers seem not equipped with the knowledge and skills that could assist them in properly identifying learners with SpLDs. One would then wonder how these children ended up in the special class.

Discussion

Here we discuss the findings and the discussion is split into thematic subheadings.

The special class model

Participants seemed to have a general understanding of the special class model. They indicated that in this model, children receive individual assistance from the teacher according to their levels of performance. Other participants also indicated that the special class teacher prepares a programme for these learners, which should not be general to all learners, as noted by Ncube and Hlatshwayo (2014). One participant referred to the model as the class with lower numbers of pupils. The level of performance and the individual attention was not highlighted by this participant. This is problematic as the special class is not only about class size. Rather, the learner should have an SpLD in order to qualify into this model (Alber, 2015). However, a manageable class size is important so that learners receive individual instruction from the teacher. It was also noted that the special class teacher teaches concepts according to the pace of the learners, as recommended by the Department of Education and Science (2007). The Department reported that concepts in the special class model are covered at a slower pace. That way, learners will have a better chance of mastering concepts that they might have initially missed.

The participants also suggested that a teacher qualified to teach children with various SpLDs should be in charge of the special class. This is also suggested by Samkange (2013), who believes that special class model teachers should be versatile enough to address the diverse needs of all learners with SpLDs. However, this was not the case with most schools as teachers in special classes had no skills or experience of teaching learners with diverse SpLDs. Samkange (2013) also observed that most teachers in Zimbabwean special classes lack relevant training to teach learners with SpLDs. The shortage of such teachers in these schools shows the challenges Zimbabwe is facing with regard to human resources. This presents a challenge in the learning outcomes of children with SpLDs as they are taught by teachers who might not be adequately equipped with the necessary skills of handling a special class.

Some participants raised concerns on the issue of the learners with SpLDs going back to the mainstream classes for other curriculum subjects as only English and mathematics are taught in the special class. They referred to the issue of large numbers in the mainstream as a contributory factor to teachers not being able to offer individual attention to learners with SpLDs or prepare individualised learning materials for them. In support, Goulandris (2009) argues that in the mainstream, class teachers might not be in a position to prepare learning media for each and every learner. Unfortunately, this compromises learner performance, leading to failure.

Learner eligibility for special class model testing

The study established that schools have ways in which they select learners eligible for special class testing. These procedures differ from school to school as some indicated that they were not aware of the laid down criteria. Hence, they devise their own ways of selecting learners for testing. This implies that the criteria used by schools in Hwange district when selecting learners eligible for the special class model is likely to differ per school. This poses a challenge for the effective implementation of this model, as standard procedures from the MoPSE seem not to be followed. Also, the issue of evaluating its success when various modes are being used could be problematic. Some selected learners at grade three as indicated by the DRT, while others selected them from grade four. Those whose selection was at grade four, indicated that grade three is a transitional level. Therefore, it might be difficult to identify a child as having an SpLD. They also indicated that at grade three, the learners are being introduced to new concepts. Hence, it becomes challenging or misleading to identify a child as having a learning difficulty. They reiterated that at grade four, it was easier to identify a child who lags behind as they would have covered major concepts from the syllabus. McCook (2006) also supports the idea of targeting grade four as learners would have covered adequate basic numeracy and literacy skills. This allows learners to reveal their strengths and educational needs in the selection tests administered by the SPS and SNE personnel.

One school indicated that they selected non-readers and non-writers for the special class model testing, which is opposed to Ncube and Hlatshwayo's (2014) view. They note that special class eligibility is based upon evidence that the learner does not achieve adequately for his or her age or meet grade level standards in one or more of the following: basic reading skills, reading fluency skills, mathematical calculations and mathematics problem solving. Hence, the selection criterion is likely to misplace learners in the special class model.

Another concern raised by participants was that some learners who were identified for special class model testing were not eligible for this class as they could improve in their respective classes. It then implies that the school authorities should monitor the selection process to ensure that suitable learners are identified so that they are provided with appropriate instruction in the mainstream settings (Fletcher *et al*, 2007). By so doing, measures would be put in place to ensure that the student's learning difficulties are not primarily the result of some form of impairment (Mafa, 2012).

Challenges in the special class model

A number of challenges were highlighted by the participants in the implementation of the special class model. These included teacher attitudes, peer attitudes as well as parental attitudes.

TEACHERS' ATTITUDES

Participants pointed out that some teachers in the mainstream held negative attitudes toward learners with SpLDs. Some of them associated these attitudes with lack of knowledge on the teaching of these children, yet some indicated that the large numbers in the mainstream classes were a contributory factor to the teachers' negative attitudes. There were concerns that these attitudes toward differences could lead to learners who might need more time under the mainstream teacher's supervision being referred for special class testing just as a means of getting rid of them. Such a teacher might not be knowledgeable on how to handle children with SpLDs. In support, Mnkandla and Mataruse (2002) established that teachers develop negative attitudes because of lack of knowledge and incompetence in teaching children with SpLDs. Hence, learners' needs are most likely ignored by the mainstream teacher due to this lack of knowledge. Chakuchichi *et al* (2003) observed that negative attitudes toward differences result in discrimination and can lead to a serious barrier to learning.

Large pupil numbers in the mainstream make it impossible for teachers to individually attend to learners with SpLDs. Participants indicated that they will be struggling with attending to learners they have in the mainstream. As a result, having those from the special class will be an added burden to an already overloaded teacher. This might be the reason why they were selecting non-readers and non-writers for referral to the special class, as a way of easing their 'burden'. These findings are similar to what Maunganidze and Kasayira (2002) established. They reported that mainstream teachers feel that they already have too much workload and having to deal with children with SpLDs would be an extra burden.

PEER ATTITUDES

Learners with SpLDs indicated that they were labelled and stigmatised by some peers and this trend has also been reported by Vignes (2009). The author noted that numerous studies have explored attitudes toward peers with SpLDs and they have shown that many primary school children with SpLDs feel rejected by their peers and are rarely chosen as friends. Such attitudes pose a challenge as these learners might end up not participating in group work. They might also be forced to end up socialising only with those learners with whom they learn in the special class. Vignes (2009) indicates that access to the mainstream class does not necessarily guarantee full participation and students with SpLDs often have limited social relationships. However, some learner participants indicated that some of their peers had the most positive of attitudes as they played with them and shared learning resources and materials, hence the need to capitalise on such relationships in order to influence other learners in accepting learners with SpLDs.

PARENTAL ATTITUDES

From the study, it is clear that negative parental attitudes impact on the achievement of children with SpLDs. Parents seemed not too keen to have their children enrolled into the special class model as they felt that their children would not benefit much. Some indicated that parents had negative attitudes toward the special class model as they did not have an understanding of the model and its benefits to their children. Thus, a vague understanding of the purpose and the benefits of the education of children with SpLDs on the part of the parents can be the main reason for holding negative attitudes toward their children's education in the special class (Somaily *et al*, 2012). Such negative attitudes affect the success of the special class model as well as the learning outcomes of children with SpLDs.

Conclusions

This chapter is based on establishing the effectiveness of the special class model on the learning outcomes of children with SpLDs in Hwange District in Zimbabwe. The background that led to the study is highlighted, as well as what other researchers have discovered pertaining to the effectiveness of the special class model. What is clear from this study is that there is lack of understanding on the special class model among teachers, parents and learners. Hence, the good intention of this model is being compromised. The idea of this model is to promote via a twin-track approach, where learners with SpLDs are withdrawn for numeracy and literacy so that they receive intense support and then re-join their mainstream class once they master the concepts. However, negative attitudes, lack of understanding and the selection criteria of learners have adversely affected the implementation of this model. Hence, the need to raise awareness and capacitate teachers, parents and learners so that such a class is not labelled; an aspect that works against improving learning outcomes. Further research might be needed at a larger scale in order to evaluate the effectiveness of this model. This would allow policy makers and implementers to come up with more effective ways of supporting learners with SpLDs.

Reflective questions

1   Based on this chapter, how effective is the special class model in effectively improving the learning outcomes of learners with SpLDs?
2   Howe best can teachers', learners' and parents' attitudes toward the special class model be changed? What are the teacher attitudes toward learners with SpLDs like?
3   What lessons can be drawn from this chapter that can assist you in understanding and implementing the special class model?
4   How can the special class model be improved in order to address the learning needs of children with SpLDs?

Acknowledgements

This chapter is based on an undergraduate research project conducted by the lead author in 2016. The second author was the supervisor.

References

Alber, R. (2015). *5 Highly Effective Teaching Practices.* Retrieved from www.edutopia.org on 18 March 2016.
Aro, T. & Ahonen, T. (2011). *Assessment of Learning Disabilities: Cooperation between Teachers, Psychologists and Parents.* Finland: Niilo Maki Institute.
Bell, J. & Waters, S. (2014). *Doing Your Research Project: A Guide for First Time Researchers in Education, Health and Social Science.* Berkshire: McGraw Hill Education.
Chakuchichi, D. D., Chiinze, M. M. & Kaputa, T. M. (2003). *Including the Excluded: Issues in Disability and Inclusion.* Harare: Zimbabwe Open University.
Coolican, H. (2014). *Research Methods and Statistics in Psychology.* New York: Psychology Press.
Department of Education and Science (2007). *Inclusion of Students with Special Educational Needs: Post Primary Guidelines.* Dublin: Stationery office.
Fletcher, J. M., Lyon, G. R., Fuchs, L. S. & Barnes, M. A. (2007). *Learning Disabilities: From Identification to Intervention.* New York: Guilford Press.
Fletcher-Janzen, E. & Reynolds, C. R. (2008). *Neurological Perspectives on Learning Disabilities in the Era of RTI.* New Jersey: Wiley.
Florian, L. & Hegarty, J. (2010). *ICT and Special Educational Needs.* Milton Keynes: The Open University Press.
Gay, L. R. & Airasian, P. W. (2002). *Educational Research: Competencies for Analysis and Applications* (7th edn). Upper Saddle River, NJ: Prentice Hall.
Goulandris, N. (2009). *Dyslexia in Different Languages.* London: Whurr.
Haslam, A. S. (2014). *Research Methods and Statistics in Psychology.* London: Sage Publications.
Hocutt, A. M. (1996). Effectiveness of special education: is placement the critical factor? *Special Education for Students with Disabilities* **6**(1), 1–26.
Horne, M. D. (2011). *Attitudes toward Handicapped Students: Professional, Peer and Parent Reactions.* New York: Routledge.
Jenjekwa, V., Rutoro, E. & Runyowa, J. (2013). Inclusive education and the primary school teacher education curriculum in Zimbabwe: the need for a paradigm shift. *The International Journal of Humanities and Social Science* **1**(3), 21–28.
Kay, J. & Yeo, D. (2003). *Dyslexia and Maths.* London: David Fulton Publishers.
Kessler, E. H. (2013). *Encyclopaedia of Management Theory.* Brunswick, NJ: Sage Publications.
Kourkoutas, E. (2012). Young children's attitudes toward peers' learning disabilities: effect of the type of school. *Journal of Applied Research in Intellectual Disabilities* **5**(2), 1–11.
Lerner, J. (2003). *Learning Disabilities: Diagnosis and Teaching Strategies.* Boston, MA: Houghton Mifflin.
Mafa, O. (2012). Challenges of implementing inclusion in Zimbabwe's education system. *Journal of Education Research* **1**(2), 14–22.
Maunganidze, L. & Kasayira, J. M. (2002). Educational integration of children with disabilities in schools in the Midlands region of Zimbabwe. *The Zimbabwe Bulletin of Teacher Education* **11**(1), 72–82.

McCook, J. E. (2006). *The RTI Guide: Developing and Implementing a Model in Your Schools*. Horsham: LRP Publications.

Ministry of Education (2011). *Resource Room Program*. Riyadh: Department of Special Education.

Mitchell, D. (2008). *What Really Works in Special and Inclusive Education: Using Evidence Based Teaching Strategies*. New York: Routledge.

Mnkandla, M. & Mataruse, K. (2002). The impact of inclusion policy on school psychology in Zimbabwe. *Educational and Child Psychology* **19**, 12–23.

Mpofu, E. (2001). *Learning Disabilities: Theories, Practices and Applications in the Zimbabwean Context*. Harare: College Press.

National Council for Special Education (2014). *Children with Special Educational Needs*. Retrieved from http://ncse.ie/wp-content/uploads/2014/10/ChildrenWithSpecialEdNeeds1.pdf on 19 March 2016.

Ncube, A. C. & Hlatshwayo, L. (2014). The provision of special education in Zimbabwe: realities, issues and challenges. *IOSR Journal of Humanities and Social Sciences* **19**(8), 72–77.

Price, G. R. & Ansari, D. (2013). Dyscalculia: characteristics, cause and treatments. *Numeracy* **6**(1), 1–16.

Rose, J. (2009). *Identifying and Teaching Children and Young People with Dyslexia and Literacy Difficulties*. Retrieved from www.thedyslexia-spldtrust.org.uk/media/downloads/inline/the-rose-report.1294933674.pdf on 27 April 2018.

Samkange, W. (2013). Inclusive education at primary school. *International Journal of Social Science and Education* **3**(4), 1–8.

Somaily, H., Al-Zoubi, S. & Rahman, M. B. A. (2012). Parents of students with learning disabilities: attitudes towards resource room. *International Interdisciplinary Journal of Education* **1**(1), 1–5.

Thomas, P. Y. (2010). *Research Methodology and Design*. Retrieved from htttp://www.uir.unisa.ac.za>bitstream>handle>so on 19 May 217.

Vignes, C. (2009). Determinants of students' attitudes towards peers with disabilities. *Developmental Medicine and Child Neurology* **51**(6), 473–479.

PART III

Inclusion in higher education

Part III brings out the challenges, opportunities and threats faced by disabled students in accessing higher education in southern Africa. Having impairments appears to be used as exclusionary criteria, yet disabled people constitute approximately 15% of the world's population.

11

WHEN RIGHTS ARE DISCRETIONARY

Policy and practice of support provision for disabled students in southern Africa

Knowledge R. Matshedisho

Introduction

Disability is a development concern in Africa. This partly stems from the exclusion of disabled people from participating in the socio-economic and political life of their respective countries. It is both a colonial legacy (Grech and Soldatic, 2015) and a post-colonial neglect of disability as a development issue. The United Nations' *Post 2015 Millennium Development Goals* do not seem to fully acknowledge the impact of the exclusion of disabled people in Africa. However, the idea of inclusion masks variations and levels of exclusion. An example of this is access to higher education for disabled people. Morley and Croft (2011) indicate that the increasing global participation rates in higher education mask the exclusion of other groups such as disabled people. Hence, since the 1990s there has been an increasing interest in research on disability and higher education in Africa as indicated by the United Nations Educational, Scientific, and Cultural Organization's (UNESCO) 1997 survey entitled *Disabled Students at Universities in Africa*. This interest should also be understood in the international context of both the *Education for All* (EFA) and the *Convention on the Rights of Persons with Disabilities* initiatives (UNESCO, 1990; United Nations, 2006). These initiatives advocated for quality education as a right for all people (including disabled people).

Some researchers across Africa argue that the right to education for disabled people is important but fraught with difficulties and exclusions (Peters & Chimedza, 2002; Kabzems & Chimedza, 2002; Matshedisho, 2007; Kochung, 2011; Emong & Eron, 2016). Hence, this chapter focuses on disability and higher education in southern Africa to suggest reasons for these difficulties and exclusions. While recognising other geopolitical definitions (e.g. Southern African Development Community definition), this chapter will only make references to Angola, Botswana, Lesotho, Malawi, Mozambique, Namibia, South Africa, Swaziland, Zambia and Zimbabwe. Some southern African countries have extreme poverty and pioneered disability activism. Zimbabwe, for example, pioneered disability activism in the 1970s and was followed by other countries in the 1980s, such as South Africa. However, 40 years later there is uneven progress in the availability of rights and services for disabled people in the region. This chapter tries to explain some of the unevenness. It begins by explaining the international and national disability rights templates that exist to situate southern African advocacy on disability and higher education. Second, it problematises disability rights, illustrating how rights can lie in tension

139

to one another and explains how neoliberal values become correlated to disability rights. The chapter then moves to illustrate how the first two parts might contribute toward the arbitrariness of implementing disability rights for disabled students in higher education. Finally, I end with some questions and ways forward for disability in higher education in southern Africa.

Situating disability educational rights in legislation and advocacy

There are various international conventions and commitments made about supporting and respecting the rights of disabled people across the world. It is customary, if not expected, that discussions about disability rights in Africa and support thereof points at the legal and advocacy strides at both international and national levels. This is also an indication of the intellectual practical templates that guide disability support across the world. With relevance to Africa, there are international legal frameworks such as the 1983 *United Nations Decade for Persons with Disabilities* and the 2006 United Nations Conventions on Rights of Persons with Disabilities (CRPD). At regional level, these include the 1987 *African Charter on Human and People's Rights*; 1993 *United Nations Standard Rules on the Equalization of Opportunity for People with Disabilities*; 1999 *African Decade for Persons with Disabilities*; the 2003 African Union Continental Plan of Action for the African Decade of Persons with Disabilities; 2009 *African Second Decade for Persons with Disabilities*; and the 2016 *Draft Protocol on the Rights of Persons with Disabilities in Africa*. All the listed instruments lay important foundations and justifications of the right to education for people with disabilities in higher education. However, in this chapter, I argue that their implementation is difficult and uneven.

One of the sub-themes of the 2016 Ninth Session of the Conference of States Parties to the CRPD was, 'Eliminating poverty and inequality for all persons with disabilities'. In this context of poverty and marginality, it is not enough to only politically sign or ratify conventions, but to constantly have disability rights advocacy for moral and intellectual justification of these rights. Article 24 Section (5) of the CRPD declares:

> States Parties shall ensure that persons with disabilities are able to access general tertiary education, vocational training, adult education and lifelong learning without discrimination and on an equal basis with others. To this end, States Parties shall ensure that reasonable accommodation is provided to persons with disabilities.
>
> *(United Nations, 2006)*

Article 11 Section 3(b) of *The Draft Protocol on the Rights of Persons with Disabilities in Africa* declares:

> Persons with disabilities are able to access general tertiary education, vocational training, adult education and lifelong learning without discrimination and on an equal basis with others, including by ensuring the literacy of persons with disabilities above compulsory school age.
>
> *(Africa Commission on Human and Peoples' Rights, 2016)*

These declarations are necessary but not sufficient to tell us about the practices of countries that have either signed or ratified some of the conventions on disability. The intellectual and political context of these disability rights needs to be analysed to partly understand their uneven implementation. Disability rights in southern Africa are typically discussed within the political economy of poverty and marginality. The Open Society Initiative for southern Africa on the status of disability rights in southern Africa, states:

Disabled people are the most marginalised people in a region where life is already diffi-cult for the majority of the population due to severe poverty, lack of development and high unemployment. In all countries, the rights of disabled people are not given any priority by their governments. Usually, any ministry dealing with disability also has to address other marginalised groups such as women and children, so disability rights and the protection of disabled people receive minimal state funding and focus.

(Kotzé, 2012, p. 1)

Then, in its conclusion, emphasises:

Currently, the people in most of the countries in the region face high levels of poverty and unemployment. The most badly affected are people with disabilities, who have the highest rates of poverty, deprivation, malnutrition, ill-health and child mortality . . . Most of the human development indicators show that people with disabilities have been worst affected by the deteriorating conditions in almost all southern African countries.

(Kotzé, 2012, p. 54)

We can list 11 national disability rights organisations in southern Africa, which in 1986 formed the Southern Africa Federation of the Disabled (SAFOD). These disability rights organisations have three common duties which have implications for disability rights in higher education in southern Africa. The first duty is to publicise the rights of disabled people and to morally appeal to the public to respect these rights. The second is to recommend the disability agenda as an impera-tive and mainstream consideration in national policies for education, employment and recreation. The final and most important duty is the immediate help and services that they offer to disabled people. Whereas these duties are justified and necessary, they inadvertently continue to repro-duce a pragmatic but simplistic approach to the establishment of disability practices in southern Africa. The first of these practices is an uncritical translation of disability rights (including those of disabled students in higher education). These organisations are also functioning within a sce-nario where disability rights are also affected by a particular economic climate affecting the way in which rights are being interpreted. This also affects why and how disability rights in higher education are implemented piecemeal. I turn to this conundrum in understanding the values and frameworks behind the interpretation of disability.

The problem of competing rights

The concept of rights within human rights and its moral framework is convincing at face value. However, there are practical problems in trying to justify or question these rights. The intel-lectually elusive question is what are rights? Freeden (1991) indicates that there is a difference between rights and human rights, and that some see rights as a subset of human rights but other observers' views are the other way round. He argues that human rights are the most basic and encompassing rights and thus defines them as:

[A] conceptual device, expressed in linguistic form, that assigns priority to certain human or social attributes regarded as essential to the adequate functioning of a human being; that is intended to serve as a protective capsule for those attributes; and that appeals for deliberate action to ensure such protection.

(Freeden, 1991, p. 7)

The above definition of rights has its intellectual foundations from classical liberal theory of philosophers such as John Locke and Thomas Hobbes who conceptualised rights as natural and inalienable. These conceptualisations are famously enshrined in the United Nations Universal Declaration of Human Rights (UDHR) (1948), in which Article 2 reads:

> Everyone is entitled to all the rights and freedoms set forth in this Declaration, without distinction of any kind, such as race, colour, sex, language, religion, political or other opinion, national or social origin, property, birth or other status.

The relevance of this definition of rights is that it is dominant in the Western world and its former colonies and thus the intellectual foundation of disability rights in southern Africa. If that be the case, then some of the problems with this version of rights need to be expounded in relation to support provision for disabled students in southern Africa.

I argue that there are four problems that disability right movements in southern Africa need to resolve in making higher education a reality for disabled people. The first problem is the argument of whether human rights are universalistic or particularistic. Gloppen and Rakner (1993) refer to the United Nation's UDHR (1948) and indicate that this is underpinned by European traditions of rights and is often at odds with regional declarations of rights, such as the 1981 African Banjul Charter and the 1994 Arab Charter of Human Rights (Enabulele, 2016; Ndahinda, 2016). The challenge for the disability rights movement in southern Africa is to make international rights to fit the regional context and translate those rights into access to higher education for disabled people. Another challenge is to situate these rights with the socio-economic priorities that have to address and frame the rights of all southern African countries and national citizens. For example, in Angola, the disability rights movement struggles with tensions in trying to secure rights for disabled people in a country emerging from colonisation and years of civil war.

The interpretation and translation of disability rights is compounded by the second problem of competing rights or a hierarchy of rights. Gloppen and Rakner (1993) list six types of human rights: personal rights; civil rights; political rights; social and economic rights; cultural rights; solidarity rights. McQuoid-Mason *et al.* (1991) categorise civil and political rights as first-generation rights and include values such as freedom from government interference and participation in political life. Social, cultural and economic rights are second-generation rights and include the right to decent standards of living and work. Cultural rights are advocated by communitarians who

> emphasise the importance of belonging to a distinctive community as an essential component of, as well as a means to, individual well-being, or 'flourishing', as it often termed (with gestural connotations). Communitarians have defended (usually with qualifications) the importance of patriotism and nationalism, which tend to be disparaged from the cosmopolitan viewpoint connoted by the idea of universal human rights, as well as from the individualistic perspective sometimes said to be fostered by the 'culture' of rights.
>
> *(Edmundson, 2004, p. 177)*

There are also third-generation rights, which are neither communitarian rights nor individual rights. These are future generations' rights and belong to humankind (Edmundson, 2004).

With competing rights in the context of poverty and marginality in southern Africa, it would be difficult and insensitive to speak even of second-generation rights when basic needs of the population have yet to be met. Moreover, access to higher education is determined by more factors than just disability support. Meritocracy, social class, gender, religion, geographical position and other forms of difference affect access to higher education in different contexts (Heap & Morgans, 2006). Thus, in southern Africa where poverty is a national concern, disability rights are bound to collide with other rights.

The problem with these types of rights is that some argue that first-generation rights are more important than other types of rights, because they create environments that are conducive for democracy. Others, however, argue for the primacy of second-generation rights. For example, Kollapen (2003) observes that human rights become insignificant when people live in squalour, are marginalised and cannot meet their specific basic rights. Albert (2004, p. 4) adds, 'In fact, access to a wheelchair or a hearing aid is a basic human right for someone who would otherwise be unable to take part in any social activity'. Thus, in an environment that prioritises rights, disabled people's organisations need to articulate the position in which they locate every right that they demand. If all the rights they demand are equally weighted, then they would still need to articulate how they would respond and mobilise against trade-offs, competing demands of other citizens and justifying their rights against criticisms, such as those laid down by Low (2001), who warns the disability rights movements against rhetoric that ignores rights other than disability rights. What then should disability rights movement do with this conundrum?

To answer the question, I turn to the third problem for consideration. Disability rights movements have to take into account that rights are value-laden or ideological. Gloppen and Rakner (1993) outline three ideological traditions in respect of rights. The first is the liberal tradition, which espouses personal and civil rights. The second is the democratic tradition, which espouses political rights. The third is the socialist tradition, which advocates social and economic rights based on distributive justice. These traditions are historical in context and reflect the political climate in which they are embedded. However, disability and its experiences are not just a context-specific category. They can be universal and cut across other social categories. Moreover, disability rights movements might be global but there are inter and intra ideological perspectives that shape their demands. Allen (2002) points out that the contemporary discourse on human rights is a synthetic product of the cold war struggles among liberal internationalists, realists and Marxists. He argues that contemporary human rights discourse is more useful for global capitalism and predictability of the markets than morally justified rights discourse that will continue to produce real outcomes for social justice. In the southern Africa context, we also see how human rights are intertwined with neoliberal economic policies in which rights are simply about recognition, access and inclusion in the mainstream economies without questioning the exclusionary tendencies of those economies in denying disability rights in the first place (Grech & Soldatic, 2015).

The final problem is that rights are not only claims, but that they must be recognised by other citizens (Machan, 1989). This process becomes problematic in what Lee (2002, p. 149) calls 'simplistic politics' in his critique of the social model of disability which has globally influenced disability right movements advocacies, policies and legislations. He asks:

> Producing evidence of this inaccessible, segregated and exclusionary world is relatively straightforward. Yet how far is the 'able-bodied' majority prepared to go in reconstructing 'its' social order so that 'it can accommodate a far wider spectrum of disability?
>
> *(Lee, 2002, p. 149)*

This observation indicates the limitations of claims and justification to rights. For rights to be effective, part of it lies in them being recognised by someone other than the right-bearer.

The above four concerns about liberal rights partly explain why disability rights in southern Africa are arbitrarily crafted and implemented. We will examine how his neoliberal emphasis on rights is expressed and what that tells us about disability support in higher education.

Disability support as charity

The main issue with disability rights is that they have always been conceptualised as a resource burden, especially in the higher education support provision. In the neoliberal fashion, disability rights have been a demand whose supply requires resources and willing helpers rather than an issue for social justice. This section illustrates this view with examples of three countries in southern Africa. In these countries, the way in which disability is viewed as charity can be illustrated by a quote from Block (2004, p. 1) who observes:

> The burden of disability is unending; life with a disabled person is a life of constant sorrow, and the able-bodied stand under a continual obligation to help them. People with disabilities and their families – the 'noble sacrificers' – are the most perfect objects of charity; their function is to inspire benevolence in others, to awaken feelings of kindness and generosity.

Even with the 'disability template' of conventions and declarations, the above quote speaks directly to the support provision for disabled students in southern Africa. South Africa is a good example of Block's (2004) observation because of its history of disability rights since the 1980s and the Department of Education and Training's (2016) *Draft Policy Framework for Disability in the Post-School Education and Training System*. It is a good example because of the shift from the charity model of the 1980s to an attempt to now legally standardise disability support in higher education.

The first formal unit for the support of disabled students in the South African higher education system was only established in 1986 at the University of the Witwatersrand through the efforts of the disability activist Kathy Jagoe. The unit was called the *Disabled Student Programme* (DSP), renamed the *Disabled Students Office* and now it is called the *Disability Rights Unit*. Kathy became a quadriplegic at the age of 15 and pursued her higher education at Rhodes University (in Grahamstown, South Africa). She was granted a Bachelor of Fine Arts in 1978, a Higher Diploma in Education in 1979, a Bachelor of Education in 1981 and an honorary degree in 1991 for her work on ensuring disability mainstreaming in South African education. In 1993, she received an honorary doctorate from the University of Cape Town (UCT), 'In recognition of her contribution to changing attitudes towards disability in South African society in making UCT, other institutions and organisations disability-friendly environments, and in making disability studies part of the mainstream curricula at UCT' (University of Cape Town *Monday Paper*, 2003).

What is noteworthy about Kathy Jagoe is not just that she was a woman and disabled, but she also had to advocate for inclusive higher education settings. Although it is now standard (though uneven) practice in South Africa to have support provision for disabled students, this had been created on the initiative of an individual who felt the need to help herself and other disabled students. The university and its management did not make disability rights an institutional policy priority like other topical national imperatives such as race, religion and gender representations. However, South African universities tend to support such initiatives once they have been initiated by individuals out of need and frustration with disability exclusion. Disabled students in other southern Africa countries do not enjoy such provisions. Some countries are only beginning to catch up with the global disability rights advocacies. If we take Angola and Mozambique as examples, we note how education inclusion in higher education is often last on the disability list of priorities. I will explain why this is the case in what follows and illustrate how rights are hierarchical and discretionary in the southern African context. Examining the history of their adoption of international conventions, it is noted: 'During the course of 2014, Angola, Burundi, the Republic of Congo, Côte d'Ivoire, and Guinea Bissau became the latest members of the African Union to ratify the Convention of the Rights of Persons with Disabilities (CRPD)' (Ngwena *et al.*, 2014, p. v).

As the latest signatory in the region, Angola is emerging from a civil war that lasted decades (1975–2002). This longstanding conflict affected all aspects of life and badly affected educational progress, training of teachers, access to primary education for girls in particular and general literacy of the population. Angola is beginning to reconstruct and is devising interventions to improve the higher education sector and ensure socio-economic status of its disabled population. With the international community, Angola's Social Welfare Ministry has drafted policies to improve access to higher education for disabled people. The process has been undertaken through the *National Council of People with Disability* which seeks to coordinate all ministries to the problem of disability in Angola. Policy making has focused on ensuring the rebuilding of the educational sector and access to education and employment, for example, for the disabled former child soldiers. Inclusion in schools and understanding specialised educational needs of disabled students was a priority before access to higher education was a focus. However, these developments should also highlight the neoliberal nature of the reforms in which 'very few Angolans have the ability to finance their studies, making access to higher learning a reserve of the privileged in society' (Langa, 2013, p. 17).

By contrast, Mozambique is also emerging from decades of civil war (1977–92) and beginning to address disability rights. First, it is focusing on alleviating the socio-economic conditions of disabled people as a result of the war and ensuring no further disablement, for example, by landmines. Second, policy has also focused on ensuring literacy through building both the primary schools system and access to adult literacy programmes for disabled people. Finally, through initiatives such as the Disability Rights Law Project at the University of Eduardo Mondlane, the disability jurisprudence is being developed. These efforts are made in the context of Mozambique's National Disability Strategy. Unfortunately, most of the provisions thereof have not yet materialised due to insufficient government resources.

Disability advocacy movements in Angola and Mozambique face challenges in terms of ensuring access to all disability rights because of lack of national frameworks and resources. With the exception of Swaziland's *Persons with Disabilities Bill* (2014) and Zimbabwe's *Disabled Persons Act* (1992), other countries in the region also do not have disability specific legislation. Instead, they apply the diversity-rights framework to support disabled students in higher education. This framework provides for disability support within a general national anti-discrimination legislation and policy. These are used to formulate specific policy for disabled students and form a legal basis to determine disability discrimination disputes in higher education. Underlying this framework is respect for human rights, diversity, equal opportunity and fair advantage for disabled students. In this framework, disability support is not enforceable by a specific disability law. Rather, institutions of higher education are expected to implement the policy of supporting disabled students and, if disputes arise, they would be resolved within the framework. Moreover, Swaziland and Zimbabwe do not criminalise disability discrimination in their legislation. They specifically protect government from litigation. Legislation without recourse to courts of law is a travesty of disability rights and its declarations in various national and international conventions.

Other countries in southern Africa face different limitations to real disability rights in accessing higher education. The right to higher education is not as straightforward as it reads from 'disability right templates'. For example, in South Africa, Botswana and Lesotho, rights are restricted by the regulations of higher education institutions in their different contexts. The typical restriction on the right to education at tertiary level is generally three-fold. First, a disabled person must be qualified to enter an institution of higher education. This right is limited by the measly participation of disabled people in general education. Second, a disabled student will receive assistance in as far as the universities can afford concomitant resources. Finally, disabled students' claims for assistance depend on choice of disclosure, lecturers' voluntary preparedness and voluntary institutional commitment. In fact much of the literature on access to higher education for disabled students heavily centres on the quotidian physical, personal and institutional restrictions (United Nations, 2006; Matshedisho, 2007; Emong & Eron, 2016).

It is at this point that (disability) rights can become discretionary in the context of competing national priorities and discretionary institutional interventions. Depending on the political context of a country, there is an uneven progress and challenges for the support provision for disabled students in higher education institutions in southern Africa. As mentioned earlier, at one end, some are reconstructing their societies after decades of civil war, thereby making disability rights hierarchical to other rights 'instead' of mainstreaming (with higher education being at lower bottom of educational priorities). At the other end, disability support provision has become an institutional policy. These unevenness and challenges are indicated by three observations.

The first points at the aspects of disability that are prioritised. In all of southern Africa inclusive education is the buzz word because of the links to international conventions such as the CRPD. For example, Namibia has the 2013 *Sector Policy on Inclusive Education*. Angola has the *National Education Development Plan 2015/2025*. Botswana has the 1997 *Education for Kgahisano*, which states that a child has the right to education without reference to – inter alia – their disability. South Africa is grappling with implementing 2001 *Special Needs Education*. Lesotho began its *Special Education Unit* in 1989 and is now supported by its Education Act of 2010. Malawi has a *National Special Needs Education Policy* of 2006. Zambia and Zimbabwe do not have a specific policy on inclusive education, but can use some of their legislations to make a case for inclusive education. In the case of Zambia it is the Persons with Disabilities Act of 1996 and the 1996 *National Education of Policy*. In Zimbabwe, it is the Education Act of 1996 and the Zimbabwe Disabled Persons Act of 1996, which can be used to promote inclusive education.

The focus on inclusive education does not mean there is satisfactory implementation thereof. For example, in Swaziland, disability rights activism is comparatively new. Hence disability support in higher education is neglected in favour of general education. The focus is on

> The National Education and Training Sector Policy, National Children's Policy, National Development Strategy and the Children's Protection and Welfare Act clearly recognise that children with disabilities are vulnerable to educational exclusion.
> *(SWANCEFA, 2014, p. 27)*

Hence, disability is mentioned only twice in the *Swaziland Education for All Review Report, 2000–2015* and implementation thereof is of low priority as the country faces other challenges such as poverty and demands for political reforms against the monarchy.

While inclusive education policies are important, the language within which they are promoted is a concern. Disability is typically understood within the 'triple vulnerability' of poverty, disability and rurality (Vergunst, 2016, p. ii), For example, in South Africa, the 1997 *Integrated National Disability Strategy* states:

Among the yardsticks by which to measure a society's respect for human rights, to evaluate the level of its maturity and its generosity of spirit, is by looking at the status that it accords to those members of society who are most vulnerable, disabled people, the senior citizens and its children.

(Mbeki, 1997, p. 1)

Inclusive education is discussed within the same language of vulnerability. In its foreword on inclusive education, UNESCO (1997, p. 1) observes:

The Dakar Framework for Action makes reference to the groups of children who are most vulnerable and disadvantaged and calls for inclusive education practices to ensure that they are included in the education process and have access to schools . . . throughout the Decade of the EFA programme the UNESCO Bangkok Office has taken action in many ways to ensure that the right to education of all children, including those with disabilities and other disadvantages, have been addressed.

This kind of language brings us to the second observation about the unevenness and challenges of disability support provision in southern Africa. As early as 1997 UNESCO observed the following about disability support in African universities:

Universities consider accessibility the biggest problem in accommodating disabled students. This occurs all around campuses: lecture halls, students' restaurant, accommodation and even movement within the campus are not designed to be accessible for students who may have different types of specific needs . . . Another big problem for universities is the lack of equipment or other types of support services for disabled students . . . Third type of problem reflects attitudes towards the disabled. It is experienced that attitudes, in general, among students and lecturers make it difficult to accommodate disabled students into the academic world.

(UNESCO, 1997, p. 6)

Within the same arguments, Ndlovu and Walton (2016) reiterate these challenges experienced by disabled students studying toward professional degree certificates in South Africa. These challenges inform research into support provision for disabled students in southern Africa. To date, the research still highlights challenges of access, resources and attitudes. Maguvhe (2015) discusses findings about challenges faced by blind students in studying mathematics and science. Effectively, scholarship on disability and higher education in southern Africa is entirely dominated by the availability and challenges of support provision for disabled students. The challenges include access, advocacy, recruitment, disclosure, retention and attitudes by lecturers.

What accounts for these challenges is not only a question of resources, advocacy and political commitment. Part of the problem is the language of vulnerability that renders disability in higher education to be uneven and altogether discretionary. Making an example of Lesotho,

The Ministry of Health and Social Welfare, through its National Disability and Rehabilitation Policy 2011, straddles two paradigms, having adopted the social model with its one foot in the deficit and medical model. In the process, people with disabilities are constructed as 'ambiguous'.

(Leshota, 2013, p. 6)

Similarly:

> The provision of support for disabled students in South Africa finds itself in a contradictory position of espousing disability rights and the social model of disability yet being embedded in the practice and legacy of benevolence. This position is evident from the challenges that disability support services face and the lack of political commitment to disability issues by government and higher education management structures.
>
> *(Matshedisho, 2007, p. 697)*

In taking the issue of inclusive education and research on support provision in southern Africa, one recognises that, in principle, inclusive education and disability support in higher education are natural progressions. This might apply relatively well in high-income countries because schooling for children with disabilities has gradually been mainstreamed to prepare pupils for higher education. In contrast to low-income countries within southern Africa, most pupils with disabilities are educated to a limited extent in order to qualify for vocational training rather than higher education. To exacerbate the situation, the school participation rates for disabled children in southern Africa is generally low and uneven (Langa, 2013). For example, the Human Rights Watch (2015) reports the failure of the South African government to provide for disabled children's education. It estimates that 500,000 disabled children are excluded from the South African schooling system even though South Africa has national policies and international conventions in place. Yet in 2016, the South African government published a gazette proposing to standardise disability reporting, support and services for post-secondary education.

This brings us to the final observation on unevenness and challenges of support provision for disabled students in southern Africa. Research on higher education has invariably meant focus only on universities, yet there are other forms of post-secondary school education such as colleges and polytechnics. Basically, it means even in instances where there is some support provision for disabled students, there are those who are excluded because they are not pursuing their studies at a university.

> In Lesotho such institutions include: Lesotho College of Education, Machabeng College, Centre for Accounting Studies, Lerotholi Polytechnic and the National University of Lesotho. However, the policy recognises the National University of Lesotho, and the Lesotho College of Education.
>
> *(Matlosa & Matobo, 2007, p. 195)*

This applies to all countries in southern Africa whereby other forms of post-secondary education are excluded from disability support interventions unless non-governmental organisations decided to do so. Disability rights have inadvertently produced their own hierarchies of disabilities that are reminiscent of Stewart's observation that:

> Disability hierarchies position certain impairments as more or less disabling than others, with the idea that some impairments are 'better' or less severe than others. The fact that many disabled people believe in a hierarchy of disability only perpetuates the social exclusion and stigma felt by all persons with disabilities.
>
> *(Stewart, 2004, p. 113)*

The above challenge should not be isolated from how inclusive education has ended up being synonymous with disabled children's education as argued by Wapling (2016, p. 5):

> Inclusive education therefore has had something of a mixed beginning . . . it was not part of the original EFA [Education for All] agenda but rather emerged from debates within the special education sector. It is in this sense that inclusive education has continued to retain its focus on the education of disabled children, despite the original desire to move beyond this, and in turn the education of disabled children continues to be regarded as something different to EFA.

This applies to support provision for higher education in southern Africa. The intention to support disability rights has been reduced to international declarations with ad hoc and discretionary implementation thereof. Even though South Africa has a longer history of disability rights and support provision in higher education, it continues on the rhetoric declaratives which suggest a paternalistic approach to 'help' disabled people. In its *White Paper on the Rights of Persons with Disabilities (WPRPD)*, the government reiterates that the primary responsibility for disability equity lies with national, provincial and local government; and other sectors of society but also allocates responsibilities to persons with disabilities and their families. The vision of the WPRPD is the creation of a 'free and just society inclusive of all persons with disabilities as equal citizens' (Republic of South Africa, 2016, p. 28). One cannot help but read the dominance of the government in this promise, which then places such rights in the political debates of competing rights as argued by Low (2001).

Such declarations and recommendations belie the continuous tensions between progressive discourses, paternalistic practices and disregard for southern Africa contexts. Even in the broader sphere of welfarist disability support, Devereux (2013) observes the importance of context when he states:

> Social grants are designed to reach non-working vulnerable groups such as the young (the CSG), older persons (the Old Age Pension) and people with disabilities (the Disability Grant) – but many unemployed or underpaid adults end up depending on these grants: in other words, they become dependent on dependents. This is not the intention, but it is the inevitable consequence of a hybrid blend of neoliberal economic policies and progressive social policies. In other southern Africa countries where non-contributory social pensions have been introduced, including much poorer countries such as Lesotho and Swaziland, dependence of working-age adults on these transfers has also been observed.
>
> *(Devereux, 2013, p. 18)*

This not only embeds disabled students into the complex political economy of disability but leaves a lingering question on the future of disability rights for disabled students in higher education.

Conclusion

This chapter has outlined the contested contexts of disability rights that contribute to the uneven support for disabled students as rationalised in the voluntarist language of disclosure, affordability and advocacy. While they are important, these practices undermine the opportunity to contextually advance disability rights and practices because of simplistically taking national and international declarations at face value. A lot more analysis and choices need to be made in converting these declarations into substantive support and inclusion of disabled students and other disabled populations in general. This requires realistic consideration of specific histories of countries and their current political challenges linked to the neoliberal context. While southern Africa is trying to recognise disability rights in general, it has an opportunity to learn from challenges of other disability rights movements elsewhere. Attending to these challenges by raising the profile of disability rights and services seems to be the correct direction for southern Africa.

Reflective questions

This chapter opened by situating the issues with disability rights to higher education. It then illustrated the problem of neoliberal foundations of disability rights. Even as an arguably the epitome of neoliberal ideology, the United States is grappling with the problem of rights for disabled students. Gabel *et al.* (2016) uncover the deficit model of disability at the California State University. Hirschmann (2016) and Liasidou and Symeou (2016) expound on the lack of concern for social rights, social justice and diversity in the discourse of disability for disabled students in the United States and Cyprus, respectively. Two lingering questions that remain for this chapter are:

1   Can southern Africa overcome the dominant ideological foundation of disability rights?
2   How will southern Africa re-conceptualise its disability rights in the era of global neoliberalism?

Perhaps part of the answers might begin with the *Disability Rights and Law Schools Project in Africa* run by the Centre for Human Rights at the University of Pretoria, South Africa and supported by the Open Society Foundation. The project was established in 2010, 'born in response to the alarmingly low levels of discourse and advocacy on disability rights in Southern Africa' (Centre for Human Rights, 2016, p. 1). It is a law education project comprising: (a) Chancellor College Malawi; (b) Eduardo Mondlane, Mozambique; (c) Makerere University, Uganda; (d) Midlands State University, Zimbabwe; (e) University of Botswana; (f) University of Dodoma, Tanzania; (g) University of Nairobi, Kenya; (h) University of Namibia; and (i) University of Zambia. Although the project has identified the problem of disability rights in Africa, Rafudeen (2016, p. 246) warns us that in South Africa, 'Human rights discourse partakes of the same paradigm that supports commodification. This lends this discourse an indeterminate character and, as such, it can be used to both challenge and protect hegemonic interests.'

Therefore, two more questions need to be asked:

3   What forms of institutions and discourses can promote disability rights in southern Africa?
4   How can such institutions and discourses initiate and improve support provision for disabled students in its member universities?

References

African Commission on Human and Peoples' Rights (2016). *Draft Protocol on the Rights of Persons with Disabilities in Africa*. Addis Ababa: African Union.
African Union (2003). *Continental Plan of Action for the African Decade of Persons with Disabilities (1999–2009)*. Addis Ababa: MCBS.

Albert, B. (2004). *Briefing Notes: The Social Model of Disability, Human Rights and Development.* Retrieved from www.enil.eu/wp-content/uploads/2012/07/The-social-model-of-disability-human-rights-development_2004.pdf on 20 October 2016.

Allen, H. M. (2002). Globalisation and contending human rights discourses. *HRC Quarterly Review*, April, 69–77.

Block, L. (2004). *Stereotypes about People with Disabilities.* Retrieved from http://www.disabilitymuseum.org/dhm/edu/essay.html?id=24 on 3 October 2016.

Centre for Human Rights (2016). *Disability Rights and Law Schools Project in Africa.* Retrieved from www.chr.up.ac.za on 22 April 2016.

Department of Education & Training (2016). *Draft Policy Framework for Disability in the Post-School Education and Training System.* Pretoria: Government Printers.

Devereux, S. (2013). Trajectories of social protection in Africa. *Development Southern Africa* **30**(1), 13–23.

Edmundson, W. A. (2004). *An Introduction to Rights.* Cambridge: Cambridge University Press.

Emong, P. & Eron, L. (2016). Disability inclusion in higher education in Uganda: status and strategies. *African Journal of Disability* **5**(1). Retrieved from www.ajod.org, DOI: 10.4102/ajod.v5i1.193 on 29 August 2017.

Enabulele, A. O. (2016). Incompatibility of national law with the African Charter on Human and Peoples' Rights: does the African Court on Human and Peoples' Rights have the final say? *African Human Rights Law Journal* **16**(1), 1–28.

Freeden, M. (1991). *Rights.* Milton Keynes: Open University Press.

Gabel, S. L., Reid, D., Pearson, H., Ruiz, L. & Hume-Dawson, R. (2016). Disability and diversity on CSU websites: a critical discourse study. *Journal of Diversity in Higher Education* **9**(1), 64–80.

Gloppen, S. & Rakner, L. (1993). *Human Rights and Development: The Discourse in the Humanities and Social Sciences.* Bergen: Chr. Michelsen Institute.

Grech, S. & Soldatic, K. (2015). Disability and colonialism: (dis)encounters and anxious intersectionalities. *Social Identities Journal for the Study of Race, Nation and Culture* **21**(1), 1–5.

Heap, M. & Morgans, H. (2006). Language policy and SALS: interpreters in the public service. In B. Watermeyer, L. Swartz, T. Lorenzo, M. Schneider & M. Priestly (eds) *Disability and Social Change: A South African Agenda* (pp. 134–147). Cape Town: Human Science Research Council Press.

Hirschmann, N. J. (2016). Disability rights, social rights, and freedom. *Journal of International Political Theory* **12**(1), 42–57.

Human Rights Watch (2015). *'Complicit in Exclusion': South Africa's Failure to Guarantee an Inclusive Education for Children with Disabilities.* Johannesburg: Human Rights Watch.

Jagoe, K. (1987). *Establishment of a Disability Unit at the University of Cape Town.* Unpublished papers at the Disability Unit Resource, University of Cape Town.

Kabzems, V. & Chimedza, R. (2002). Development assistance: disability and education in Southern Africa. *Disability & Society* **17**(2), 147–157.

Kochung, E. J. (2011). Role of higher education in promoting inclusive education: Kenyan perspective. *Journal of Emerging Trends in Educational Research and Policy Studies (JETERAPS)* **2**(3), 144–149.

Kollapen, J. (2003). Human rights meaningless without change. *Cape Time*, 20 March.

Kotzé, H. (2012). *Status of Disability Rights in Southern Africa.* Johannesburg: Open Society Foundation for Southern Africa.

Langa, P. V. (2013). *Higher Education in Portuguese Speaking African Countries: A Five Country Baseline Study.* Somerset West, Cape Town: African Minds.

Lee, P. (2002). Shooting for the moon: politics and disability at the beginning of the twenty-first century. In C. Barnes, M. Oliver & L. Barton (eds) *Disability Studies Today* (pp. 139–161). Oxford: Blackwell Publishers.

Leshota, L. P. (2013). Reading the National Disability and Rehabilitation Policy in the light of Foucault's technologies of power. *African Journal of Disability* **2**(1), 1–6.

Liasidou, A. & Symeou, L. (2016). Neoliberal versus social justice reforms in education policy and practice: discourses, politics and disability rights in education. *Critical Studies in Education.* Retrieved from www.tandfonline.com, DOI: 10.1080/17508487.2016.1186102 on 29 August 2017.

Low, C. (2001). *Controversial Speech by British Activist: Have Disability Rights Gone Too Far?* Retrieved from http://unipd-centrodirittiumani.it/public/docs/29743_rights.pdf on 20 October 2016.

Machan, T. R. (1989.) *Individuals and Their Rights.* La Salle, IL: Open Court.

Maguvhe, M. (2015). Teaching science and mathematics to students with visual impairments: reflections of a visually impaired technician. *African Journal of Disability* **4**(1), 1–5.

Matlosa, L. & Matobo, T. (2007). The education system in Lesotho: social inclusion and exclusion of visually impaired and hearing-impaired persons in the Institutions of Higher Learning. *ROSAS* **5**(1&2), 190–211.

Matshedisho, K. R. (2007). Access to higher education for disabled students in South Africa: a contradictory conjuncture of benevolence, rights and the social model of disability. *Disability & Society* **22**(7), 685–699.

Mbeki, T. (1997). Preface. *Integrated National Disability Strategy*. Pretoria: Government Printers.

McQuoid-Mason, D., O'Brien, E. & Greene, E. (1991). *Human Rights for All: Education towards a Rights Culture*. Cape Town: David Phillip.

Ministry of Education and Training in Swaziland (2016). *Swaziland Education for All Review Report, 2000–2015*. Retrieved from http://unesdoc.unesco.org/images/0023/002327/232703e.pdf on 3 October 2016.

Morley, C. & Croft, A. (2011). Agency and advocacy: disabled students in higher education in Ghana and Tanzania. *Research in Comparative and International Education* **6**(4), 383–399.

National Disability Rights Summit (2016). *Irene Declaration*. Conference held in St George's Conference Centre, City of Tshwane, 10–12 March.

Ndahinda, F. M. (2016). Peoples' rights, indigenous rights and interpretative ambiguities in decisions of the African Commission on Human and Peoples' Rights. *African Human Rights Law Journal* **16**(1), 29–57.

Ndlovu, S. & Walton, E. (2016). Preparation of students with disabilities to graduate into professions in the South African context of higher learning: obstacles and opportunities. *African Journal of Disability* **5**(1), 1–7.

Ngwena, C., Grobbelaar-du Plessis, I., Combrinck, H. & Kamga, S. D. (2014). Editorial. *African Disability Rights Yearbook* **2**, 1–4.

Peters, S. & Chimedza, R. (2000). Conscientization and the cultural politics of education: a radical minority perspective. *Comparative Education Review* **44**(3), 245–271.

Rafudeen, A. (2016). A South African reflection on the nature of human rights. *African Human Rights Law Journal* **16**(1), 225–246.

Republic of South Africa (2016). *White Paper on the Rights of Persons with Disabilities*. Pretoria: Government Printers.

Stewart, R. (2004). The really disabled: disability hierarchy in John Hockenberry's Moving Violations. *Review of Disability Studies: An International Journal* **1**(2), 113–116.

Swaziland Network Campaign for Education for All (2014). *Strengthening the Participation of Children with Disabilities in Education in Swaziland: Policy Analysis Report*. Mbabane: SWANCEFA.

UNESCO (1990). *World Declaration on Education for All*. New York: UNESCO.

UNESCO (1997). *Disabled Students at Universities in Africa*. Harare: UNESCO Sub-Regional Office for Southern Africa.

United Nations (2006). *Convention on the Rights of Persons with Disabilities*. Retrieved from www.un.org/development/desa/disabilities/convention-on-the-rights-of-persons-with-disabilities.html#Fulltext on 9 March 2017.

University of Cape Town (2003). 'Ready . . . steady . . . cap'. *Monday Paper* **22**(38), 9 December. Retrieved from www.uct.ac.za/mondaypaper/archives/?id=4246 on 30 September 2016.

Vergunst, R. (2016). *Access to Health Care for Persons with Disabilities in Rural Madwaleni, Eastern Cape, South Africa*. Unpublished thesis, University of Stellenbosch, Stellenbosch.

Wapling, L. (2016). *Inclusive Education and Children with Disabilities: Quality Education for All in Low and Middle Income Countries*. Bensheim: CBM (Christian Blind Mission).

12

ACCESS, EQUALITY AND INCLUSION OF DISABLED STUDENTS WITHIN SOUTH AFRICAN FURTHER AND HIGHER EDUCATIONAL INSTITUTIONS

Anlia Pretorius, Diane Bell and Tanya Healey

Introduction

Despite increased enrolment numbers of students with disabilities in the post-secondary education and training (PSET) sector, the throughput rate and numbers of graduates are low (Swart & Greyling, 2011). There are many reasons for this, but in essence, the failure to enforce existing legislation related to human rights, equality and accessibility is one of the primary causes. This chapter is informed by the current state of access, equity and inclusion for students with disabilities within the PSET sector, including Higher Education Institutions (HEIs), Technical and Vocational Education Training (TVET) and Community Education and Training (CET) colleges in South Africa. The following aspects are presented in this chapter: defining the concept 'disability'; disability and decolonisation; prevalence of students with disabilities; provision of support services and reasonable accommodation; roles and responsibilities of disability rights units (DRUs); and sharing the 'lived' experiences of students with disabilities. Although the transition of students with disabilities to the labour market after graduation is not addressed in this chapter, it forms an interesting area for further research. While some progress has been made in mainstreaming disability, this chapter argues that a consolidated framework needs to be implemented in the sector in order to ensure and regulate access, equality and full inclusion for all students with disabilities in South Africa.

Background

For many years, equality issues such as race and gender have received attention while disability inclusion in HEIs in South Africa has not. Access and inclusion of students with disabilities received very little attention and resources, leading to a low number of students with disabilities entering and graduating from the PSET system. More recently, however, increased numbers of institutions are addressing the need to provide services to students with disabilities and have policies in place to ensure equal access (Foundation of Tertiary Institutions of the Northern Metropolis [FOTIM South Africa (SA)], 2011). FOTIM, a South African higher education academic consortium formed in 1995 (dissolved in 2011), with the aim of promoting collaboration among its members. It had a membership of nine universities and universities of technology in the Gauteng, Limpopo and North West provinces. FOTIM encouraged debate, best practice and capacity building through the sharing of knowledge and commitment to academic excellence in the region (FOTIM SA, 2011). However, the current gap in comprehensive inclusion across the PSET sector and in South African society, tells the story of a failure to enforce existing accessibility legislation. A major shift in the attitude of society is needed in order to make significant progress. The South African Constitution has set the stage for the removal of barriers and integrating vulnerable groups as participating members of society. Of the main pillars of the national transformation agenda of South Africa, disability has been acknowledged as the area where change has not kept pace with other areas (Department of the Presidency SA, 2012). It has been lagging behind in spite of legislation. Of critical importance is that disability is appropriately addressed along with all other areas of transformation, such as race and gender, within the PSET system.

Some effort has been made in raising disability on the national agenda. In January 2014, the South African Ministry of Higher Education launched the White Paper for Post-School Education and Training (Department of Higher Education and Training [DHET SA], 2013), which aims to build an expanded, effective and integrated PSET system. The policy document emphasises the need for expanded disability support. A recommendation was made for a national policy framework 'to guide the improvement of access to and success in post-school education and training institutions' including private institutions, for people with disabilities (DHET SA, 2013). Subsequently, in December 2014, the Higher Education Minister proceeded to appoint a ministerial committee to develop a Strategic Policy Framework for Disability in the PSET system. Further evidence of the national commitment to advancing the 'disability agenda' in South Africa can be found in the establishment of the Presidential Working Group on Disability, the inaugural meeting of which was held on 10 March 2016, chaired by President Jacob Zuma. Commitment is required at all levels of government, and needs to be built into new and existing legislation, standards, policies, strategies, and plans; as well as business and society in general.

Theoretical framework and approach

The struggle to define disability in a way that accurately and realistically encompasses the lived experience of persons with disabilities is a historical one, characteristic of power dynamics, prejudice and social exclusion of those who do not 'belong' (United Nations, 2006). Thus, defining disability for the purposes of legislation and policy requires a contextualisation of the above description with the aim of specifying who the exact target group within the disabled population is for purposes of that precise piece of legislation and/or policy.

Narrow definitions of disability, located within the medical model, focus on impairment and treatment in a medical sense and are used, pragmatically, for a specific purpose such as eligibility for a disability-related benefit, as is the case in South Africa, for eligibility for the Disability Grant (The South African Government, 2017). The medical model produces low estimates of disability prevalence, as they only consider people with very severe impairments. Thus, narrow definitions lead to exclusive measures that give rise to underestimates of the population of people with disabilities. This has historically been the case in South Africa (Pretorius & Lawton-Misra, 2011).

In contrast, broad definitions, found in the social model of disability, emphasise the importance of the environment. The Convention on the Rights of Persons with Disabilities (CRPD) (United Nations, 2006) recognises the role of both individual and environmental factors in creating the experience of disability, and promotes the notion that disability is a universal experience and not that of a marginalised group. The social model of disability includes people with mild difficulty through to extreme difficulty or 'unable to do an activity'. This leads to a more inclusive measure of disability and much higher prevalence estimates.

Evaluating the above, it is clear that a functional definition is needed to provide a more balanced approach. A functional concept of disability defines a disability as any long-term limitation in activity resulting from the interaction between health conditions and contextual factors, both personal and environmental (World Health Organization [WHO], 2001). It is the recommended international standard for data collection on disability. The use of this standard ensures that the results are comparable with those from other countries. The World Disability Report describes a 'bio-psycho-social model' based on the International Classification of Functioning, Disability and Health (ICF) (WHO & World Bank, 2011).

The bio-psycho-social model offers a coherent explanation of disability. It is an interactive and individual-centred framework that takes into account the person, the biological problem and social contextual influences (Waddell & Aylward, 2010, p. 23). It combines and balances the medical and social models and introduces a personal dimension. Thus, from a bio-psycho-social perspective, disability originates from a health condition, but is influenced by 'an individual (with a health condition) and that individual's contextual factors (environmental and personal factors)' (Leonardi *et al.*, 2006 cited in WHO & World Bank, 2011, p. 4).

Furthermore, in the South African context, a human rights and developmental approach has the potential to be a catalyst for change. A rights-based approach refers to the provision of all human and socio-economic rights enshrined within the Constitution of South Africa (The South African Government, 1996). It also provides a set of performance standards against which governments and other institutions can be held accountable. This approach reinforces commitment, participation and mainstreaming of human rights as the central core in the formulation, implementation, review, monitoring and evaluation of disability-related policies and programmes (WHO, 2015). In addition, it emphasises social justice; a minimum standard of living; equitable access; equal opportunity to services and benefits; and a commitment to meeting the needs of all South Africans with a special emphasis on the needs of the most disadvantaged. It is through the bio-psycho-social lens, framed by the human-rights-based approach, that access and inclusion in the PSET sector in South Africa are viewed in this chapter.

Disability and education

It is self-evident that all students deserve nothing less than quality education and training that provides them with opportunities for lifelong learning, the world of work, and meaningful participation in society as productive citizens. Inclusive education in the PSET sector is non-negotiable and long-term commitments from all stakeholders are needed, including an enabling teaching and learning environment which promotes student access and success. Education and training provide knowledge and skills that people with disabilities can use to exercise a range of other human rights, such as the right to political participation; the right to work; the right to live independently and contribute to the community; the right to participate in cultural life; and the right to raise a family. Moreover, ensuring that all children (persons) with disabilities have access to quality education will help South Africa meet its employment equity goals.

Despite major initiatives that have been undertaken in recent years in South Africa, the improvement of the well-being of students with disabilities in the post-school sector remains a major challenge. The importance of establishing best practice and minimum standards with regard to accommodating students with disabilities thus remains of critical importance. Research aimed at enhancing insight into the prevalence and needs of students with disabilities is needed across the continent.

According to the 2011 FOTIM Report and the White Paper for Post School Education and Training (DHET SA, 2013), most universities currently offer assistance and deliver services to students with disabilities in accordance with the South African Constitution (FOTIM, 2011), Education White Paper 6 (DOE SA, 2001), guidelines set in the National Plan for Higher Education (DHET SA, 2001a), CRPD (United Nations, 2006), White Paper for Post-School Education and Training (DHET SA, 2013) and other legislation. These documents, however, do not address specific needs in terms of the higher education context and are not seen as binding policies to guide the granting of specific accommodations. There is unfortunately very little evidence of progress in supporting students with disabilities in the rest of the PSET sector, that is, TVET and CETcolleges.

Post-school prevalence of students with disabilities

The majority of persons with severe difficulties across all functional domains aged between 20 to 24 years do not attend university in South Africa, with only about one-fifth of them gaining access. Attendance was also highest among the white population group and lowest among black South Africans (Department of Social Development SA, 2014).

According to both Higher Education Management Information System (HEMIS) 2013 data, and institutional feedback provided to the ministerial committee, there is an increase in the numbers of students with disabilities every year attending university, yet there is minimal growth when compared to the general (or total) intake and the increase that occurred in the PSET sector over the last five years. Accurate and up-to-date data on the number of post-school students with disabilities are not readily available. Data received from HEMIS as reported by the 23 public universities show that in 2011, 5,856 students with disabilities were enrolled in HEIs out of a total population of 938,201, accounting for only 0.6% of the total enrolment. In 2012, student numbers increased to 6,277 out of a total enrolment of 953,373, accounting for 0.7%. Furthermore, in 2013, student numbers increased to 7,110 out of a total enrolment of 983,698, accounting for 0.7% at the 23 universities (HEMIS, 2013).

Figure 12.1 depicts the yearly increase of students enrolled at all 23 universities in South Africa. The biggest category of impairment according to HEMIS statistics over the period of 2011 to 2013 is visual impairment, followed by mobility impairment. TVET colleges also show a yearly increase of students enrolled at all public colleges in South Africa, despite them not receiving adequate support provisions. Notwithstanding this steady increase, the average number of students with disabilities still remains low and accounted for only 0.72% of the total student population in 2013 as illustrated in Figure 12.1.

It is important to draw attention to the discrepancy between HEMIS data (2013) and reported data received from universities. In general, DRU's report higher numbers than the HEMIS system. One reason for the discrepancy might be the time of reporting, which occurs at the beginning of the academic year. The fact that students do not indicate their impairments could be indicative of a lack of trust or fear of disclosing information such as impairment-specific status on their application forms that would be captured on the HEMIS system. Some students from rural areas might not even be aware of hidden impairments such as learning

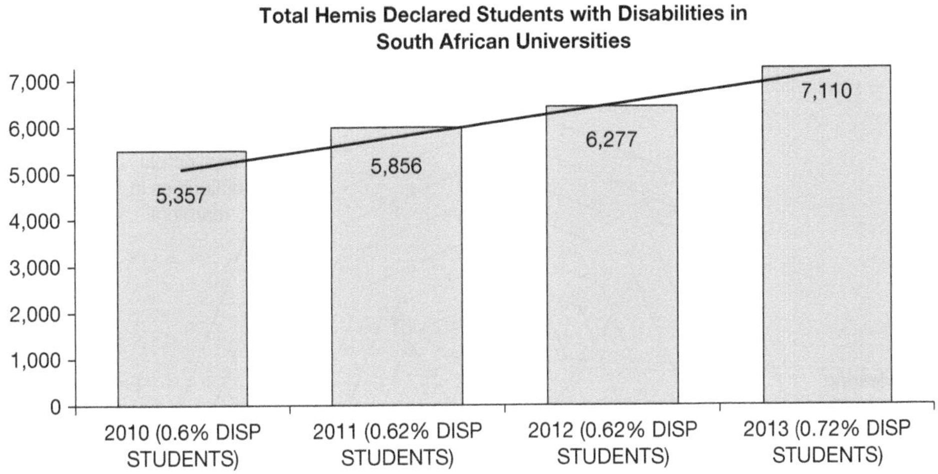

Total Hemis Declared Students with Disabilities in South African Universities

Figure 12.1 Students with disabilities in South African universities, 2010–2013

HEMIS (2013) database, extracted on 15 April 2015

difficulties, and are only diagnosed when struggling with their academic work at tertiary education level. Even taking into account the data received from institutions, the number of students with disabilities in the PSET sector is still well below the national prevalence of people with disabilities. According to the White Paper on Post-School Education (2013), this can be an indication that barriers still exist and that people with disabilities are still discouraged from entering universities. Under-representation is clearly a South African reality and if some individuals with disabilities do not feel comfortable to disclose their impairments based on fears of rejection, unfair treatment or even pity, then this clearly highlights social attitudinal problems around disability issues. If this is not adequately addressed, unreliable statistical data will remain the reality in South Africa, and will delay proper support structures being implemented and hinder efforts to obtain funding.

Turning to impairment types, universities in South Africa reported an increase in students reporting learning difficulties (such as dyslexia), and more recently, also an increase in disclosure of psychiatric disabilities (such as depression). Visual and physical impairments are also well represented but there is still a small percentage of Deaf or hearing-impaired students in the PSET sector (HEMIS, 2013). Further research into the reasons for this is necessary, but some reasons include the lack of subjects available up to Matric level (or secondary school level) in schools for the Deaf; lack of adequate teachers to equip Deaf students with learning; as well as the lack of support services based on the prohibitive cost of highly individualised support (e.g. sign-language interpreters).

The proper classification of impairments and reporting of students is vital because this informs the type of support needed. It is recommended that standardised nomenclature be used and that the 'classification' of students be uniform across institutions in the PSET sector for ease of reference when referring to a particular disability type. This will assist with the provision of reasonable accommodation and other support services.

Figure 12.2 depicts in detail annual specific impairments. Over the period 2010 to 2013, there was no change in terms of the actual numbers of the specific impairments. The communication (talking/listening) impairment figures also remains very low over the four-year period. An explanation for this could be that it is unclear what impairments should be classified

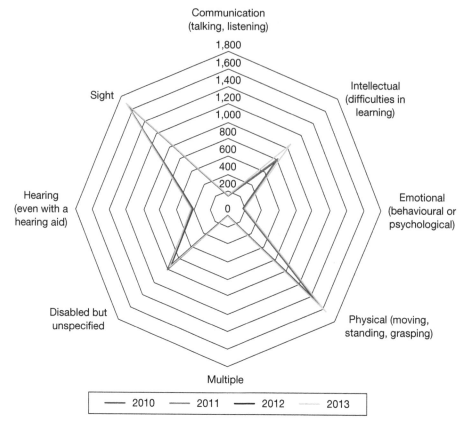

Figure 12.2   South African university students with disabilities per specific impairment
HEMIS (2013) database, extracted on 15 April 2015

under this code. Similarly, the code 'intellectual, difficulty in learning' is also problematic. These two examples highlight the challenges and the urgency of implementing a user-friendly and appropriate coding system, as the present system of capturing disability-related statistics is not adequate. Figure 12.2 summarises the statistics of South African university students with disabilities per specific impairment.

Disability rights units

The role of DRUs is to ensure full participation by students with disabilities at their chosen place of learning. Although most universities now have some type of formalised services available to students with disabilities, there is no consistency in what type of support/reasonable accommodation is offered or what minimum support standards are adhered to. TVETs and CETs in comparison with universities are lagging behind in formalised services for students with disabilities. To add to the dilemma, where services are offered, they are also 'known' under different names. This illuminates the bigger problem of non-standardisation which is a 'major concern'. There needs to be uniformity in terms of nomenclature for services provided. Consistent with the human rights perspective, it is recommended that the name disability rights units be used for all such centralised support services in the PSET sector.

One consolidated framework, which takes into account legislation and policies, needs to be in place to ensure that all students in the PSET sector can access the necessary support and experience equal access and potential success (Pretorius *et al.*, 2013).

Application of legislation and policies to DRUs

The situation in South Africa is different from international models where there is strong emphasis on adhering to and enforcing national legislation (e.g. the Americans with Disability Act). In South Africa, the level of enforcement in the different universities is currently defined by the 'buy-in' from the different HEI's senior management. A stronger emphasis on the power and influence or negotiating skills of a 'disability activist/champion' regarding disability taking its rightful place on the transformation agenda is needed to ensure that all PSET institutions comply with SA legislation.

In line with the autonomy of institutions, most universities with DRUs have their own policies to guide the work done in the field of disability support. The policies, however, differ greatly, with some not addressing all the core areas and others that are not underpinned by the CRPD (United Nations, 2006) and other government policies. In many instances, there is also a gap in terms of the implementation of the policies, where costing and budget allocation are not taken into account. Greater emphasis is needed on the development of plans to guide policy implementation.

In terms of TVETs and CETs, work needs to begin from the ground up, and in many instances, people in charge of the ad hoc services are not knowledgeable or equipped to do the work or write a policy that is holistic and addresses all areas from a human rights perspective. Disability awareness and sensitisation is required to ensure that disability is taken into account when considering changes, or when new institutional policies/strategies are implemented. This will ensure that disability matters are mainstreamed throughout the fabric of the institution.

Services provided by DRUs: availability and quality

DRUs should be adequately capacitated to support all different types of impairments in the sector. That is, learning, psychiatric/social-related and communication-related impairments (e.g. stuttering). Future plans should involve the public health sector in concrete ways; for example, making use of the new International Statistical Classification of Diseases and Related Health Problems (ICD11). ICD is the diagnostic classification standard used globally in the identification of health trends and statistics. It defines diseases, disorders, injuries and other related health conditions (WHO, 2001).

Disability has many intersections and for a large number of students, public healthcare services are crucial if their chances of success are to be maximised. In many instances, neither students nor DRUs have the funds available to provide the necessary support.

The White Paper 6 on Special Needs Education: Building an Inclusive Education Training System (DHET SA, 2001b, p. 28) called for 'regional collaboration' among HEIs when addressing disability, to allow for institutions in regions to specialise in particular disabilities. This strategy is exclusionary as students who wish to attend a specific higher or further education institution will not be able to exercise their democratic right of freedom of choice. The White Paper for Post School Education and Training (DHET SA, 2013, p. 44) acknowledges that such regional collaboration is 'restrictive in terms of access because it implies that institutions only cater for certain disabilities, even if students live nearby'. The South African disability sector has clearly articulated that although it is cost intensive to cater for all types of impairments, it is neither feasible nor in line with the human rights approach that certain universities should 'specialise' in particular types of impairments.

At universities, in general, similar services are provided across the different DRUs. The variation is more in terms of the number of different services provided, with some DRUs only providing a few services and the more established DRUs providing many more. The more established and longstanding the DRU, the longer the list of services rendered and the more types of impairments are supported. In these DRUs, services to students are tailor-made to serve each individual student's needs, however unique and complex.

Most universities are able to provide services to students who are visually or physically impaired, with some also providing services to learning-impaired and psychologically impaired students. There are, however, some great inconsistencies with regard to support, for example, the lack of support for students who are Deaf (making use of South African Sign Language (SASL)) and/or who have a hearing impairment (making use of technology and spoken language), as well as more specialised services where caregivers and assistants are required. Because of the high cost, and no other financial support apart from the institutional budget to the DRUs being received, many institutions are reluctant to enrol students requiring specialised and highly individualised support, such as SASL interpreters and full-time caregivers. This reluctance highlights the importance of a funding stream directly from the DHET or the National Student Financial Aid Scheme (NSFAS) to DRUs.

Table 12.1 illustrates the core services of well-functioning and well-resourced DRU.

Table 12.1 Core services of well-functioning disability rights units

General and administrative	• Pre-registration services • General enquiries and registering with the Disability Service; assessment for relevant support • Designated disabled parking • Assistance with registration and bursary applications
Access solutions	• Mobility training and specialised campus orientation • Accessible residential assistance • Access solutions to inaccessible venues • Accessible transport between residences and lectures • Assistance at graduation ceremonies
Advocacy	• Advocacy and counselling on disability issues; play an advisory role, e.g. awareness drives • Prospective students, orientation • Disability bursary applications • Advocacy events and disability research • Liaison with SRC and Disabled Students Movement
Teaching and learning support	• Training and educating of academic and support staff re disability matters • Access to study material in alternative formats (Braille, audio, electronic text), and to assistive technologies and assistive furniture • Scribing and note-taker support • Student Volunteers Support Team • Disability service computer lab (including specialised hardware and software); maintenance • Test and exam accommodations (including venues)
Learning disability support and extra time	• Extra time applications • Accommodations around tests and exams • Counselling

Location and size of DRUs

Regarding the location and size of the DRUs, consistency across the sector is lacking, and each DRU is differently structured and capacitated. More generally, DRUs report to either student affairs/services or in some cases to the registrar or the deputy-vice chancellor. This results in different levels of responsiveness and, in many instances, has a great impact on the functioning, power, influence and status of the DRUs. If the human rights-based approach is accepted, and disability is seen as a human rights issue, the recommendation is that the location of DRUs must be at a high level within institutional structures (for example, the DRU leader should be part of the senior executive teams responsible for allocating resources). DRUs need to function in an integrated way across the entire institution, forming strong links with various functional areas, e.g. admissions, examinations, residences, facilities, fees offices, etc. The physical location of DRUs must also be considered, as the location must be fully accessible and be placed in a physical space which is easy to access for all.

Status of DRUs

As previously discussed, most South African universities now have formal institutional disability policies in place that serve as written commitment to admit and support eligible students with disabilities. Different universities, however, determine ad hoc measures, rules, regulations and policies to adhere to in order to give structure to the very complex environment of disability support. This results in diverse implementation of accommodations (quality and type) and dissatisfaction within institutions and between institutions, and even between DRUs and faculties within institutions.

In 2009, 11 universities had established DRUs (FOTIM, 2011). During the 2012–13 Road Shows to universities conducted by the Department of Women, Children and Persons with Disabilities (DWCPD), 17 universities had established units although some were not yet fully functional. From information collated by the DWCPD Road Show, as well as from returned questionnaires to the ministerial committee, the observation is that there is no consistency in terms of the services offered, the policies governing the services, names of units, budget allocation or staff component and reporting lines. The most marked differences are in the older or earlier established units (post-1986) and those more recently established (post-2005).

The picture is unfortunately worse for TVET colleges, with very few institutions able to support students with disabilities. Staff members indicated that they were not trained nor did they have any background in the field of disability. For example, in some instances, they were co-opted from a lecturing position. It seems as if there is recognition that specialised support is needed, but it is also evident that there is a lack of knowledge about how to go about this, as well as a lack of funding to operationalise. This creates great uncertainty and concerns for the staff members tasked with this function. The same scenario is true for TVETs and CETs. There is an urgent need for the staff tasked with establishing and running DRUs to be equipped to implement effective services. Currently support is being provided through regional meetings, training workshops and a few accredited short courses.

Access and infrastructure

In ensuring an accessible environment, Universal Access principles should be applied. Universal Access is a concept encompassing an integrated philosophy by observing inclusion and accessibility as key components of developing barrier-free environments. The United Nations (2006) defines universal access as the design of products, environments, programmes and services to be usable by all people, to the greatest extent possible, without the need for adaptation or specialised design. In South Africa, the DHET from time to time calls for proposals for funding to make university campuses more accessible. This same funding model should be implemented across the entire PSET sector as TVETs and CETs have been excluded.

The DHET highlights the importance of using universal access criteria by all when doing audits to ensure the same standards are adhered to. An access audit provides best practice guidelines to improve the university compliance with the building regulations; provides guidelines and solutions that are usable by and accessible to the widest range of people; and develops and provides universal design standards for future upgrades, refurbishments, construction of new buildings and expansions of the university.

The accessibility of the physical environment remains a big challenge for universities and colleges, with many buildings being old with historical status. If the physical environment is not accessible, it belies the point of creating an accessible learning and teaching environment. Although physical access issues are often considered, some might never be implemented due to misconceptions that the cost is too high to cater for only a small number of users. If accessibility audits to identify and remove potential environmental barriers are done at the beginning of development, an inclusive, safe and secure environment is ensured, and costs are saved by minimising the need for expensive modifications later.

The significance of assistive technologies, including assistive products, also needs to be recognised (Christian Blind Mission, 2012). Provision of a device at an early stage could prevent a mild impairment from becoming severe or leading to complications. Assistive devices enable people with disabilities to participate on equal terms. An assistive product is any equipment or tool that is designed or adapted to enable persons with disabilities to participate in activities, tasks or actions. They can include mobility aids (such as wheelchairs, prostheses and crutches); communication aids (such as hearing aids); sensory aids (such as white canes); and technology aids (such as computers for alternate and augmentative communication, screen readers, magnifiers) (WHO, 2015).

Advocacy for the post-secondary education and training sector

Advocacy for PSET is crucial to ensuring the participation of persons with disabilities in higher education in South Africa. To that effect, the Higher and Further Education Disability Services Association (HEDSA) is an advocacy and rights-based non-profit organisation representing disability services in Higher and Further Education Institutions in South Africa. It is recognised and endorsed by the DHET, and accepted as a community of practice by universities in South Africa. HEDSA strives to ensure equal opportunities (including access and support) for all students with disabilities (Bell, 2013). It is a key stakeholder in the field of disability services, and is often consulted by state organisations such as NSFAS around funding for students with disabilities. However, HEDSA is not a statutory body and therefore does not hold the necessary power to enforce the required minimum standards of support. It can, however, serve as an entity to oversee monitoring and evaluation of support provisioning in the sector (Bell, 2013).

Post-secondary education and training funding
for students with disabilities

There is currently no uniform funding model for the entire post-school sector in South Africa. The current scenario for universities is that eligible students can apply for NSFAS funding, including a one-off payment for an assistive device. From time to time, the DHET also calls for proposals based on accessibility access audits to improve accessibility to infrastructure and facilities. Apart from this, universities do not receive additional funds to support students with disabilities above the general funding received by universities per student enrolment numbers.

This funding stream works differently in the TVET sector with NSFAS funding going directly to the institutions. This creates challenges as few TVET colleges have dedicated DRUs to provide sufficient support to the students in need. Planning is done in the previous year using the projected enrolment numbers on which funding will then be based. TVET colleges also submit periodic reports of students with disabilities, after which funding is allocated accordingly. CET colleges also have little in place regarding funding for students with disabilities. The recently appointed ministerial committee was tasked to review the national norms and standards for funding further education and training colleges (DHET SA, 2014).

Currently, students with disabilities studying at universities are eligible to apply for funding through NSFAS provided they meet certain criteria. This funding covers fees for tuition, university accommodation and also a single payment for assistive products. At TVET colleges, however, the institution applies for funding and the different colleges then administer the funds received from NSFAS. The amended National Norms and Standards for Funding Technical and Vocational Education and Training Colleges mention multiple times the dedicated funding for students with disabilities studying at TVET colleges. Under the heading 'Redress principles for public funding' (DHET SA, 2014, p. 19), it is stipulated that funding of public TVET colleges must contribute toward the redress of past inequalities.

It is important to point out that it costs significantly more to educate a student with a disability than a student who does not have a disability. Often, families falling within the middle socio-economic income bracket (the 'missing middle'); struggle to fund the studies of their children in the post-school sector. Funding formulae currently being used in the sector, e.g. university subsidies, NSFAS funding, do not make allowances for this 'group', resulting in exclusionary practices.

The cost of human support such as sign-language interpreters, carers, note-takers and tutors needs to be included as it is a significant support mechanism for students with specific needs. Often these needs are overshadowed by an emphasis on assistive technologies and products, but it is crucial to address the needs of students adequately and realistically to ensure academic success. In addition, to broaden the group of students able to benefit from the funding, relationships with other role-players such as the Department of Social Development and the Department of Health need to be explored.

The funding of DRUs also differs within the PSET sector. University DRUs are funded by the individual HEIs – mainly for salaries and the general running of the unit. Additional fundraising is also done to acquire extra services and enhanced assistive devices and technologies. In the TVET sector, funding can be requested from different governmental and external sources. Setting up a DRU is cost intensive and seed funding for TVETs and CETs might be a requirement to ensure that proper facilities can be established. The high cost of licencing and upgrades of computers also necessitates DRU funding.

Some DRUs still do not get dedicated funding from their institutions. There is thus a need for ring-fenced funding for the adequate resourcing of DRUs from the DHET for the PSET sector. Provision of funding for all institutions is needed to commence, continue and improve the work in the field. Vice chancellors and principals need to channel funding directly to the DRUs so that it is not allocated elsewhere in the institution. There should also be a separate allocation for staffing and other resources, namely, assistive products and human support. The provision of government funding such as NSFAS, does not take away the individual institutions' responsibility to source external funding. Funding received through fundraising should supplement institutional funding. This will also help to address the delivery of services to all different categories of impairment and encourage institutions to broaden their intake of such students.

The White Paper for Post School Education and Training (DHET SA, 2013), reports that there is less funding for and resourcing of DRUs at historically black institutions compared to historically white institutions. Currently, a differentiated approach to funding has been implemented through the provision of funding to all universities to conduct infrastructure audits, and this should also be implemented in TVET and CET colleges.

Decolonising education and disability

Universities throughout South Africa are currently grappling with decolonising the curriculum. The colonial model of academic organisation of the university was entrenched during the apartheid era and has not been significantly redressed. Le Grange (2016, p. 6) suggests that decolonisation involves a process of change that 'does not necessary involve destroying Western knowledge but in decentring it or perhaps deterritorialising it (making it something other than what it is)'. Hollinsworth (2013) concludes his article (which looks at Indigenous disability in Australia) by recommending that the dominant social model of disability needs to be contested based on acknowledgement of our shared history of racism and recognition of the diversity of Indigenous perspectives on disability. For relevant changes to be made in South Africa, inclusion should be closely examined by the PSET sector, and disability be included in the curriculum in a structured way.

Monitoring, evaluation and enforcement

There are many reasons for the slow progress toward transforming the disability sector in South Africa, including the absence of effective monitoring of compliance with national and international obligations; lack of effective coordination mechanisms; absence of enforcement mechanisms and, together with this, the lack of accountability and consequences for non-compliance (Department of Social Development SA, 2014). Discrimination against persons with disabilities continues since there are no consequences for failing to implement the legislation and policies, with the effect that mainstreaming of disability in all areas of life is lagging behind (ibid.).

Monitoring to track progress regarding the promotion and protection of the rights of persons with disabilities within the PSET environment will ensure compliance and implementation of minimum standards. Implementation of the envisaged Policy Framework on Disability in Post-School Education and Training is thus important and will enable students with disabilities to participate fully and equally in education and as members of the community.

Student experiences and perceptions

For students with disabilities, the PSET sector, especially higher education, offers an opportunity for possible economic empowerment and is thus considered a means for truly impacting their quality of life (Fuller *et al.*, 2004; Shaw, Madaus & Bannerjee, 2009). Unfortunately, in reality, students with disabilities often face a series of barriers to learning and participation at university. The barriers they face are mainly attitudinal (i.e. negative attitudes), structural (i.e. architectural barriers), inaccessible curricula and resource-related (human and financial).

Research has been conducted in South Africa regarding the provision for students with disabilities, focusing specifically on their 'lived' (own) experiences (Howell, 2005, 2006; Howell & Lazarus, 2003; Matshedisho, 2007a, 2007b; Pretorius & Yates, 2014). The research indicates that first, *personal characteristics* (denoting intra-personal qualities) and *self-determination* (knowledge, skills and beliefs that enable them to become independent) help students with disabilities to transition to university; students with disabilities need to take ownership and communicate their needs (practising self-advocacy). Practical and emotional *support from peers* is important with the overall campus climate of a university being central to both personal happiness as well as academic success. Although students with disabilities expressed a firm belief in their own ability and inherent potential, yet their *perceptions of others' beliefs* influenced their own beliefs concerning support and adaptations. Students with disabilities are typically not a homogeneous group and thus their support requirements differ and can change over time. They experience difficulties related to awareness and attitudes of lecturers, physical space in the classroom, assessment accommodations, curriculum delivery and the provision of user-friendly handouts (Swart & Greyling, 2011).

Second, the understanding of disability and the focus on and strategy of inclusion have mostly been influenced by personal interest and disciplinary requirements; often due to the large amount of curriculum content to be covered, often the focus is on the impairment, with the societal and attitudinal causes of disability receiving less attention (Ohajunwa, McKenzie, Hardy & Lorenzo, 2014).

A number of studies have been conducted in South Africa concerning the improvement of the 'situation' for students with disabilities. Various recommendations have been made, including the need for information and orientation sessions for students with disabilities (Morina, Lopez-Gavira & Molina, 2016). Participation will be enhanced if students with disabilities develop self-determination (Swart & Greyling, 2011). Support should aim not to change students with disabilities but to enable them – they learn differently but have the same ideals as any other student (Swart & Greyling, 2011). Accessible, flexible, appropriate and responsive curricula and learning spaces are crucial if the learning needs of a diverse student population are to be met (Ohajunwa *et al.*, 2014; Howell & Lazarus, 2003; Bell, 2013). All physical structures should be made fully accessible (Howell & Lazarus, 2003). Academic staff should be trained on achieving universal design in instruction, first as part of a formal teaching qualification and second, as part of their continuous learning requirements (FOTIM SA, 2011). The role of support staff (including the educational psychologists) needs to change to being more strategic in developing support and inclusive practices in higher education (Lyner-Cleophas *et al.*, 2014).

Through paying attention to the voice (lived experience) of students with disabilities and the implementation of the above-mentioned recommendations, PSET institutions could be made more welcoming and equitable for students with disabilities (Pretorius & Lawton-Misra, 2012).

Conclusion

Having sketched a picture, albeit bleak, of the current state of access, equality and inclusion of students with disabilities in further and higher education (PSET sector) in South Africa, the main question that arises is 'So where to from here?' Although some progress has been made in addressing the needs of students with disabilities, especially in the university environment, much still needs to change to ensure access, equality and full inclusion. It is therefore encouraging to note that the DHET seems to be taking the provision of services seriously. One positive and proactive step has followed from the recommendations made in the White Paper for Post-School Education and Training (DHET SA, 2013) where it was clearly articulated that a strategic policy framework for the PSET environment is necessary to guide the improvement of access to, and success in, post-school education and training (including private institutions) for people with disabilities. The work on the policy framework was completed by the ministerial committee and it is now in the process of being approved by cabinet. Once implemented, the framework will create an enabling and empowering environment across the entire PSET system that will provide direction and guidance to institutions in terms of implementation and adherence to disability policies; setting of minimum norms and standards for the DRUs; identifying best practices that can be shared with newly established DRUs; prescribing the provision of services to DRUs to meet the needs of every student with a disability in the institution; and encouraging all PSET institutions to employ people with disabilities and provide assistance and support to them where needed.

Thus, once in place, the current state of access, equity and inclusion for students with disabilities within further and HEIs in South Africa will improve, and students with disabilities will be able to enter the PSET environment with the academic ability and all the necessary support provisioning to be able to compete on an equal level with their non-disabled peers.

Reflective questions

1 In order to improve the well-being and educational outcomes of students with disabilities, how should the PSET sector operationalise the establishment and implementation of best practice, as well as minimum standards with regards to accommodating students with disabilities across the sector?
2 How could the establishment of DRUs at TVET colleges be expedited?
3 In which ways could the professionalisation of all DRU staff be strategically approached for maximum impact?
4 How should the recommendations be prioritised and implemented to ensure greatest returns and impact for students with disabilities in further and higher education?

References

Bell, D. (2013). *Investigating Teaching and Learning Support for Students with Hearing Impairment at a University in the Western Cape*. Unpublished PhD Thesis, University of Stellenbosch, Cape Town. Retrieved from http://scholar.sun.ac.za/handle/10019.1/80004 on 29 August 2017.
Christian Blind Mission (2012). *A human rights-based approach*. Retrieved from www.cbm.org/article/downloads/54741/A_human_rights-based_approach_to_disability_in_development.pdf on 20 March 2017.
Department of Education [DOE] (2001). *White Paper 6: Special Needs Education: Building an Inclusive Education and Training System*. Pretoria: Government Printer.
Department of Higher Education & Training [DHET SA] (2001a). *National Plan for Higher Education*. Pretoria: Government Printer.
Department of Higher Education & Training [DHET SA] (2001b). *The White Paper 6 on Special Needs Education: Building an Inclusive Education Training System*. Pretoria: Government Printer.
Department of Higher Education & Training [DHET SA] (2013). *White Paper for Post School Education and Training*. Pretoria: Government Printer.
Department of Higher Education and Training [DHET SA] (2014). *Call for Comments on the Draft Amendments to the National Norms and Standards for Funding Further Education and Training Colleges (NSF-FET Colleges)*. Pretoria: Government Printer.
Department of the Presidency (2012). *National Development Plan 2030: Our Future – Make it Work (Executive Summary)*. Pretoria: Government Printer.

Department of Social Development (2014). *Draft White Paper on the Mainstreaming of the Rights of Persons with Disabilities to Equality and Dignity (National Disability Rights Policy)*. Pretoria: Government Printer.

Foundation of Tertiary Institutes of the Northern Metropolis [FOTIM] (2011). *Disability in Higher Education Project Report*. Retrieved from www.uct.ac.za/usr/disability/reports/annual_report_10_11.pdf on 18 September 2016.

Fuller, M., Healey, M., Bradley, A. & Hall, T. (2004). Barriers to learning: a systemic study of the experience of disabled students at one university. *Studies in Higher Education* **29**(3), 303–318.

Higher Education Management Information System (HEMIS) (2013). *HEMIS Database*. Data extracted April 2015.

Hollinsworth, D. (2013). Decolonizing Indigenous disability in Australia. *Disability & Society* **28**(5), 601–615.

Howell, C. (2005). *Higher Education Monitor: South African Higher Education Responses to Students with Disabilities*. Pretoria: Council for Higher Education.

Howell, C. (2006). Disabled students and higher education in South Africa. In B. Watermeyer, L. Swartz, L. Lorenzo, M. Schneider & M. Priestley (eds) *Disability and Social Change: A South African Agenda* (pp. 164–178). Pretoria: HRSC Press.

Howell, C. & Lazarus, S. (2003). Access and participation for students with disabilities in South African higher education: challenging accepted truths and recognising new possibilities. *Perspectives in Education* **21**(3), 59–74.

le Grange, L. (2016). Decolonising the university curriculum. *South African Journal of Higher Education* **30**(2), 1–12.

Lyner-Cleophas, M., Swart, E., Chataika, T. & Bell, D. (2014). Increasing access into higher education: insights from the 2011 African Network on Evidence-to-Action on Disability Symposium – Education Commission. *African Journal of Disability* **3**(2), Art.#78, 3 pages.

Matshedisho, K. R. (2007a). Access to higher education for disabled students in South Africa: a contradictory conjuncture of benevolence, rights and the social model of disability. *Disability & Society* **22**(7), 685–699.

Matshedisho, K. R. (2007b). The challenges of real rights for disabled students in South Africa. *South African Journal of Higher Education* **21**(4), 706–710.

Morina, A., Lopez-Gavira, R. & Molina, V. M. (2016). What if we could imagine an ideal university? Narratives by students with disabilities. *International Journal of Disability, Development and Education*. Retrieved from http://dx.doi.org/10.1080/1034912X.2016.1228856 on 8 August 2017.

Ohajunwa, C., McKenzie, J., Hardy, A. & Lorenzo, T. (2014). Inclusion of disability issues in teaching and research in higher education. *Perspectives in Education* **32**(3), 104–117.

Pretorius, A. & Lawton-Misra, N. (2011). Disability: continued marginalisation! *Paper presented at AFSAAP Africa Conference*, 30 November – 2 December 2011, Flinders University, Adelaide, Australia.

Pretorius, A. & Lawton-Misra, N. (2012). Adjustment to university and its psychological impact on disabled student. *Paper presented at the International Congress of Psychology (ICP) Conference*, 22–27 July 2012, Cape Town.

Pretorius, A. & Yates, D. (2014). Inclusion: mapping the achievements and challenges for students with disabilities in higher education. *Paper presented at the Bellavista Conference on Dyslexia*, February 2014, Johannesburg.

Pretorius, A., Yates, D., Ramaahlo, M. & Wolfensburger-Le Fevre, C. (2013). If Freud worked in a disability unit: perspectives from three disability units in Higher Education Institutions (HEIs). *Paper presented at the Psychological Society of South Africa Conference*, 24–27 September 2013, Johannesburg.

Shaw, S. F., Madaus, J. W. & Banerjee, M. (2009). Enhance access to postsecondary education for students with disabilities. *American Annals of the Deaf* **44**: 185–190.

South African Government (1996). *Constitution of the Republic of South Africa, 1996*. Retrieved from www.gov.za/sites/www.gov.za/files/images/a108-96.pdf on 20 March 2017.

South African Government (2017). *Disability Grant*. Retrieved from www.gov.za/services/social-benefits/disability-grant on 19 March 2017.

Swart, E. & Greyling, E. (2011). Participation in higher education: experiences of students with disabilities. *ActaAcademica* **43**(4), 81–110.

United Nations (2006). *The Convention on the Rights of Persons with Disabilities and Optional Protocol*. New York: United Nations. Retrieved from www.un.org/disabilities/documents/convention/convoptprot-e.pdf on 7 September 2016.

Waddell, G. & Aylward, M. (2010). *Models of Sickness and Disability Applied to Common Health Problems.* London: Royal Society of Medicine Press.

World Health Organization (2001). *International Classification of Functioning, Disability and Health.* Geneva: WHO.

World Health Organization & World Bank (2011). *World Report on Disability.* Geneva: WHO.

World Health Organization (2015). *Concept Note: Opening the GATE for Assistive Health Technology: Shifting the Paradigm.* Retrieved from www.who.int/phi/implementation/assistive_technology/concept_note.pdf on 20 March 2017.

World Health Organization (2016). *International Classification of Diseases.* Retrieved from http://apps.who.int/classifications/icd10/browse/2016/en on 29 August 2017.

PART IV

Disability, employment, entrepreneurship and CBR

Part IV presents employment and entrepreneurship issues affecting disabled people and the relevance of community-based rehabilitation in promoting sustainable development.

13

COMMUNITY-BASED REHABILITATION FOR INCLUSIVE SOCIAL DEVELOPMENT IN SOUTHERN AFRICA

Kayi Ntinda, Elias Mpofu, Helen Dunbar-Krige,
Messiah R. Makuane and Veronica I. Umeasiegbu

Introduction

Persons with disabilities face numerous social and economic barriers to participation in typical community activities (World Health Organization [WHO] & World Bank, 2011). They experience significant human development challenges from social stigma, prejudice, discrimination, poverty, lack of access to health services, including rehabilitation, education and workforce participation (van Rooy *et al*, 2012; Eide *et al*, 2015). This is particularly the case in the countries of the Southern African Development Community (SADC), which has comparatively lower resources for disability social inclusion. Citizens with disabilities from the SADC member countries are at elevated risk for social exclusion and poverty compared to non-disabled others from the impact of the underdevelopment of the SADC national economies on the availability of disability-inclusive programmes and services. For instance, less than 10% of children living with disabilities in developing or emerging countries have access to education making it very unlikely they will achieve the human development index criterion of being knowledgeable (International Disability Alliance [IDA], 2010). The reciprocal relationship between disability and poverty is well established (Hoogeveen, 2005; Coleridge, 2007; Filmer, 2008; Mitra & Sambamoorthi, 2008; Croft, 2010; Groce *et al*, 2011; Mitra, Posarac & Vick, 2011; Mpofu *et al*, 2017). This is explained by the fact that poverty is likely to result from lack of education, social marginalisation and barriers to employment (Hartley *et al*, 2009). Unmitigated poverty would make it unlikely for citizens to meet the human development index criteria of healthy living and a satisfying quality of life. In order to end the poverty–disability cycle among persons with disabilities there is need for their inclusion in all aspects of society and in every development initiative or activity in the SADC region (Miles, 1996; Lang, 2009; Mitra *et al*, 2011).

We consider community-based rehabilitation (CBR) as a disability-inclusive approach for sustainable community development. First, the chapter begins with a review of disability prevalence in some SADC member countries. It defines the concept of disability inclusivity for sustainable development. Next, the chapter addresses conceptions of inclusive CBR from the WHO (2003, 2010a, 2010b) perspective. In doing so, the chapter considers CBR for sustainable community development with illustrative examples from some SADC countries. Moreover, it makes the argument for CBR programmes to be expanded, strengthened and used as a service delivery model for persons with disabilities. The chapter also discusses issues prospective to CBR for inclusive social development in the SADC region. Finally, the chapter concludes with suggestions for enhanced disability-inclusive community development in the SADC region for poverty reduction.

Disability prevalence

About 15–25 million southern African citizens have some form of impairments, making persons with disabilities the largest minority population group in the region (United Nations Secretary General, 2009). For example, according to the 2011 Botswana national census about 2.9% (59,103) of the country's estimated total population of two million people have a form of impairment (Republic of Botswana, 2011; Hlalele *et al*, 2014). Statistics South Africa (2015) estimated the mid-year national population as 54.96 million, with about 2.9 million or 7.5% of the population being persons with disabilities. In Swaziland, the national population census was projected at 1,018,449 (Central Statistical Office Swaziland & Macro International, 2008). Accordingly, persons with disabilities in Swaziland are estimated at 16.8% of the population [171,347] (Mavundla, 2015).

Zambia, with a population of approximately 13 million, has approximately two million, which is 15% of the country's population, with disabilities as estimated by WHO and World Bank (2011). Lower estimates of the proportion of persons with disabilities in some SADC countries are likely to be from inadequate data collection or built-in limitations with the census surveys. All national and local government authorities in the SADC region subscribe to disability inclusion in development policies and across the political, economic, social and cultural life domains (United Nations, 2010). SADC national governments are also signatories to the Convention for Rights of Persons with Disabilities (CRPD) (United Nations, 2006) and the WHO Community-Based Rehabilitation Guidelines (WHO, 2010a, 2010b), which are disability-inclusive policy documents.

Disability inclusion

Disability inclusion is when persons with disabilities are engaged in ordinary activities of their communities in ways in which they self-perceive to be: (1) respected and appreciated as valuable members of their communities; (2) participating in recreational activities in their neighbourhood settings; (3) working at jobs in the community that pay a competitive wage and have careers that use their capacities to the fullest (Institute for Community Inclusion [ICI], 2016). Thus, disability inclusion has the potential of increasing community participation in socially expected life roles and activities of persons with disabilities. For example, disability inclusion makes it possible for persons with disabilities to benefit from the same health promotion and prevention activities as citizens without any impairment (Courtney-Long *et al*, 2014).

Where disability-inclusive policies are backed with implementation resources, CBR programmes have requisite monitoring and evaluation tools for them (Madden *et al*, 2013), as a development strategy aims to reduce socio-economic disparities in communities (Hartley, 2006; Kahonde, Mlenzana & Rhoda, 2010; Mpofu *et al*, 2017). Hence, the inclusion of persons with disabilities in poverty-reduction initiatives promotes equality, equity and improved economic wellbeing; thus, promoting sustainable community development (Mwendwa, Murangira & Lang, 2009; Mitra *et al*, 2011).

CBR as a disability-inclusive approach

The WHO (2003, 2010b) defined CBR as a strategy to ensure the full social and economic inclusion of people with disabilities with the same access to regular services and opportunities as their ordinary community members. CBR as a community-development approach includes people with disabilities in everyday activities of their communities and in roles similar to their counterparts without impairments (Centers for Disease Control and Prevention [CDCP], 2016). It includes people with disabilities in the mainstream activities and services as opposed to their community participation in separate facilities. By design, CBR programmes facilitate equal opportunities for access to education, employment and health services (including rehabilitation) to people with disabilities (Mpofu, 2004). For instance, about 80% of rehabilitation needs of people with disabilities could be addressed at community level. The remaining 20% are likely to need referral to some specialist facilities (Miles, 1996; Gel & Rule, 2008; Mpofu *et al*, 2011). Therefore, it is important to pull resources for community development for disability-inclusive collaborative partnerships from governments, non-governmental organisations and communities. These activities could include, for instance, education and counselling programmes that promote improved nutrition or reduce the use of alcohol or drugs. Disability-inclusive CBR aims to provide both opportunities and support for people with disabilities to participate in society on an equal basis with others members of their community (Chappell & Johannsmeier, 2009; WHO, 2010a) and in the context of mainstream development programmes, strategies and initiatives (Gel & Rule, 2008).

As a community-development strategy, CBR aligns with other global agendas that aim to address development and poverty to the current Sustainable Development Goals (SDGs) (Sachs, 2012). The SDGs aim at addressing all three dimensions of sustainable development (environmental, economic and social). Disability is referenced in numerous parts of the SDGs and specifically parts related to education, growth and employment, inequality, accessibility of human settlements, as well as data collection and monitoring. In line with the CBR guidelines, five key areas of socio-economic participation are critical to community development: health, education, livelihood, social and empowerment (WHO, 2010b). CBR activities aligned to each of these key areas of community living also serve to enhance success in related domains. For example, people with disability with education and health support are more likely to achieve superior livelihoods and social and economic empowerment.

Although CBR objectives have somewhat evolved over the decades following the seminal Alma-Ata declaration in 1978, it remains true to the aspirational goal of providing inclusive rehabilitation services 'close to people with disabilities, especially in low-income countries' (WHO, 2010b, p. 23). As noted previously, CBR aims at (1) meeting the basic needs of people with disabilities; (2) reduction of poverty; and (3) access to health, education, livelihood and social opportunities of people with disabilities (WHO, 2010b).

CBR principles are premised on supporting the human rights of individuals as outlined in the CRPD (United Nations, 2006). Thus, CBR (1) promotes and protects human rights; (2) creates equal opportunities; (3) makes the best use of scarce resources; (4) empowers individuals to take action to improve their own lives; and (5) facilitates access to relevant information and ideas from outside the community (Hartley *et al*, 2009; Kuipers & Doig 2010; WHO, 2010b; Harley *et al*, 2015). Such initiatives allow people with disabilities to be welcomed, valued and embraced as equal members of their communities. As previously discussed, disability inclusion is about placing disability issues and people with disabilities in the mainstream activities rather than as an afterthought (Kassah, 1998; Evans *et al*, 2001; Albert, Dube & Riis-Hansen, 2005; Mutepfa, Mpofu & Chataika, 2007).

Sustainable CBR programmes for social development are designed to last beyond the immediate life of the specific or individual community-development initiatives (Mpofu *et al*, 2017). Thus, sustainability is likely when CBR programmes are targeted at educating, empowering and equipping people with disabilities as allies in the community, resulting in improved quality of life. This is because CBR for sustainable development seeks to promote personal agency, accessibility to resources and opportunities for participation (Kuipers & Doig, 2010; Heinicke-Motsch, 2013).

CBR as a strategy for sustainable development seeks to create an enabling environment for people with disabilities to access education and training opportunities for micro and macro income-generation opportunities. In emerging or low-income countries, CBR for sustainable development engages disabled people's organisations (DPOs) at national and international levels when addressing discrimination and exclusion of people with disabilities from mainstream development programmes (Lang, 2011). Such strategies have the potential of realising the rights of people with disabilities and, eventually, improved community and national development participation (United Nations, 2006, 2011).

Also, disability-inclusive CBR for sustainable development entails ensuring that all marginalised and excluded groups are stakeholders in the development process. Currently, many groups are excluded from development in the SADC region due to gender, ethnicity, age, sexual orientation and impairment (Eide *et al*, 2015; Mpofu *et al*, 2017). The effects of such exclusion contribute to rising levels of inequality in the region. By implication, it becomes difficult to promote national development and poverty reduction unless all groups participate in national development through all-stakeholder decision-making processes. Thus, the need for disability-inclusive development in the SADC region through promoting inclusive societies, which embrace diversity, cannot be overemphasised.

Accessibility and disability inclusion within SADC countries

Lack of accessibility has been a major barrier to the participation of people with disabilities in the sustainable development of their communities (Schneider, 2006; Eide & Kamaleri, 2009; Eide & Jele, 2011; van Rooy *et al*, 2012; Eide *et al*, 2015). For instance, people with disabilities face barriers ranging from physical access to environmental and built structures, communication and programme design. Physical access here refers to the ability to use the built-in environment and other natural geo-structural amenities within the community (Rule, Lorenzo & Wolmarans, 2006).

Physical access challenges

People with disabilities in the rural SADC settings often find it difficult to move around their homes and communities due to inaccessible buildings and environments. They also experience difficulties accessing community facilities such as wells and latrines and they are often excluded from disaster management activities. Regardless of habitat (rural vs. urban), people with disabilities in the SADC region experience public transportation problems from lack of provision by governments and local authorities, which hampers their community participation on an equal footing with citizens (Mji *et al*, 2013). Poor environmental access by people with disabilities increases their risks for health challenges from poor sanitation and poor water quality within their communities. It also hampers access to educational opportunities. For instance, a person with disability who uses a wheelchair might be unable to attend school if it has no ramps for classroom access. Similarly, poor access to livelihood resources can seriously impair the quality of life of people with disabilities. Case study 13.1 is illustrative of the challenges people with disabilities encounter in a SADC country:

Case study 13.1 Donna

Donna is a 60-year-old South African woman with quadriplegia. She lives in a care home in Johannesburg, South Africa. All the inhabitants of the house need full-time care and support. Her disability pension does not cover all expenses and she cannot afford physiotherapy to alleviate the stiffness in her body. Donna would like to have access to public transport and be able to move around and be part of the local community. Unfortunately the public transport buses do not provide access to wheelchairs. Access to buildings is also often a problem. She uses her electric wheelchair to drive to church on the same road as cars as there are no pavements for her to drive on and she is in danger of being run over by a car or bus at any stage when she moves into the street.

Donna's case is typical of the experience of many people in SADC countries with musculo-skeletal conditions. They live with severe physical, financial and social limitations. Health care for people with disabilities in the SADC region is compromised due to limited or lack of funds targeting impairment-specific interventions. Mobility of people with disabilities is limited due to poor infrastructure, which does not accommodate assistive technology such as wheelchairs. This eventually limits their participation in social activities that are crucial for inclusion promotion (United Nations, 2006).

Communication access challenges

People with disabilities in the SADC countries experience significant communication access barriers in not having the same access to information in formats that can enhance their involvement in community activities (Scheer *et al*, 2003). Communication access barriers mean that people with disabilities experience limited participation, thus compromising their quality of life and engagement in community-development activities. Communication access is often difficult due to inaccessible information. For example, lack of sign-language interpreters in health and legal centres.

Social access challenges

People with disabilities from SADC countries experience social access challenges with accessing ordinary community services compared to their non-disabled peers (Smith *et al*, 2004; Kroll *et al*, 2006; Eide *et al*, 2015). Social access is about delivery of public services, facilities and amenities to intended user groups. Attitudes by service providers and community at large pre-vent people with disabilities from participating in community programmes for their social develop-ment. Case study 13.2 illustrates the social access difficulties people with disabilities and their families might experience.

Case study 13.2 Panga Muntu

Panga Muntu, a teenage Zambian girl, has cerebral palsy and multiple co-morbidities. She sought the services of a local health clinic, which was a one-hour drive each way. The clinic was the only health service provider in the district and for Panga Muntu to access it, required close family support and assistance; not only with the travel but talking to the rehabilitation services team about Panga Muntu's needs. They were concerned by her community social inclusion as a person with cerebral palsy living in a rural remote village. Panga Muntu's parents had experienced some communication difficulties with a staff person at the clinic and wanted to be assisted by someone different. Panga Muntu needed surgery to one of her legs to enhance her mobility. For that, she needed to attend pre-surgery clinic, tendon transfer surgery and follow-up appointments. Panga and her family did not know of anyone in the health service sector or organisation that would be of assistance. As a family, they lacked any preparatory education on resources from the public services they could access for Panga's health care consultations or appropriate assistive technology due to lack of occupational therapists and physiotherapists with expertise in wheelchair assessment and spasticity management in the vicinity.

Panga's case study is a clear example of how health care restrictions for people with disabilities in some SADC countries marginalise people with disabilities and their families. People with disabilities might need access to specialist management for co-morbidities and the requisite expertise is mostly lacking in most SADC countries (Kahonde *et al*, 2010). If available, it would be in distant urban centres and unaffordable to the typical people with disabilities.

Disability-inclusive social development programmes in SADC countries

There has been little evaluation of CBR services in the contexts of development policies in most SADC countries (Ndawi, 2000; Mpofu *et al*, 2007; Ngoma, 2007; Mji *et al*, 2013). However, many SADC countries appear to have elementary programmes for the full community inclusion of people with disabilities. For that reason, countries with relatively public or transparent accountability of national resources (e.g. Botswana, South Africa) have verifiable instruments for the practical implementation of the inclusive MDGs by state and regional governments compared to others with less transparent systems or failed economic policies (e.g. Lesotho, Malawi, Zimbabwe).

In the SADC region, disability-inclusive livelihood programmes typically include income-generating activities such as gardening or small land-holder farming arrangements. This is because most people from SADC countries earn their livelihood by working on the land carrying out subsistence farming (Devereux, 2002). Social protection programmes for people with disabilities are also widely utilised as livelihood support systems. These include social assistance in the form of cash transfers and food baskets and are increasingly recognised as important components of poverty reduction and development in low-income countries (Gooding & Marriot, 2009). For example, the Botswana government's social protection programme provides for cash transfer and food baskets to ensure food security of the people with severe impairments (Republic of Botswana, 2015). These social protection livelihood programmes are often means-tested. The South African government provides a disability grant for the purposes of assisting individuals with disabilities to afford basic amenities of living.

The criteria and eligibility for social protection programmes vary across SADC countries, and poorly designed social protection programmes may lack in disability inclusion by having the unintended effects of creating dependency. To minimise the risk of dependency, access must be flexible and participation in livelihood must be pivotal and central to increase self-sustenance and the resource base for the SADC region.

Families have been the linchpin of sustainable disability-inclusive CBR in the SADC region. For example, in Zambia, families have come together to form organisations such as the Association of the Parents for Children with Disabilities. This emerged with the mandate of overseeing issues affecting children with disabilities. Also there are the Zambian Association of Disabled Women and the Zambia Federation of Disability Organisations, which promote and advocate for the rights of people with disabilities in communities across the country (Zambia Federation of Disability Organisations, 1990).

In Zimbabwe, the Jairos Jiri Association and Council for the Blind provide vocational training for people with disabilities, with the intention of promoting self-sustenance (Jairos Jiri Association, 1996). The Botswana government has several disability-inclusive sustainable social development programmes (Republic of Botswana, 2002, 2013). An example is the Citizen Enterprise Development programme aimed at supporting citizens to develop small, medium and large scale enterprises with soft loans. Thus, the above programmes are intended to improve the livelihood of people with disabilities, although they encountered several challenges, including lack of funding.

The fragmentation of services for disability inclusion-oriented services has been a barrier to the success of CBR in the SADC region countries. In recognition of this limitation, the government of Botswana in 2009 established the office of the coordinator for disability at the Office of the President. This was done with the mission to coordinate the implementation of disability policy through development of strategies and programmes to empower people with disabilities.

In Swaziland, disability-inclusive social policies are sparsely developed and implemented. However, the Ministry of Health and Social Services oversees disability issues in the country through a national disability unit (Eide & Jele, 2011). The mandate of the unit is to prioritise important improvements in the standard of life for people with disabilities. Additionally, the Ministry of Home Affairs offers vocational rehabilitation services for inclusion of people with disabilities in the communities across the country.

The Government of Namibia developed a policy for mental health in 2004 (Ministry of Health and Social Services, 2004). The policy aimed at promoting participation, integration and equalisation of opportunities for people with disabilities in the country's disability-inclusion initiatives. In 2006, the Government of Malawi published the National Policy on Equalisation of Opportunities for People with Disabilities (NPEOD) (Ministry of Social Development and People with Disabilities, 2006). The NPEOD disability-inclusive policy's mandate is to promote the rights of people with disabilities to enable them to actively and fully participate in society.

The disability-inclusion regulatory policies in South Africa are the National Rehabilitation Policy (Department of Health, 2000), WHO Community-Based Rehabilitation Guidelines (WHO, 2010a, 2010b) and the CRPD (United Nations, 2006). The mandate of the polices and guidelines is to provide the goals for effective and accountable rehabilitation services that take into account the full participation of people with disabilities in planning, monitoring and evaluation of services for disability inclusion (Mji *et al*, 2013). Additionally, organisations such as the National Council for People with Physical Disabilities in South Africa run services and advocacy programmes to support the integration of people with disabilities in society and help them gain more independence. South Africa raises awareness of the rights of people with disabilities annually between 3 November and 3 December, the practical benefit of which, for people with disabilities, is unknown (Mji *et al*, 2013).

Family carers are generally the major contributors to the care and support of people with disabilities in SADC countries. Families are typically the ones to initiate and facilitate access to all health care and social services for their members with disability. Family carers themselves can develop secondary health conditions from their carer roles as well as social exclusion caused by the demands of caring for a member with disability with little support by the public welfare programmes. For instance, back problems are particularly prevalent in carers of people with significant physical disabilities, and stress-related illnesses are also common. Exclusion from, or lack of availability of, services causes additional strains on health and wellbeing. Effective support for family carers is crucial to ensure that their own health needs are met which also would enhance the social access and development of their members with disability (Caldwell, 2008; Ntinda & Nkwanyana, 2017). This would require the development and implementation of individual health care and social protection management plans in conjunction with patients, their families and/or social workers. These support systems are either solely lacking in many SADC countries or, if in place, they are poorly implemented due to lack of resource allocation by the national governments (Mji *et al*, 2013; Ndawi, 2002).

SADC country citizens with age-related impairments are among the most vulnerable to social exclusion and marginalisation (United Nations, 2010; United National Development Programme, 2015; Gretschel, 2016) as illustrated in case study 13.3.

Case study 13.3   Mr Boyi Zwelibanzi

Mr Boyi Zwelibanzi is a 90-year-old Zimbabwean male with chronic chest pain in geriatric care. Due to severe thrombocytopenia from African indigenous herbal medication, he could not be treated with anti-coagulation when he initially went to the local health centre with a clinical record that parts of his heart system were dying (ST elevation myocardiac infarction). However, supportive care with anti-platelets helped sustain his circulation although his physical endurance deteriorated significantly. To make matters worse, Mr Boyi Zwelibanzi had hospital-acquired pneumonia (HAP), which further debilitated him. His family (wife and daughter) had him admitted to the district hospital and had complaints including delay in changing incontinence aids during ongoing diarrhoea exacerbated by taking antibiotics. With improved function, Mr Zwelibanzi was regarded by the treatment team to be safe to be discharged home with family care. However, there was fierce resistance from his family who believed that Mr Zwelibanzi was being discharged home to die. The family expected and demanded functional recovery to pre-morbid state. Understandably, they had difficulty in adjusting to Mr Zwelibanzi's illness as he had been healthy and independent up until chest congestion complaints at the age of 90.

Incomplete communication by the treatment team was an issue for the family to be better prepared to provide home-based care for their elderly family member. For instance, family members were not consulted about treatment decisions and goals or about the irreversibility of ischaemic damage so they could accept the medical condition. Thus, adoption of guiding principles in dealing with family concerns for the support of members with disabilities by SADC national governments, including communication access with appropriate disclosure, commitment to positive social outcomes, responsiveness, transparency and accountability, would go a long way to the inclusive social development of people with disabilities in the sub-region.

Furthermore, there is lack of knowledge about disability issues among decision makers in most SADC countries which perpetuates the social exclusion of people with disabilities from mainstream community programmes, adding to the poverty–disability cycle among this population (Miji *et al*, 2013; Mitra, 2004). Case study 13.4 is illustrative of the lack of knowledge about disability issues by an educator.

Case study 13.4 Mainstreaming girls with mobility impairments

Three girls with mobility impairments attended an ordinary South African primary school. They were between 8 and 9 years of age and attending Grade 3. For a certain period each morning, the class would stand and recite poems and times tables. All three girls had physical impairments that made it difficult for them to stand. For this reason, the principal of the school allowed these three girls to sit and do the recitations. However, the class teacher refused to allow the girls to sit. Unfortunately, during the recitations, one or more of the girls would fall over and the other children in the class would laugh. The teacher punished these girls for not standing by threatening to send them to a special school. The principal became aware of the problem when one of the girls came to complain about the teacher. The principal initiated a workshop for all teachers in the school to address the attitudes of teachers toward learners with disabilities. The workshop also provided information that enabled teachers to understand the impact of impairments on children.

Thus, people with disabilities may be mistreated by people in leadership positions because they do not have an understanding of the disability issues. There is need to create awareness among communities and decision makers on the rights of people with disabilities and how to better include them in activities in communities without embarrassing them. Creation of awareness on rights and advocacy by people with disabilities will allow for their issues to be prioritised and thus promote their inclusion in their communities and beyond.

Summary and conclusion

CBR is a widely adopted strategy by SADC countries for providing opportunities for people with disabilities and their families in mainstream activities to live meaningful lives. However, its implementation is patchy and seriously under-resourced as reflected in the presented case studies. Consequently, livelihood support of people with disabilities, including social protection programmes is often inadequate. For these reasons, people with disabilities are denied their human rights as well as equal opportunities to participate and contribute to their societies. Furthermore, legislative and programmatic interventions for the social development inclusion of people with disabilities in the region are under-developed on a daily basis. The resourcing of CBR for sustainable development in the SADC region requires inter-organisational, intra-organisational and social organisation for the appropriation of national resources, which prioritise the interests and wellbeing of average citizens (including people with disabilities). Lessons on inclusive community development from some SADC countries suggest that successful CBR implementation depends on the extent to which the appropriation of national resources prioritises the interests and wellbeing of ordinary citizens.

Reflective questions

1 Define CBR and its requirements for successful implementation in a community you are familiar with.
2 What is disability-inclusive social development? Discuss strategies of inclusive social development that would optimise the livelihood of people with disabilities.
3 Outline three types of access that need to be addressed for disability-inclusive development?
4 With reference to your context, how might government and civic community organisations partner for disability-inclusive community development?

References

Albert, B., Dube, A. K. & Riis-Hansen, T. C. (2005). *Has Disability Been Mainstreamed into Development Cooperation?* Disability KaR Programme: UK.
Caldwell, J. (2008). Health and access to health care of female family caregivers of adults with developmental disabilities. *Journal of Disability Policy Studies* **19**(2), 68–79.
Census (2011). *Profile of People with Disabilities in South Africa Report.* Pretoria: Statistics Office.
Centers for Disease Control and Prevention (2016). *CDC 24/7: Saving Lives, Protecting People.* Retrieved from www.cdc.gov.ncbddd/disabilityandhealth/disability-inclusion.htm on 29 August 2016.
Central Statistical Office Swaziland & Macro International (2008). *Swaziland Demographic and Health Survey.* Mbabane: Central Statistical Office.
Chappell, P. & Johannsmeier, C. (2009). The impact of CBR as implemented by community rehabilitation facilitators on people with disabilities, their families and communities in South Africa. *Disability and Rehabilitation* **31**, 7–13.
Coleridge, P. (2007). *Economic Empowerment: Disability and Inclusive Development.* London: Leonard Cheshire International.
Courtney-Long, E., Stevens, A., Caraballo, R., Ramon, I. & Armour, B. S. (2014). Disparities in current cigarette smoking prevalence by type of disability, 2009–2011. *Public Health Reports* **129**(3), 252–260.
Croft, A. (2010). Including Disabled Children in Learning: Challenges in Developing Countries. CREATE Pathways to Access. *Research Monograph No. 36.*
Department of Health (2000). *Rehabilitation for All: National Rehabilitation Policy.* Pretoria: Government Printers.
Devereux, S. (2002). Can social safety nets reduce chronic poverty? *Development Policy Review* **20**(5), 657–675.
Eide, A. H. & Jele, B. (2011). Living conditions among people with disabilities in Swaziland: a national, representative study. *SINTEF Report No. A 20047.* Oslo: SINTEF.
Eide, A. H. & Kamaleri, Y. (2009). Living conditions among people with disabilities in Mozambique: a national representative study. *SINTEF Report No. A 9348.* Oslo: SINTEF.
Eide, A. H., Mannan, H., Khogali, M., Van Rooy, G., Swartz, L., Munthali, A., *et al.* (2015). Perceived barriers for accessing health services among individuals with disability in four African countries. *PLoS One* **10**(5), e0125915.
Evans, P. J., Zinkin, P., Harpham, T. & Chaudury, G. (2001). Evaluation of medical rehabilitation in community based rehabilitation. *Social Science & Medicine* **53**(3), 333–348.
Filmer, D. (2008). Disability, poverty, and schooling in developing countries: results from 14 household surveys. *The World Bank Economic Review* **22**(1), 141–163.
Gel, H. F. & Rule, S. (2008). Integrating community-based rehabilitation and leprosy rehabilitation services into an inclusive development approach. *Leprosy Review* **79**, 83–91.
Gooding, K. & Marriot, A. (2009). Including persons with disabilities in social cash transfer programmes in developing countries. *Journal of International Development* **21**(5), 685–698.
Gretschel, D. (2016). *Levels of Community Integration Achieved by Adults with Disabilities Post Discharge from a Specialised In-patient Rehabilitation Unit in the Western Cape.* Unpublished PhD Thesis, Stellenbosch University, Stellenbosch.
Groce, N. E., Kembhavi, G., Wirz, S., Lang, R., Trani, J. F. & Kett, M. (2011). Poverty and Disability: A Critical Review of the Literature in Low and Middle-income Countries. *Leonard Cheshire Disability and Inclusive Development Centre Working Paper Series 16.* London: Leonard Cheshire Disability.

Harley, D., Mpofu, E., Scanlan, J., Umeasiegbu, V. I. & Mpofu, N. (2015). Disability social inclusion and community health. In E. Mpofu (ed.) *Community-oriented Health Services: Practices across Disciplines* (pp. 207–222). New York: Springer.

Hartley, S. (2006). *CBR as Part of Community Development: A Poverty Reduction Strategy.* London: University College London/Centre for International Child Health.

Hartley, S., Finkenflugel, H., Kuipers, P. & Thomas, M. (2009). Community-based rehabilitation: opportunity and challenge. *The Lancet* **374**(9704), 1803.

Heinicke-Motsch, K. (2013). Community-based rehabilitation: an effective strategy for rights-based, inclusive community development. In G. Musoke & P. Geiser (eds) *Linking CBR, Disability and Rehabilitation* (pp. 18–23). Kyambogo University, Uganda: CBR Africa Network.

Hlalele, T. R., Adeola, R., Okeowo, A., Muleta, D. B. & Njiti, L. U. (2014). Country report: Botswana. *African Disability Rights Year Book* **2**, 151–226.

Hoogeveen, J. G. (2005). Measuring welfare for small but vulnerable groups: poverty and disability in Uganda. *Journal of African Economies* **14**(4), 603–631.

Institute for Community Inclusion (2016). *Promoting the Inclusion of People with Disabilities: What We Mean When We Talk about Inclusion.* Boston: University of Massachusetts.

International Disability Alliance (2010). '*Overcoming Invisibility: Making the MDGs Inclusive of and Accessible for People with Disabilities*'. Contributions to informal interactive hearings of the General Assembly with non-governmental organisations, civil society organisations and private sector, 14–15 June 2010. Retrieved from www.internationaldisabilityalliance.org/resources/overcoming-invisibility-making-mdgs-inclusive-and-accessible-persons-disabilities on 12 September 2016.

Jairos Jiri Association (1996). *External Evaluation Report.* Jairos Jiri Association Headquarters, Bulawayo.

Kahonde, C. H., Mlenzana, N. C. & Rhoda, A. (2010). A people with physical disabilities' experiences of rehabilitation services at community health centres in South Africa. *South African Journal of Physiotherapy* **66**(2), 1–6.

Kassah, A. K. (1998). Community-based rehabilitation and stigma management by physically disabled people in Ghana. *Disability and Rehabilitation* **20**(2), 66–73.

Kroll, T., Jones, G. C., Kehn, M. & Neri, M. T. (2006). Barriers and strategies affecting the utilisation of primary preventive services for people with physical disabilities: a qualitative inquiry. *Health & Social Care in the Community* **14**(4), 284–293.

Kuipers, P. & Doig, E. (2010). Community-based rehabilitation. *International Encyclopaedia of Rehabilitation [serial online].* Retrieved from http://cirrie.buffalo.edu/encyclopedia/en/article/362 on 16 January 2016.

Lang, R. (2009). The United Nations Convention on the Right and Dignities for Persons with Disability: a panacea for ending disability discrimination? *ALTER-European Journal of Disability Research/Revue Européenne de Recherche sur le Handicap* **3**(3), 266–285.

Lang, R. (2011). Community-based rehabilitation and health professional practice: developmental opportunities and challenges in the global North and South. *Disability and Rehabilitation* **33**(2), 165–173.

Madden, R., Hartley, S., Mpofu, E. & Baguwemu, A. (2013). The ICF as a tool to support **CBR** planning and management. In G. Musoke & P. Geiser (eds) *Linking CBR, Disability and Rehabilitation* (pp. 72–89). Bangalore: Africa Network.

Mavundla, S. D. (2015). Country report: Swaziland. *African Disability Rights Year Book* **3**, 245–264. Retrieved from http://dx.doi.org/10.17159/2413-7138/2015/v3n1a11 on 8 August 2017.

Miles, S. (1996). Engaging with the Disability Rights Movement: the experience of community-based rehabilitation in southern Africa. *Disability & Society* **11**(4), 501–518.

Ministry of Health and Social Services (2004). *National Policy on Mental Health.* Windhoek: MoHSS.

Ministry of Social Development and People with Disability (2006). *National Policy on Equalisation of Opportunities for People with Disabilities.* Lilongwe: Ministry of Social Development and People with Disability.

Mitra, S. (2004). Viewpoint: disability – the hidden side of African poverty. *Disability World.*

Mitra, S. & Sambamoorthi, U. (2008). Disability and the rural labor market in India: evidence for males in Tamil Nadu. *World Development* **36**(5), 934–952.

Mitra, S., Posarac, A. & Vick, B. C. (2011). Disability and poverty in developing countries: a snapshot from the World Health Survey. *Social Protection Discussion Paper No. 1109*, World Bank. Retrieved from http://siteresources.worldbank.org/SOCIALPROTECTION/Resources/SP-Discussion-papers/Disability-DP/1109.pdf on 14 August 2017.

Mji, G., Chappell, P., Statham, S. B., Mlenzana, N., Goliath, C., De Wet, C. & Rhoda, A. (2013). Understanding the current discourse of rehabilitation: with reference to disability models and rehabilitation policies for evaluation research in the South African setting. *South African Journal of Physiotherapy*, **69**(2), 4–9, doi:10.4102/sajp.v69i2.22.

Mpofu, E. (2004). Learning through inclusive education: practices with students with disabilities in sub-Saharan Africa. In C. de la Rey, L. Schwartz & N. Duncan (eds) *Psychology: An Introduction* (pp. 361–371). Cape Town: Oxford University Press.

Mpofu, E., Jelsma, J., Maart, S., Levers, L. L., Montsi, M. M., Tlabiwe, P., *et al.* (2007). Rehabilitation in seven sub-saharan African countries: personnel education and training. *Rehabilitation Education* **21**(4), 15–32.

Mpofu, E., Levers, L. L., Makuwire, J., Mpofu, K. & Mamboleo, G. (2017). Community-based rehabilitation in sub-Saharan Africa. In A. Abubakar & F. van de Vijver (eds) *Handbook of Applied Developmental Science in Sub-Saharan Africa* (pp. 335–345), New York: Springer.

Mpofu, E., Ukasoanya, G., Mupawose, A., Harley, D., Charema, J. & Ntinda, K. (2011). Counseling people with disabilities. In E. Mpofu (ed.) *Counseling People of African Ancestry* (pp. 294–309). New York: Cambridge University Press.

Mutepfa, M. M., Mpofu, E. & Chataika, T. (2007). Inclusive education in Zimbabwe: policy, curriculum, practice, family, and teacher education issues. *Childhood Education* **83**(6), 342–346.

Mwendwa, T. N., Murangira, A. & Lang, R. (2009). Mainstreaming the rights of persons with disabilities in national development frameworks. *Journal of International Development*, **21**(5), 662–672.

Ndawi, O. P. (2000). The role of legislation in facilitating CBR in Zimbabwe. In S. Hartley (ed.) *Community-based Rehabilitation (CBR) as a Participatory Strategy in Africa* (pp. 97–105). New York: Cornell University Press, New York.

Ngoma, M. S. (2007). *An Overview of Rehabilitation Services in Zambia*. Unpublished manuscript.

Ntinda, K. & Nkwanyana, S. (2017). Resources for resilient caregiving by parents of children with schizophrenia in Swaziland: a multiple case study. *Journal of Psychology in Africa*, **27**(1), 88–92.

Republic of Botswana (2002). *Revised National Policy on Destitute Persons*. Gaborone: Government Printer.

Republic of Botswana (2009). *Guidelines for Livestock Management and Infrastructure Development Programme Phase 11*. Gaborone: Ministry of Agriculture.

Republic of Botswana (2011). *Population & Housing Census: Preliminary Results Brief*. Statistics, Gaborone.

Republic of Botswana (2013). *Guidelines for Integrated Support Programme for Arable Agriculture Development (ISPAAD)*. Gaborone: Ministry of Agriculture.

Republic of Botswana (2015). *Disability Cash Transfer Guidelines*. Gaborone: Ministry of Local Government and Rural Development.

Rule, S., Lorenzo, T. & Wolmarans, M. (2006). Community-based rehabilitation: new challenges. In B. Watermeyer, L. Swartz, T. Lorenzo, M. Schneider & M. Priestley (eds) *Disability and Social Change: A South African Agenda* (pp. 273–290). Pretoria: HSRC Press.

Sachs, J. D. (2012). From millennium development goals to sustainable development goals. *The Lancet* **379**(9832), 2206–2211.

Scheer, J., Kroll, T., Neri, M. T. & Beatty, P. (2003). Access barriers for persons with disabilities: the consumer's perspective. *Journal of Disability Policy Studies* **13**(4), 221–230.

Schneider, M. (2006). Disability and the environment. In B. Watermeyer, L. Swartz, T. Lorenzo, M. Schneider & M. Priestley (eds) *Disability and Social Change: A South African Agenda* (pp. 8–18). Pretoria: HSRC Press.

Smith, E., Murray, S. F., Yousafzai, A. K. & Kasonka, L. (2004). Barriers to accessing safe motherhood and reproductive health services: the situation of women with disabilities in Lusaka, Zambia. *Disability and Rehabilitation* **26**(2), 121–127.

Statistics South Africa (2015). Mid-year population estimates. Pretoria, South Africa: Statistics South Africa.

United National Development Programme (2015). *Human Development Index Report*. Geneva: United Nations.

United Nations (2006). *Convention on the Rights of People with Disabilities and Its Optional Protocol*. Geneva: United Nations. Retrieved from www.un.org/disabilities/ on 12 October 2016.

United Nations (2010). *United Nations Enable Rights and Dignity of People with Disabilities: The Millennium Development Goals and Disability*. Retrieved from http://www.un.org/disabilities/default.asp?id=1470 on 18 October 2016.

United Nations (2011). *Disability and the Millennium Development Goals: A Review of the MDG Process and Strategies for Inclusion of Disability Issues in Millennium Development Goals Efforts.* New York: United Nations.

United Nations Secretary-General (2009). *Realizing the Millennium Development Goals for Persons with Disabilities through Implementation of World Programme of Action Concerning Disabled Persons and the Convention on Rights of Persons with Disabilities.* Report of the Secretary-General. A/64/180. General Assembly Distribution 27 July 2009. Retrieved from www.un.org/esa/socdev/documents/reports/MDG%20and%20Disability.pdf on 27 April 2018.

van Rooy, G., Amadhila, E. M., Mufune, P., Swartz, L., Mannan, H. & MacLachlan, M. (2012). Perceived barriers to accessing health services among people with disabilities in rural northern Namibia. *Disability & Society* **27**(6), 761–775.

World Health Organization (2003). *International Consultation to Review Community-based Rehabilitation CBR.* Helsinki, 25–28 May.

World Health Organization (2004). *CBR: A Strategy for Rehabilitation, Equalization of Opportunities, Poverty Reduction and Social Inclusion of People with Disabilities. Joint Position Paper 2004.* Geneva, Switzerland.

World Health Organization (2010a). *United Nations Educational, Scientific and Cultural Organization, International Labour Organization, International Disability and Development Consortium. Community-based rehabilitation: CBR guidelines.* Geneva: World Health Organization, 459–468.

World Health Organization (2010b). *Community-based Rehabilitation: CBR Guidelines: Towards Community-based Inclusive Development: Introductory Booklet.* Geneva, Switzerland.

World Health Organization and World Bank (2011). *World Report on Disability.* Geneva: WHO.

Zambia Federation of Disability Organisations (1990). *Midyear Report.* Lusaka: ZAFoD.

14

EMPLOYMENT, ENTREPRENEURSHIP AND SUSTAINABLE DEVELOPMENT ISSUES IN SOUTHERN AFRICA

John Charema

Introduction

Disabled people are greatly under-represented and disadvantaged in the workplace throughout the world. They often face discrimination by employers and, most of the time, are not effectively served by training institutions and vocational rehabilitation systems, whose primary purpose is to get disabled individuals to acquire the necessary skills and requisites for employment. Relevant equipment and qualified personnel to train disabled people in industrial vocational skills are often not a priority in many low-income countries, particularly in Africa where there is an acute shortage of financial resources (International Labour Organization [ILO], 2015; World Bank, 2014). Additionally, many disabled individuals face discrimination and/or fear of becoming a liability to business owners. It is southern African countries' responsibility to create entrepreneurship programmes for disabled people in order to counteract these barriers. In turn, this would promote empowerment and facilitate economic self-sufficiency for disabled people. Such programmes would include, among other skills, how to write business proposals and plans, company formation, business mentoring, technical assistance, start-up business grants, and assistance from a business incubator or advisor. In addition to the core programme components, there would be programme coordinators who monitor and evaluate project progress to ensure programme sustainability. The social and the eco-systematic models underpin the bases of the arguments in this chapter.

The current status of disabled people in low-income countries

Creating a world where everyone enjoys human rights, self-respect, equal opportunities, social inclusion and dignity, economic empowerment and many other rights, is an ideal situation that does not exist, particularly in the lives of disabled people. Hence, the need to create awareness and to empower all beings against any kind of abuse, through isolation, neglect, discrimination and denial of opportunities and resources by a society to a particular group just because the group is perceived as different. Disabled people, particularly in low-income countries, in some cases, have been ignored, abused, neglected and considered a burden to the society and they have not been able to enjoy any human rights (Craig & Bigby, 2010; Cox, 2012). Many have spent the best part of their lives in institutions, where conditions have not been the best, if not inhuman (Cox, 2012). Institutionalisation is not a phenomenon of the dim and far distant past at all. All over the world in both high- and low-income countries, as recently as the 19th and 20th centuries, disabled people were, and in some cases, are still ordered to live in institutions where, in some cases, they were/are often mistreated and denied the opportunity to make basic choices about how they live (International Labour Organization [ILO], 2011; Independent Living Institute, 2014). Thus, they lack control over the most basic aspects of their lives and have no freedom of movement. Before the 19th century, institutionalisation was considered the best option other than leaving disabled people in restricted homes where they were neglected and viewed as objects of pity. Grunewald (2003) asserts that although criticisms of residential care grew in the mid-19th century, there was ironically an expansion of segregation of disabled people, particularly in low-income countries. Up to the present moment most low-income countries, particularly in southern Africa, (Zimbabwe, Zambia, Malawi, Botswana) still have disabled people (mostly students) living in institutions, boarding and community homes (World Bank, 2014; United Nations, 2015). One example is the Jairos Jiri Association in Zimbabwe, which has a number of institutions running different programmes in different provinces of the country. However, with the dawn of civilisation, awareness and more education, inclusive and independent living, has become the ideal. The move toward widespread inclusive independent living in the community is a relatively recent development.

The present situation depicts high rates of unemployment in the Southern African Developing Community (SADC) countries, with Zimbabwe topping the list with an unemployment rate of 95%; Democratic Republic of Congo, 49%; Swaziland, 40%; and with Namibia, Angola, South Africa, Lesotho and Botswana ranging from 20% to 28% (WHO & World Bank, 2011; Chamberlin, 2014; World Bank, 2016). These are general unemployment rates for each country's population, including disabled people. Among the unemployed, disabled people are the most affected, with the highest percentage in both high- and low-income countries (United Nations, 2015; World Bank 2016). Those who are employed often suffer job insecurity (temporary work, irregular job availability or part-time work) and receive low income (Jang *et al.*, 2014). Most disabled people in southern African countries (for example, Zambia, Zimbabwe, Malawi, Lesotho, Swaziland and Namibia) live on handouts (World Bank, 2016). Those who try to engage in self-help activities find themselves competing with everybody else on the open market. Disabled people in these countries live in abject poverty and generally have low literacy levels such that they often resort to street begging as a means of survival, which is not sustainable. With limited skills due to either the impact of their impairment, poor or lack of training, lack of appropriate equipment to use and shortage of resources, they end up producing products that are of poor quality (ILO, 2011). When the products are of good quality sometimes they (disabled people) are short-changed and offered very little money which they only accept out of desperation.

According to the Independent Living Institute (2014), most low-income countries have extremely high levels of unemployment among disabled people, mostly attributed to: low skills level due to inadequate education; economic status of a country; discriminatory attitudes and practices; less habitable environments; ineffective employment policies;fewer enabling mechanisms to promote employment opportunities; inaccessible public transport; inadequate provision and poorly funded vocational training centres; inadequate access to information; and ignorance in society. It is most likely that dependency dis-empowers disabled people and isolates them from the mainstream of society, preventing them from accessing fundamental social, political and economic rights.

The challenge today continues to be the marginalisation of disabled people in many spheres of life, from employment to education to the allocation of resources such as housing and land. In a study conducted by Mitra *et al.* (2012) in 30 low-income and 40 high-income countries, research results indicate that in both cases the majority of disabled people had significantly lower educational attainment and lower employment rates than non-disabled persons. In Zimbabwe, a survey on living conditions established lower literacy rate among disabled people when compared with non-disabled people (UNICEF, 2013). The survey also established similar trends on access to health, education, information and other related facilities and services. Furthermore, in the majority of countries, the difference in employment rates is worse for disabled people due to lack of necessary skills, funding, access to information or networking opportunities (Mitra *et al.*, 2012).

Those who are involved in community-based rehabilitation (CBR) programmes are much better off in the sense that they are in a community and are fully included, involved and engaged in the natural day-to-day routine life. Research shows that what disabled people need most is to earn a living and live a natural 'independent life' (Cox, 2012; Craig & Bigby, 2014; Independent Living Institute, 2014). A change is needed for the betterment of disabled people and this can only be achieved by change of attitude, implementing inclusive education and redesigning our training and vocational centres to equip them with the necessary skills for entrepreneurship.

Policy initiatives

While the political and policy implications for disabled people from the CRPD (United Nations, 2006) are favourable, low-income countries experience different challenges that include, among others, civil wars, social and economic factors and unequal distribution of already limited resources. Such factors limit the progress of employment and business opportunities for disabled people. Majola and Dhunpath (2016) claim that the employment of disabled people has been challenged, slowed down and hampered by the slow development of policies regarding their employment in South Africa. Where policies are available they seem to be either silent or vague and lack specificity when it comes to the employment of disabled people. Most countries have well-documented policies sitting on shelves which are rarely implemented, maybe due to lack of resources or will power.

Legislation and a number of laws and Acts in Zambia and Zimbabwe for example, articulate inclusion in terms of employment, self-employment and entrepreneurship programmes, unfortunately with no implementation of policies (ILO, 2015). The focus has been on inclusive education and formulating legislation to encourage and implement inclusion in almost every country, unfortunately at the expense of policies that pinpoint and give direction on what to do concerning the employment of disabled people. In their research on workplace accommodations in the United States of America, Vedeler and Schreuer (2011) interviewed 29 employed Americans and Norwegians with mobility impairments. They noted similarities and differences in experiences with accommodation provision. As a whole, the results indicate that most obstacles were from the employer or agent who slowed down the process. Similarly, in low-income countries, sometimes the process of employing or providing for disabled people is chocked or blocked by corrupt officials who buy time and eventually divert resources meant for disabled people elsewhere.

Most disabled people were politically and technically excluded from the land redistribution exercise, which benefited 'most' Zimbabweans. It appears disabled people, especially the youths, did not benefit from the youth fund disbursed by the Zimbabwe government for entrepreneurship development (Mpofu & Shumba, 2013). Also, the authors indicated that most disabled youths did not know about the entrepreneurial policies in their country and those who were involved had poor business networking. The country, for a long time, did not have a financial inclusion policy, but there is now a national financial inclusion strategy of 2016. However, the challenge is on the extent to which the policy is being translated into practice as this has been a challenge in most low-income countries as disability issues seem not to be on their priority list (WHO & World Bank, 2011). Disabled people have, for a long period, been regarded as benevolence recipients without enjoying their rights like their non-disabled counterparts.

Jang *et al.* (2014) point out that effective disability policies and proper implementation could reduce public expenditure and disability benefits in countries where disabled people are offered benefits. In their study, carried out in South Africa, Dubihlela and Rundora (2014) indicate that poverty was increasing and spreading despite the expansion of expenditure on grants in terms of what was distributed to those already identified, which included disabled people and the new poor who joined the list. Typically, the point in question is what should be done to reduce poverty where unemployment is looming among disabled people? One possible solution is for government policies to embrace and point toward entrepreneurship. If developing countries could purposely formulate, support, drive and implement policies that encourage entrepreneurship with a bias for disabled people, social and economic sustainability could be achieved. It is time to change and make sure that policies are specific and clearly articulate what should be done to accommodate and provide resources for small businesses for disabled people.

It is very clear that in low-income countries, particularly in sub-Saharan Africa, provision for disabled people and the poor has never been adequate to sustain them (WHO & World Bank, 2011; World Bank, 2016; United Nations, 2015; Majola & Dhunpath, 2016). It would appear that the national cake in developing countries is shrinking while the population of the poor and disabled people is increasing. A study conducted by the Independent Living Institute in South Africa (2015) estimates that 99% of disabled people in South Africa have no job and depend on social security benefits for survival purposes. In Zimbabwe the ever increasing and looming number of disabled people seen begging in Harare and other cities bears testimony to the high rate of unemployment.

According to WHO and World Bank (2011), more than one billion of the world's population live with some form of impairment. The real number could be much higher since most low-income countries do not have the capacity and resources to carry out research regularly for reliable statistics. While the issue of employment for disabled people has received considerable attention in theory worldwide, the implementation and practical aspect remains at a considerable remote distance. Hence, the call for entrepreneurship programmes for disabled people.

Policy developments affect employment prospects for disabled people. Therefore, policymakers are encouraged to formulate policies that promote business creation for disabled people and cite any success stories (Avendano & Berkman, 2014). Such examples might inspire other disabled people to become entrepreneurs and demonstrate that business creation and self-employment can be achieved. Successful entrepreneurs and self-employed disabled people can be included in broader awareness and promotional campaigns related to entrepreneurship and self-employment. This would not only benefit disabled individuals, but also serve to address negative stereotypes and societal attitudes toward disability (European Union, 2014). Governmental departments in both low-income and high-income countries need to continuously monitor, assess and update employment policies that deal with work-related accommodations, accessibility, work environment and fair practices. Once favourable policies that promote the advancement and creation of employment for disabled people are put in place, the role of governmental institutions is to monitor and enforce implementation.

Educational institutions

The education system in every country should remain relevant to support the economic needs of that country through different sectors of the industry. Sound educational policies backed by the development of fine-tuned, health, industrial and technological practical skills promote development, sustainability and better living conditions for all citizens, including disabled people.

187

Educational institutions should embrace the ideology of inclusion, and focus on the demands of different industrial sectors and community participation, in order to offer relevant and useful educational skills. The use of flexible teaching methods and employing more training and practical activities would accommodate different learning styles for disabled people. It is of paramount importance that educational institutions focus on education for sustainability, changing students' mind sets from being educated to be employed to being educated to employ. Therefore, there is a need for a shift from teaching students a lot of outdated theory that has very little to do with development, to practical knowledge that creates opportunities for employment. While there are particular students who take subjects for entrepreneurship, exposure of every student to the business world would prepare them for real-life situations. Sustainability and self-reliance should be at the core of every education system to promote political, social and economic freedom. Disabled students should be equipped with skills that prepare them for social inclusion, accommodations, workplace environment management, adaptations and adjustments in order to participate and function effectively (Caldwell *et al.*, 2016). Realistic education should help disabled people understand limitations imposed by their impairments and also their strengths in order for them to make informed decisions and choices about employment and entrepreneurship, if they want to venture into business. It is through positive teaching that disabled students develop the confidence to be entrepreneurs.

Education should promote in students creativity, innovation and enterprising minds that further promote implementation. The new Zimbabwe curriculum framework (2015–22) has entrepreneurship and business components to be taught to all learners including learners going through the Life Skills Orientation Programme (Ministry of Primary & Secondary Education, 2015). This is a very positive development. However, such developments can only be successful to serve all people if the curriculum is inclusive and stipulates the transition path for all learners with different types of impairments into adulthood and employment.

Entrepreneurship could be one of the most important programmes run in high schools, colleges, vocational training centres and other tertiary institutions to prepare students for the business world. If disabled students are exposed early to entrepreneurship programmes, when it comes to taking up small businesses, they are likely to be ready and confident. Entrepreneurship education might be the solution to the problem of unemployment for disabled people. Youth could be taught and prepared through real-life situations and experiences to be responsible, accountable, disciplined and enterprising, such that they can become entrepreneurial thinkers who can take risks, manage the results and learn from the outcomes (ILO, 2009). For disabled youth to be fully included in entrepreneurship education programmes, it is important to consider accommodations and financial resources. Governments can commit themselves fully and support such programmes, which could be a huge saving in the future as compared to providing handouts (which are not easy to come by in low-income countries). Entrepreneurship could be made as practical as possible to allow all disabled students to be involved.

The government could set up a fund to support students doing practical and business subjects at secondary and tertiary levels. A practical subject levy could be charged to promote the development of future business in the making. Students could fund their projects by making and designing different furniture or clothing articles, which they advertise, and sell to the community. They would have among them persons that do sales, marketing, book keeping and accounting as part of preparing them for entrepreneurship in future. They could also be allowed to run small tuck shops, keep chickens, rabbits, and many other viable projects. Students would learn in real-life situations. At adult and employment levels, disabled youths could be given their quarter of funding and some grants to pay back with the establishment of the businesses. Mentoring and monitoring could be done continuously to ensure good returns and success in the businesses.

Self-employment and entrepreneurship

Disabled people, on average, are more likely to experience adverse socio-economic outcomes than non-disabled persons, such as lower rates of education, worse health outcomes, less employment, and higher poverty levels (World Bank, 2011). Disability is both a cause and an effect of poverty. According to the ILO (2011), poor people are likely to acquire impairments because of the conditions in which they live. Hence, when their impairments interact with disability conditions, they are also likely to result in poverty due to limited opportunities for skills development and employment. To change the economic landscape for disabled people, considering the barriers they experience, possible viable options are self-employment and entrepreneurship.

Before embarking on entrepreneurship for disabled people, it is important to make a distinction between self-employment and entrepreneurship. Renko *et al.* (2016) posit that self-employment is creating a job for a particular individual with the goal of becoming financially self-reliant. They go on to point out that in the business literature self-employment is considered to be an alternative to salary or wage toward employment. Entrepreneurship is starting one's own business with the hope of making profit and expanding to the point of even hiring other people to work on the company, thus creating employment (Renko *et al.*, 2016). Basically, self-employment is employing oneself and entrepreneurship is creating a business that one owns, manages, expands if possible, employs workers and makes profit. However, for the purposes of this chapter, both are under discussion for the sustainable development of disabled people. In most southern African countries, a greater percentage of people, including people with disabilities, are self-employed mostly in sheltered workshops, at bus ranks, designated market places, edges of town buildings where they sell a variety of commodities, including food. Self-employment and entrepreneurship are possible ways of securing employment and self-sustainability. Entrepreneurship has the potential to further significantly reduce poverty and create employment for many people.

Typically, entrepreneurship has the potential to address the challenges of unemployment and under-employment that further impoverishes disabled people (Renko *et al.*, 2016). Disabled people represent a significant percentage of the working-age population, which makes employment for disabled people a cause for concern and a key issue (Majola & Dhunpath, 2016; Mitra *et al.*, 2012). There is research evidence suggesting that the percentage of unemployed disabled people is much higher than that of unemployed non-disabled people (Majola & Dhunpath, 2016). Despite gazetted legislation and labour laws that encourage employing disabled people in most sub-Saharan countries, there continue to be fewer employment opportunities and no guarantees of any positive changes (WHO & World Bank, 2011; Majola & Dhunpath, 2016). It is against this background that low-income countries should change their mind sets, help set up, support and encourage, entrepreneurship for disabled people. Entrepreneurs who partnered and purposed to engage disabled people experienced positive benefits morally, financially and socially (ILO, 2011). At the same time, disabled employees can help the community and enterprises understand and meet the needs of a wider and important increasing customer population of disabled people and their families. Of interest is the fact that research (European Union, 2014; Independent Living Institute, 2014) indicates that customers, both disabled and non-disabled, prefer to deal with businesses that employ a mixture of groups, whom they claim to have a better understanding of all types of different people in society, which gives them a competitive edge in today's world that advocates for inclusion.

Due to a variety of expertise, talent, innovation and experiences, disabled people are likely to produce quality products to prove a point, and can only be limited by society's perceptions of who society thinks they are (Renko *et al.*, 2016). Society's attitude toward disabled people can also change by recognising them as job creators and employers contributing to national development, and not as beggars who live on handouts. However, it does not pay just to set up entrepreneurship programmes without equipping disabled people with the necessary knowledge and skills to run successful businesses. In most low-income countries, entrepreneurship has not been a success (ILO, 2006). However, there have been sporadic individual success stories in some southern African countries and many others. Accordingly, in Malawi, there is an individual's company 'General Vision Screen Printers'; in South Africa, there is 'Motswako Office Systems'; in Namibia, a 'skincare business'; in Uganda, a number of retail trade businesses started well, but most of them closed due to a number of already cited reasons (Namatovu *et al.*, 2012; Entrepreneurs Malawi, 2015; United Nations, 2015; World Bank, 2014).

The same authors (Namatovu *et al.*, 2012) in the Trust Africa report further pointed out that within the body of literature on entrepreneurship there is little scholarly research on disabled entrepreneurs, despite a number of them being self-employed with some success in their businesses. It is interesting to note that there is increasing positive talk and written policies and programmes on and about entrepreneurship in almost all low-income countries. However, theoretical development in understanding the entrepreneurial environment, business ethics, knowledge on accountability and expansion of businesses, attitudes and growth aspirations and many other relevant factors are still lacking as illustrated in case study 14.1.

Case study 14.1   Kabelo Mahoso

Kabelo is a disabled 23-year-old Motswana lady, who received assistance from the government to start a Body Shop business. She is trained in beauty therapy and is confident that most young ladies will support her business. She set up her business in one of the shopping malls on the outskirts of Gaborone, the capital city of Botswana. Body Shop Beauty Queens as it is named, is a retail shop that sells beauty therapy products: which include, among other things, facials, soaps, perfumes, gels and many other related products. Kabelo does not have trained personnel because the business is not yet in a position to pay professional salaries. The business intends to offer top quality services and a friendly environment. In order to expand her business, Kabelo has plans to move to the inner city where she can attract a bigger population of quality customers.

1   What should Kabelo do to have her business established?
2   Discuss what Kabelo needs to consider for her to become a successful entrepreneur.
3   Discuss the challenges that Kabelo is likely to meet and suggest possible solutions.

Entrepreneurship education and training

In recent years, there has been awareness throughout the world, in terms of disability-related policies and legislation; but many of these laws have not yet been implemented (e.g. 2006 CRPD). Most low-income countries have formulated positive Acts, policy documents and laws to equalise opportunities for disabled persons, however, there is still a long way to go when it comes to equal distribution of resources, employment, social and political rights, which are closely linked to economic empowerment (ILO, 2006).

Disabled people face several barriers, which hinder their full participation in society due to economic and social reasons. Some have acquired at different levels, skills, abilities and interests, but they experience economic and social exclusion resulting from negative societal attitudes (ILO, 2015; Mitra *et al.*, 2011). Knowledge and skills are necessary tools to make informed decisions and perform either at a workplace or at a small-scale enterprise, in order to run businesses effectively and successfully. However, there is a strong link between lack of education, poverty and disability; aspects that marginalise disabled people (World Bank, 2010). Thus, disabled people have a higher risk of being exposed to more disabling conditions, thereby becoming poor by being excluded from participating in developmental activities. Some of the main obstacles faced by disabled people to successful entrepreneurship include but are not limited to: lack of business knowledge, management skills, funding, equal opportunities and accountability (Renko *et al.*, 2015). A study carried out in a rural community in Zimbabwe by Mpofu & Shumba (2013) indicates that most disabled young people lacked entrepreneurial skills and their training needs were not incorporated in most entrepreneurial skills training. They also lacked business networking skills. Thus, disabled people need training in business skills in order to break the cycle of poverty through engaging in entrepreneurship programmes that benefit individuals, the community and the country at large.

A study on entrepreneurial entry by disabled people that was conducted by Caldwell *et al.* (2016) in the United States of America, established that one of the largest barriers was access to entrepreneurship education and training opportunities. It is vital that training takes into consideration the necessary required skills, the nature and severity of the impairment of individual disabled people to be trained and the skills of the trainers. Trainers must be made aware of different people's potentials and personal limitations imposed by their impairments. With different experiences and educational back grounds, trainees must be encouraged to work as a team to help one another. The training curriculum must address any disabling limitations, economic factors, business demands and the needs of disabled entrepreneurs. These guidelines will help trainees to choose businesses they can operate successfully.

In most low-income countries, there has been little or no commitment by government departments to address the social and economic needs of disabled people (WHO & World Bank, 2011). Training of disabled people should include, among other things: access to information, writing business proposals, application for funding, advertising, basic accounting skills, management skills, business ethics, processing orders, sales and distribution of products. Realistically, training disabled people in ICT must be a priority since such skills can change their lives, especially for the purposes of electronic banking, marketing, advertisements, distribution of products, importing and exporting. Training sessions should create a business-like atmosphere that encourages mentorship, networking for exchange and cross-pollination of business ideas. The government, families and society at large could support such programmes so as to wean disabled people off handouts from government or non-governmental organisations (NGOs). Disabled people could be encouraged to form cooperatives and work in groups, sharing ideas and skills according to individual abilities. A link between disabled people and enterprise suppliers, micro-financial organisations and training centres could help them get supplies, secure loans and have well-trained personnel. This would further enhance their status and make their businesses more viable.

Some of the skills that could be taught as part of entrepreneurship education, to both young non-disabled people and those who are disabled, would include organisational skills, time management, leadership development and interpersonal skills, all of which are highly transferable skills sought by employers (ILO, 2015; Renko *et al.*, 2015). Such programmes would be viable if governments were to set aside a budget for entrepreneurship in schools and other training institutions. Through a small business or institution-based enterprise, disabled people can lead, act and experience different roles. Such projects would afford them the opportunity to learn to communicate their ideas, accept other people's contributions, tolerate differences and influence others effectively through the development of self-advocacy and interpersonal skills. It would also give them a chance to become team players, and to engage in problem-solving and critical thinking, skills that are highly valuable in the competitive business world (Mitra *et al.*, 2012). Business mentors could be assigned to small groups to assist in developing the necessary relevant competencies. Disabled youths could be trained to have the ability to set goals, manage time, money and other resources, which are critical entrepreneurship skills necessary to run a successful business. Urban and rural craft artists could be employed to train disabled people and offer apprenticeships to prepare them for entrepreneurship. In 2016, the Namibia University of Science and Technology graduated 16 disabled people in capacity building initiatives that equipped them with the necessary skills of running successful businesses and making meaningful contributions toward the local economy (Shubiak & Kauffman, 2016). Such initiatives are likely to empower disabled people residing in southern Africa.

The benefits of entrepreneurship are numerous if disabled people are well trained and equipped with the necessary skills. It is an employment strategy that can lead them to economic self-sufficiency. Some can venture into self-employment, which will provide them with income for self and family sustainability. Research regarding the impact of entrepreneurship education on disabled people shows a number of benefits that include opportunity to exercise leadership, interpersonal skills and the ability to develop business planning, financial management, financial literacy and basic accounting (Caldwell *et al.*, 2016). Some of the identified benefits comprise: participation in the mainstream economy, promotion of economic growth, promotion of attitudinal change, improved quality of life, accommodations and flexibility and integration and social participation (Harris, Renko & Caldwell, 2014). These are some of the motivating positive key factors that entrepreneurship can bring. However, like any other business venture, entrepreneurship has a number of challenges to be overcome as illustrated in case study 14.2.

Case study 14.2   Kaimba Mulungu

Kaimba Mulungu is a disabled young man aged 28 years. He studied ICT at school and he is talented in that area. An NGO funded him to start a business. Kaimba's home area is in Mazabuka, in Zambia. He moved to Livingstone, a bigger town for better business initiatives. Kaimba started a printing business, printing on clothes; T-shirts, caps, banners, bags, posters and other related items. He also does photocopying and scanning of documents. Kaimba employs one trained printer and two more people who do the general work. He gets limited orders and sometimes he travels to Lusaka in search of business. His business has potential to grow.

1   What do you think are the major challenges in Kaimba's business? Suggest possible solutions.
2   What advice would you give to Kaimba to grow his business?
3   Discuss the necessary skills needed in Kaimba's business.
4   What do you think Kaimba should do, to become a successful entrepreneur?

Entrepreneurship challenges encountered by disabled people

Entrepreneurship is not for every person who is disabled as this might not be realistic for those with profound, severe and multiple impairments. However, it is still a possible option for many disabled people (European Union, 2014). Disabled people do not necessarily have the same experiences even though they might operate in a similar environment. The nature and severity of their impairments impose various limitations that might hinder their full participation in society on an equal basis with others (Harris *et al.*, 2013). In most low-income countries, major problems are more pronounced in rural areas where education and training services are limited and hard to access. Rural training centres are scarce, in most cases without trainers or with only semi-qualified trainers, ill-equipped facilities, without the necessary assistive technology, and the methods used do not necessarily cater for learners' diverse needs (ILO, 2009, 2011, 2015).

The International Labour Organization (2011) points out that in some low-income countries, for example in Malawi and Tanzania, having impairments doubles the probability of children never getting an opportunity to attend school. Government departments have not always been forthcoming in providing the necessary equipment for disabled people to function effectively. Unfriendly environmental factors due to limited resources and financial constraints within the community and poor access to information, can limit access for disabled people to participate fully in community activities. Most of these barriers are indicated in the Zimbabwe's living conditions survey conducted in 2013 (UNICEF, 2013). Transport is generally unsuitable and not easy to access for disabled people to move from one area to another, particularly in the rural areas where some of the roads are impassable. It is important to ensure that environments are accessible through rehabilitation of roads. Where necessary, adaptations and accommodations should be made to allow disabled people to function effectively.

Expectation barriers created by society (that disabled people need help and a lot of support) can further create inadequate facilities to help disabled people toward being entrepreneurs (Harris, Renko & Caldwell, 2014). Lack of confidence to work or stand on their own can also create psychological barriers. There is a general feeling among non-disabled people that it is difficult for them to be successful business owners. That myth needs to be dispelled because it affects those who provide funding, training and eventually disabled people themselves. A higher percentage of disabled people live in rural areas where access to basic services is limited (WHO & World Bank, 2011). It is the role of the family, government departments and society to support and encourage disabled people to start small businesses and be entrepreneurs. In their research, Caldwell *et al.* (2016) interviewed entrepreneurial disabled people and they noted that stigma associated with impairment produced attitudinal barriers that impacted entrepreneurs in a variety of ways. One entrepreneur noted that getting into a bank on a wheelchair or on crutches attracted negative looks or stares. Although some of the disabled entrepreneurs were doing very well, generally they experienced that they were not considered competent, and not equal to their non-disabled counterparts, but treated like some form of charity (Caldwell *et al.*, 2016).

Summary and conclusion

In low-income countries, southern Africa included, disabled people are marginalised and have no easy access to education, transportation, vocational training, employment, decent living and good medical health services. Poverty is looming in most low-income countries and worse situations are experienced by the disabled population. Unemployment is on the upward trend and further impoverishes disabled people, the major proportion of whom are unemployed. Jobs offer opportunities for social engagement and inclusion that often elude a disabled person and a chance to earn money, which facilitates greater independence (Woods Resources, 2016). There is dignity in work. It contributes to an individual's self-worth and self-respect and offers a sense of purpose and accomplishment. The establishment and implementation of entrepreneurship programmes in high schools, institutions of higher learning, vocational centres and training institutions could be the answer to the ever soaring unemployment rates. Unfortunately research studies and available literature in southern Africa and most low-income countries, are sporadic and limited.

This chapter explored self-employment and entrepreneurship options to alleviate unemployment among the disabled people. It further examined the present status of disabled people, policy initiatives, entrepreneurship education and training, the role of governmental institutions, the family and society in supporting entrepreneurship programmes. The benefits and challenges of entrepreneurship together with possible intervention strategies were also discussed. With proper planning, self-employment and entrepreneurship have the potential to reduce poverty and unemployment and sustain the disabled population in developing countries.

Reflective questions

1 How can unemployment among the disabled people be addressed in low-income countries?
2 Examine the benefits of self-employment and entrepreneurship.
3 What are the major challenges that disabled people encounter when they work for themselves or run their own businesses?
4 In what ways can institutions prepare disabled people to become entrepreneurs?
5 What is the role of government, family and the community in supporting disabled people's engagement in business?
6 What policy initiatives can be put in place to make small enterprises viable?

References

Avendano, M. & Berkman, L. F. (2014). Labor markets, employment policies and health. In L. F. Berkman, I. Kawachi & M. M. Glymour (eds) *Social Epistemology*, 2nd edn (pp. 357–384). Oxford University Press, New York.

Caldwell, K., Harris, S. & Renko, M. (2016). Social entrepreneurs with disabilities: exploring motivational and attitudinal factors. *Canadian Journal of Disability Studies* **5**(1), 212–243.

Chamberlin, B. (2014). *Creating employment opportunities for people with significant disabilities*. Retrieved from www.maine.gov/dhhs/oads/docs/Employment-Individuals-Significant-Disabilities.doc on 20 March 2017.

Cox, G. (2012). *Why employing disabled people is the most difficult form of social enterprise*. Retrieved from www.theguardian.com/social-enterprise-network/2012/jul/03/social-enterprises-employing-disabled-people on 15 July 2017.

Craig, D. & Bigby, C. (2010). Social isolation and exclusion. *Journal of Intellectual and Developmental Disability* **11**(29), 239–254.

Craig, D. & Bigby, C. (2014). Supporting the active participation of people with intellectual disabilities. *Journal of Intellectual Disability Research* **54**,1004–1014.

Dubihlela, J. & Rundora, R. (2014). Employee training, managerial commitment and the implementation of activity based costing: impact on performance of SMEs. *International Business Research Journal* **13**(1), 28–38.

Entrepreneurs Malawi (2015). *Disability Not Inability in Entrepreneurship*. Malawi: Lions Africa.

European Union (2014). Report on the Implementation of the UN Convention on the Rights of Persons with Disabilities (CRPD). Brussels: European Union.

Grunewald, K. (2003). *Close the institutions for the intellectually disabled: everyone can live in the open society*. Retrieved from www.independentliving.org/docs7/grunewald2003.html on 6 October 2016.

Harris, S., Caldwell, K. & Renko, M. (2014). Entrepreneurship by any other name: self-sufficiency versus innovation. *Journal of Social Work in Disability & Rehabilitation* **13**(4), 1–33.

Harris, S., Renko, M. & Caldwell, K. (2013). Accessing social entrepreneurship: perspectives of people with disabilities and key stakeholders. *Vocational Rehabilitation* **38**, 35–48.

Harris, S., Renko, M. & Caldwell, K. (2014). Social entrepreneurship as an employment pathway for people with disabilities: exploring political-economic and socio-cultural factors. *Disability & Society* **29**(8), 1275–1290.

Independent Living Institute (2014). *Promoting the Self-determination of Disabled People.* Sweden: Storforsplan.

Independent Living Institute (2015). *Promoting the self-determination of people with disabilities.* Independentliving. org. Retrieved from: www.independentliving.org/docs1/ilanrp2015.html on 24 August 2017.

International Labour Organization [ILO] (2006). *Promoting the Employability and Employment of People with Disabilities through Effective Legislation (Southern Africa),* Cornell University, Gladnet.

International Labour Organization [ILO] (2009). *Rural Skills Training: A Generic Manual on Training for Rural Economic Empowerment.* Geneva: ILO.

International Labour Organization [ILO] (2011). *Disability Elements in Training for Rural Economic Empowerment.* International Labour Laws. Geneva: ILO.

International Labour Organization [ILO] (2015). *Disability inclusion: good for business.* Retrieved from www.ilo. org/wcmsp5/groups/public/@asia/@ro-bangkok/documents/genericdocument/wcms_149586.pdf. on 6 October 2016.

Jang, Y., Wang, Y. & Lin, M. (2014). Factors affecting employment outcome for disabled people who received disability employment services in Taiwan. *Journal of Occupational Rehabilitation* **24**, 11–21.

Majola, B. K. & Dhunpath, R. (2016). The development of disability-related policies in the South African public service. *Problems and Perspectives in Management* **14**(1), 150–159.

Ministry of Primary & Secondary Education (2015). *Zimbabwe New Curriculum.* Zimbabwe Government.

Mitra, S., Posarac, A. & Vick, B. (2011). *Disability and poverty in developing countries: a snapshot from the world health survey* (English). Social Protection Discussion Paper; no. SP 1109. Washington, DC: World Bank. Retrieved from http://documents.worldbank.org/curated/en/501871468326189306/Disability-and-poverty-in-developing-countries-a-snapshot-from-the-world-health-survey on 16 March 2017.

Mitra, S., Posarac, A. & Vick, B. (2012). *Disability and poverty in developing countries: a multidimensional study.* World Development. Retrieved from http://dx.doi.org/10.1016/j.worlddev on 12 June 2017.

Mpofu, J. & Shumba, O. (2013). Disabilities and entrepreneurship in Makonde rural community in Zimbabwe. *Studies of Tribes and Tribals* **11**(2), 135–144.

Namatovu, R., Dawa, S., Mulira, F. & Katongole, C. (2012). Entrepreneurs with disability in Uganda. *Trust Africa,* Makerere University Business School, Kampala.

Renko, M., Harris, S. & Caldwell, K. (2015). Entrepreneurial entry by people with disabilities. *International Small Business Journal* **13**(4), 505–518.

Renko, M., Harris, S. & Caldwell, K. (2016). Entrepreneurial entry by disabled people. *International Small Business Journal* **34**(5), 555–578.

Shubiak, P. & Kauffman, C. (2016). Social enterprise: creating employment opportunities for people with disabilities. *Journal of Social Innovations 28.* Retrieved from www.socialinnovationsjournal.org/...social-innovations/2148-social-enterprise-creatin on 21 March 2017.

UNICEF (2013). *Zimbabwe Living Conditions among Persons with Disability Survey.* Zimbabwe: Ministry of Health and Child Care.

United Nations (2015). Global Status Report on Disability and Development. New York.

Vedeler, J. S. & Schreuer, N. (2011). Policy in action: stories on the workplace accommodation process. *Journal of Disability Policy Studies* **22**(2), 95–105.

Woods Resources (2016). *Social enterprise: creating employment opportunities for people with disabilities.* Retrieved from www.woods.org/http:/server4.kproxy.com/servlet/redirect.srv/slxv/sbnzaj/slmn/p1/social-enterprise-creating-employment-opportunities-people-disabilities/on 13 May 2017.

World Bank (2010). *Disability, politics and poverty in a majority world context* (pp. 771–782). Retrieved from https://doi.org/10.1080/09687599.2010.520889 on 1 November 2016.

World Bank (2014). *World Development Indicators.* Washington, DC: World Bank.

World Bank (2016). *Trading Economic Indicators.* Washington, DC: World Bank. Retrieved from www. tradingeconomicsindicators/unemployment/rates on 6 October 2016.

World Health Organization & World Bank (2011). *World Report on Disability.* Geneva: WHO.

15

ENHANCING REALISTIC HOPES AND ASPIRATIONS TOWARD VOCATIONAL CHOICES

Focus on deaf secondary students in Zimbabwe

Phillipa C. Mutswanga

Introduction

This chapter's thrust is to empower deaf secondary school students in making realistic vocational choices by inserting a tick against the preferred vocational choices using Becker's (1988) Reading-Free Vocational Interest Inventory. Deaf denotes a deficiency in auditory perception which may cause fluctuating or permanent hearing loss depending on various variables such as hearing loss type and age of onset just to mention a few. The hearing loss, whether mild or profound has the potential to negatively impact on the speech and language development of an individual. Shield (2006) reinforces this by defining deafness as a qualitatively known difficulty in hearing normal conversations and/or quantitatively known as unaided hearing threshold in levels of mild, moderate, severe and profound, denoting a deficiency in auditory perception which could be congenital (born with) or acquired after birth but is serious enough to interfere with normal development and maintenance of speech communication skills and concept formation.

Against this background, the study recommends the Reading-Free Vocational Interest Inventory as an appropriate means of data collection, because use of pictures addresses the participants' language shortcomings. A mixed method comprising of the quantitatively analysed vocational interests of deaf students was qualitatively augmented by data generated from the insights of purposively selected secondary school teachers from Harare with experience in deaf education. The chapter emphasises inclusive practices, despite their impairments, and that justify the focus of career guidance. This chapter further enhances the importance of rights of people with disabilities to optional employment, entrepreneurship and sustainable development. The chapter is also informed by informal conversations with secondary school teachers and the author's desire to transform African societies so that they view people with disabilities as people who can make realistic vocational choices after exposure to guidance and counselling.

The study informing this chapter took place in two Harare urban secondary schools, where deaf students learned under inclusive practices, which this study recognises as schools A and B. School A is a high school five kilometres away in the northern part of Harare city centre along Upper East and Mount Pleasant drive while school B is a high school six kilometres away in the north-west of Harare. Inclusive practice is a system where disabled people learn alongside their non-disabled counterparts under well-resourced and provisioned conditions. Harare is the capital city of Zimbabwe. Zimbabwe is a landlocked area in southern Africa with Mozambique to the east; Botswana to the west; South Africa to the south; and Zambia to the north. As a central place many factors are likely to control issues of career guidance.

Factors influencing the hopes and aspirations of deaf people toward employment

Deafness is an impairment that can manifest congenitally (before birth) or can be acquired in later life. Deaf students are people like any other students, and thus are equally expected to make career paths as noted by the World Health Organization (WHO, 1990). This justifies the application of the person-first philosophy of which this chapter is conscious. Aspirations are strong desires for a career path of interest. However, Kintrea, St Clair and Houston (2011) feel that it is not enough to just aspire, but there is a need to navigate the paths of the goals. Navigating career paths is in most cases a struggle for deaf people due to the impacts and attitudinal problems associated with deafness.

Out of the 15% world population of disabled people, WHO and the World Bank (2011) reported the prevalence of deaf people as 5.3% (360 million). This is a significant figure that should cause concern in any educational systems. In support, Lorenzo (2011) asserts that education is the foundation to a career although most secondary school systems lacked that focus. Donaldson, Hinton and Nelson (2006, n.p.) quoted Bill Clinton's 1994 related statement: 'We are living in a world where what you earn is a function of what you learn.' This implies that there ought to be a relationship between one's education and the career paths of interest. Such practices and links seem lacking in most developing countries, including Zimbabwe. Inclusive provisions should play a pivotal role in allowing every individual to fulfil life plans regardless of the country's status. Thus, Lorenzo (2011) proposes that participation of disabled people in the world of work should remain a human rights issue. That, then, places the responsibility for solutions within the domain of civil society; rehabilitation; guidance and counselling. Secondary schools are ideal places for equipping both people with and without disabilities with sound academic teaching matching their vocational dreams. Based on my experiences as an educationist, deaf students seem to continue to experience challenges in matching their academic subjects to vocational interest despite efforts by the education system of exposing them to 'career days'. The preparations do not cater for the communication needs of deaf students in their midst, thus the events are considered in Mutswanga (2016) as deaf-unfriendly and lagging in helping their deaf students make realistic vocational choices. The issue seems to remain a deprivation for people with disabilities.

Likewise, Madzivanzira (2015) posits that childhood deprivation imposes long-lasting limits in making realistic vocational choices in any context. In other words, the emphasis is on early individual career preparation. Education is therefore seen as the ideal avenue for entry into the world of work, although according to my experience as an educationist, career preparation is given little focus in Zimbabwe. This could be a future survey worthy investigating. In Zimbabwe, churches have played leading roles in the education of disabled people but their career choice preparation seems to be given little or no attention. Additionally, despite influences of robust conventions and policies on human rights that Zimbabwe affiliates to, such as Education for All (EFA) (Inter-Agency Commission, 1990) and the Convention on the Rights of Persons with Disabilities (CRPD; United Nations, 2006), issues of vocational choice preparation seem to be lagging and that prompted this study.

Continuously reported dearth of knowledge by other studies from the African perspective also prompted this study. Carnevale, Smith and Strohl (2010) argue that today's economy demands a better and more educated workforce than ever before and jobs in this new economy require more complex knowledge and skills than the jobs in the past. The 2016 outgoing President Obama set a goal that ensured every American access to postsecondary training to gain skills needed to rebuild the economy and meet market demands through smoothed transition to post-secondary success. True, students need guidance and counselling in making realistic career plans. Unfortunately, President Obama's goals are currently not undertaken as planned because many secondary schools in America have recently been forced to cut school counsellor positions due to budgetary constraints (Carnevale *et al.*, 2010) making the phenomenon under study a global cause of concern. Although the American Public law 94-142 in Warnock (1978) emphasises that education systems should meet the career interests of all people with disabilities in the same manner, systems seem to still continue to short-change deaf students' vocational aspirations.

Despite the fact that many African countries endorsed the eight Millennium Developmental Goals (MDGs) which Zimbabwe ratified in September 2013 to uphold principles of human rights, issues of informed vocational choices preparation seem to remain a dream for most deaf people at secondary schools in Zimbabwe. The major reasons for creating MDGs is to free the world from poverty, but the absence of issues of disability in these goals created little difference to the reduction of poverty. The MDGs were improved to Sustainable Development Goals (SDGs) (United Nations, 2012) after the realisation that set goals were not achievable without including people with disabilities which came to pass in 2010 but still issues of vocational preparations remained under-utilised and not given full focus. The observed gaps prompted the development of this book chapter with a view to seek ways of reducing the challenges.

Zimbabwean secondary schools claimed attempts to address the challenge through teaching practical subjects but the matter still remained an issue as many deaf students continued to engage in unrealistic choices as evidenced in Mutswanga and Chakuchichi's (2014) study where one deaf individual moved, of her own free will, from a secretarial job to street vending where talking and listening were not a prerequisite. The Ministry of Education, Sports and Culture (1991, n.p.) describe *Education for Living* syllabus 'as a laboratory where pupils focus on their own lives as well as on health and environmental issues'. The syllabus covers topics such as human development, health risks and problems, social development, food and nutrition and career guidance, just to mention a few. This document emphasises exposing all people to the world of work matching their academic performance but while these facts appear noble on paper, they are largely absent in practice, especially with regard to people with disabilities. Additionally, the Zimbabwean system expects schools, as indicated by the Ministry of Education, Sports and Culture (1991) syllabus, to carry out once a week, guidance and counselling session on any issues of concern under selected interested mentors who are not necessarily skilled counsellors. All these circumstances prompted this study with a view to remind all educational systems in Africa of the relevance of career guidance counsellors to any country's workforce.

As emphasised by the Ministry of Education, Sports and Culture (1991), the Zimbabwean secondary schools made attempts to expose deaf and hearing students to vocational aspirations through skills teaching. Based on the author's experience as an educationist, this system is criticised for unsystematic focus and funding toward practical education. These are possible indicators driving some schools to continue to under-estimate career counselling by considering composition writing on preferred jobs after exiting secondary education as enough preparation yet the system never pursues the students' actual vocational interests thereafter. On the other hand, deafness imposes receptive and expressive language communication limitations in both oral and written work. Indicators are, then, that deafness might cause further complex and pervasive limitations on concept formation, especially where listening and talking are prerequisites. This study, then, observes with concern why some inclusive practices continue to use modes of communication where listening and talking are prerequisites with deaf students. The next question is, 'Do deaf students benefit under such systems? It is because of such actions that the majority of deaf students are assumed to excel in practical work and not in academics (Shield, 2006; Punch, Hyde & Creed, 2004), an issue that Agro (2014) argued against. Furthermore, the current Zimbabwean curriculum is academic-oriented thus the practical subjects are likely undertaken with *ad hoc* provisions and that is likely to compound deaf students' efforts in making realistic vocational choices.

In the context of the Zimbabwe Education Act of 1987 amended in 2006, education is the birthright of every child in Zimbabwe. This policy accords education to every school going age child in Zimbabwe irrespective of colour, creed, religion or biological constitution. This, therefore, means that every child has the right to education in Zimbabwe. The major question of concern in this chapter is whether the existing educational facilities benefit deaf students in making informed and realistic vocational choices. The 1996 Disabled Persons Act (DPA) prohibits discrimination against career selection by people with disabilities. The idiopathic deaf merely have sensory impairment, which does not necessarily interfere with physical access. Rehabilitation International (1990) proposes that the systems need to realise the legitimacy of vocational dreams of deaf students and enhance them through career guidance and counselling, yet counsellor positions are generally absent in Zimbabwean systems.

In support WHO (1990) suggests that deaf students could be assisted to make informed vocational choices from the 1,260 professions and trades where hearing is not a prerequisite. Agro (2014) urges the systems to consider it as a human rights issue. The WHO (1990) and Rehabilitation International (1990) note that deaf students have the humanity right to learn but the problem is with their societies which have not yet learned to fully protect these rights due to stereotypes. This makes most deaf students fail to extend their horizons in the same way as their hearing counterparts. According to my experiences Zimbabwean systems lack specific focus on vocational choice preparation for all students. The preceding evidence prompted this study with a view to establishment of permanent career guidance positions in Zimbabwe's systems because preceding studies considered them relevant in producing a market alert workforce that is likely to contribute to sustainable economic development. A mixed methods study using quantitative and qualitative approaches was utilised to explore the vocational interests of deaf students which were respectively augmented by teachers' narrative experiences to support the relevance of career guidance counsellors in Zimbabwe's educational systems.

The research process

Becker (1988) provided a Reading-Free Vocational Interest Inventory used to collect the vocational interests of deaf students. This was appropriate because it addressed these respondents' communication shortfalls through use of pictures to enhance voices of deaf students in vocational choices. The sample was drawn from 50 secondary deaf students under inclusive practices and six teachers experienced in deaf education. Participants' consent was sought after explaining issues of confidentiality and the purpose of the study. Becker's 29-page Reading-Free Vocational Interest Inventory was completed by ticking one vocational interest from each of the 55 rows from three different job pictures. The number of ticked interests were quantitatively used to obtain the vocational interests of deaf students from two high schools in Harare urban, known as schools A and B in this study. Narratives from six teachers experienced in deaf education augmented the obtained vocational choices of deaf students. Following the standards of research, quantitatively collected data presented in Table 15.1 and qualitatively analysed generated emerging patterns, and themes were compared and contrasted. Becker's (1988) Reading-Free Vocational Interest Inventory was the best method to collect vocational choices of deaf students because it allowed them to make their choices without verbally labouring. This is in favour of the 2006 CRPD's advocacy on deaf people's right to Sign Language as their natural language, which is missing in Zimbabwe although it ratified this convention in September 2013, indicating that Zimbabwe needed to adhere to its obligations.

The voices of deaf students and teachers on vocational choices

Table 15.1 shows a cross tabulation bivariate analysis of data collected using Becker's (1988) 29-page Reading-Free Vocational Interest Inventory.The inventory was appropriate for this study because it enabled the comparison to establish deaf students' vocational choices vis-à-vis their class subjects of specialisation without constraining them linguistically. The main issue was to cross-check whether their areas of study matched or mismatched their vocational choices. The relationships and variances were determined against the frequencies and percentages. In support Wyse (2012) defines cross-tabulation as a tool that allows comparison of the relationship between variables. Cross-tabulation analysis allowed a descriptive comparison of the two (multiple) variables which are deaf students' vocational interests against their secondary school subjects of specialisation. Cross-tabulation is a statistical tool that is used to analyse categorical data. Categorical data are data or variables that are separated into different categories that are mutually exclusive from one another. Table 15.1 provides information on class subject and vocational choices of deaf students.

The cross-tabulation analysis in Table 15.1 reveals that 9.1% deaf students who undertook commercial subjects chose automotive, building trades, housekeeping, laundry services and material handling. Another 18.2% from the same subject area expressed vocational interests in animal care, patient care and personal services, which did not match the commercial subjects they were studying. Other preferred vocational choices included patient care which was mismatched to commercial subjects while those in commercial classes had no interest in clerical work; others were interested in food services and horticulture yet their subjects matched clerical work.

Table 15.1 further reveals that 8.3% deaf students from arts classes preferred automotive and clerical jobs, while 16.7% of them had patient care and housekeeping interests which were quite

Table 15.1 Class subjects and vocational choices of deaf students

Vocational choices of deaf students	Subject areas of deaf students									
	Commercials		Arts		Sciences		Vocational		Totals	
	Nos	%	Nos	%	Nos	%	Nos	%	Nos	%
Automotive	1	9.1	1	8.3	1	7.7	1	5.3	4	7.3
Building trade	1	9.1	0	0	0	0	4	21	5	9.1
Clerical	0	0	1	8.3	2	15.4	3	15.8	6	10.9
Animal care	2	18.2	0	0	2	15.4	1	5.3	5	9.1
Food service	0	0	0	0	1	7.7	1	5.3	2	3.6
Patient care	2	18.2	2	16.7	0	0	0	0	4	7.3
Horticulture	0	0	0	0	0	0	2	10.5	2	3.6
Housekeeping	1	9.1	2	16.7	2	15.4	0	0	5	9.1
Personal service	2	18.2	6	50	2	15.4	7	36.8	17	31
Laundry service	1	9.1	0	0	3	23	0	0	4	7.3
Material handling	1	9.1	0	0	0	0	0	0	1	1.7
Total	11	100	12	100	13	100	19	100	55	100

mismatched. How could students in arts classes select patient care? This is a good example of unrealistic vocational choices. About 50% made realistic choices by selecting personal services as their vocational preferences although they expressed less interest in building trades, animal care, food services, horticulture, laundry service and materials handling.

From science classes, 7.7% expressed vocational interests in automotive and food services; 15.4% animal care, clerical, personal services and housekeeping; while 23% preferred laundry services which was a mismatch to science classes. Science students showed no interest in building trades, patient care, horticulture or materials handling.

From deaf students' undertaking vocational subjects such as woodwork, building, food and nutrition, metalwork, computers, technical graphs and fashion and fabrics just to mention a few, 5.3% preferred automotive, animal care and food service; 10.5% horticulture; 15.8% clerical; 21% building trades; and 36.8% personal services. These group members did not have vocational interests in patient care, housekeeping, laundry services or material handling, thus, patient care was a mismatch for most deaf students' academic pursuit and career paths.

Personal services had highest vocational interests of 31%, most of which were from arts subjects followed by vocational or practical subject(s) classes and respectively included commercial and science subjects. This was followed by 10.9% clerical interest, the highest being from those studying practical subjects – sciences and arts respectively – but no indicators from those in commercials. The building trade, animal care and housekeeping gained interest from 9.1% of students and these were from varied areas of subject specialisation. Automotive, patient care and laundry services had 7.3% vocational interests mainly from those studying sciences, arts and commercial subjects. Food service and horticulture had 3.6% while materials handling had least interests of 1.7 % from commercial classes. Table 15.1 findings were then compared and contrasted with data obtained from narratives of teachers.

Study outcomes

Challenges were experienced in collecting narratives from the ten participants who had given their consent to the study because only six returned the narrative responses guided by semi-structured questions. The six participants positively responded to phone calls to verify data. The preceding section reveals that deaf participants were excluded from the yearly cluster career days that hearing counterparts attended. The majority of teachers (interviewees) commented the Zimbabwean career day system as noble commitment to vocational exposure though actual focuses on helping individuals make vocational choices was a missing link. According to participants this was evidenced by career days that excluded deaf students by making presentations without Sign Language interpreters. The majority of participants complained that only oral-aural biased presentations were given without taking care of the linguistic needs of the deaf minority students thus, most participants considered the system as insensitive to deaf education.

The majority of interviewees reported that they were under-skilled in deaf education as evidenced by two teachers who specialised in intellectually challenged learners but were misplaced at resource units for deaf students. Additionally, the other two were special needs graduates with general qualifications but without skills in practical training in any disability type, indicating the need for training institutions to equip teachers with related practical skills such as Sign Language or Braille. All these were missing links in Zimbabwe's educational systems, an issue which opens doors to further study gaps and investigate ongoing practical skills in deaf education. The majority of teachers completed their studies without practical experiences and, thus, the majority of participants proposed that they were taught Sign Language by their students, a gap that could be met through school Sign Language workshops and a call on Zimbabwean universities to incorporate varied practical courses to meet inclusive practices. Education changes the way youths and adults function in a global and industrious economy. In other words, education paves the way to a fulfilling living but when unguided its cause is likely lost, which could be the reason why deaf participants in Table 15.1 made unrealistic vocational choices, an issue that is likely to exist in other countries, though empirical evidence is still lacking. This indicates the need for readers to compare and contrast findings with their country's status. This is supported by the following excerpts:

> There are no career guidance officers at our school. Besides . . . our school faces challenges in helping students who are deaf. . . . it becomes a challenge in helping them make realistic vocational choice. This makes it hard for the deaf to explore their areas of interest in vocational training.
>
> *[Teacher 1]*

> It is difficult to determine . . . there is no time set for this but it is done in passing through classroom talks, composition writing and is a one-off feedback about their career choices.
>
> *[Teacher 4]*

> I reinforce and help them match their academic work to industrial fields . . . we do not have career guidance counsellors but . . . carry out such exercises situationally.
>
> *[Teacher 3]*

> Have no focused career education but it is generally carried out through practical subjects teaching.
>
> *[Teacher 5]*

> I tell students available markets and occasionally take them to nearby industries but this is controlled by focus on completing the syllabus in time and lack of financial support.
>
> *[Teacher 2]*

All interviewees consensually agreed that career guidance was instrumental in helping deaf students unpack vocational realities matching their interests and capabilities. Deafness is a complicated condition due to involved complexities such as: ranges of hearing loss, types of hearing loss, age of onset, just to mention a few. This is a pervasive condition and has great limitations on conceptual formation where listening and talking are prerequisites. It is for such reasons that most deaf students function with limitations in hearing environments such as verbally delivered career days. It is also for these reasons that deaf students are generally expected to excel in practical work and not in academics. That means deaf students are likely to miss the details of conversations unless otherwise taught in their natural Sign Language. However, despite the legislative recognition of the importance of career guidance as stipulated in the Ministry of Education, Sports and Culture 1993 Circular, deaf students seem to continue to be deprived of instruction in their natural language as already expressed by narrative realities. Though still lacking empirical evidence, the majority of participants felt that most African countries probably need to create positions of career guidance counsellors skilled in Sign Language. Participants also stressed that a majority of deaf students in Zimbabwe expressed not knowing where to go after exiting school. The goal is to build a bridge between the theories taught at secondary school and vocational choices. In support, Wolanin and Steele (2004) propose provision of essential enterprises such as guidance and counselling as enhancers to gainful and fulfilling vocational choices. Where such enterprises are absent deaf students might not eloquently describe their aspirations. The following qualitatively obtained data augmented the preceding quantitatively collected data:

I am not a skilled . . . counsellor but only have experience using speech reading on HIV and AIDS teaching; morals and good behaviour but I am not proficient in career guidance . . . only know a few Sign Language basics.

[Teacher 6]

Schools need career guidance officers to avoid blind choices which in most cases cause drop-outs. Schools need policies to guide them on how to do it.

[Teacher 1]

The majority of interviewees confirmed that they managed inclusive practices using ad hoc skills. They further proposed the ad hoc provisions to contribute to deaf students' unrealistic vocational choices. Career days were criticised for lack of focus on all students as advocated by EFA and the CRPD. Other excerpts depicting deaf students' under-preparedness to vocational choices included the following:

Most deaf students have mixed vocational choices while a good number still continue to live in confusion over career choices; while others dropped out very few made sustainable choices

[Teacher 5]

Many deaf students make unrealistic vocational selections or just follow choices of others, such as, medical doctor, nursing, driving, pastor and many others mismatching their school academic pursuits.

[Teacher 5]

Art is highly selected by deaf students though one dropped-out due to lack of funding. I was inspired by one of the girls who did knitting at Masasa who is currently a self-employed knitter.

[Teacher 6]

According to the preceding excerpts some teachers in inclusive schools avoid lessons on career education in order to complete the syllabi and, thus, have no time to reinforce students' career interests. As exemplified by the American vocational education though currently such posts have been reduced even in America due to budgetary constraints, the excerpts from the study propose that African states could reduce the problem by creating positions of career guidance counsellors:

There is need to have vocational education for all children to help them translate their career prospects and interests into goals and action.

[Teacher 1]

After workshopping the vocational career teachers on how to communicate with deaf learners they should be placed on secondment in deaf education to teach career guidance.

[Teacher 4]

Design a career guidance booklet with possible industries and career centres and match to various academic subjects.

[Teacher 5]

Although the Zimbabwean education system does not have inclusive systematic and mandated career plans it partially supports the ongoing global view of linking educational achievements, capabilities and limitations to one's vocational choices through career days. In support, Donaldson, Hinton and Nelson (2006) noted that all students need to be prepared to enter the job market early in their lifetime before they exit secondary studies. The majority of teacher interviewees suggested that since the world is faced with a dynamic job market every country needed to mandate inclusive career counselling to match ongoing technological changes. The technological changes were reported to increase complex management of career preparation for hearing rather than deaf students. Considering these loop-holes most participants felt that most deaf students in Zimbabwe needed career counselling guidance. One school had school-based enterprises where deaf students produced goods for sale as preparatory ground for future realistic vocational choices, but participants criticised it as inadequate. Carnevale *et al.* (2010) notes that vocational education topics prominently discussed in American education always shift with times from an agrarian to an industrial economy, a position that the Zimbabwean system should emulate and consider.

Based on preceding arguments the majority of participants proposed that Zimbabwe needed to make major reforms on career education to reshape career days by making them inclusive. The findings further proposed that career guidance counsellor positions be established and budgeted for. The reforms would need to base their jurisdiction and guidance on the CRPD's human rights thrust. This study therefore recommends that the CRPD acts as a driving force since Zimbabwe ratified it in 2013 to enhance vocational choice preparation to all member states. The CRPD is an instrumental legal framework, with an international human rights focus to increase the employment rights of people with disabilities with adequate provisions (United Nations, 2006). However, the CRPD is equally criticised for its unspecific focus on inclusive vocational choice preparation. The majority of participants proposed that through clear policies, education systems could be mandated to create career guidance counsellor positions as a through-put to functional career education in Zimbabwe.

Shield (2006) proposes that teachers should make deaf students understand the consequences of their hearing loss and stay informed on possible limitations and how that deprives their explorations. Participants proposed that all this be reinforced by using successful deaf adults as role models. Choosing an appropriate job seems to remain an issue of concern among deaf students.

Implications and conclusions

The majority of teacher interviewees suggested that although focused career guidance and counselling is absent at secondary schools in Zimbabwe, besides that found at some private schools, it is a highly needed service for students who are deaf both locally and globally. Carnevale *et al.* (2010) earlier on emphasised that President Obama supports the engagement of career guidance officers in America although financial constraints limit its implication. The majority of teacher interviewees criticised the Zimbabwean educational system for not mandating placement of career guidance counsellors at every school, thus further viewed as lip-serviced. The participants viewed the selection of unskilled counsellors as short-changing the practice and contributing to raising unrealistic aspirations. The findings also stressed that stigmatisation and cultural belief systems created limits in deaf people in defining and fulfilling their aspirations and work dreams. In support, Javaraza (2014, n.p.) provides an incidence of a deaf footballer in the B-Metro, which is a regional Zimbabwean newspaper:

> Upon finishing high school, I had big dreams but Zimbabwe like in many societies; people with disabilities are faced with social exclusion and stigmatisation resulting in their aspirations and dreams being shattered before they are even realised.

According to most participants, the placement of career guidance counsellors at schools was likely to reduce noted limitations. Participants criticised existing career guidance and counselling systems for not addressing adequately the needs of diversified groups within society. McMahon and Patton (2002) posit that the national curriculum and career assessments are not immune to such criticism. They proposed innovative and cost-effective ways of providing counselling to large groups of people. McMahon and Patton (2002) proposed increased use of group counselling to provide supportive instructional guidance activities related to student's self-knowledge along with educational and career planning to facilitate focused vocational plans.

The teachers further revealed that both hearing and deaf students made unrealistic vocational choices because of inadequate preparation, lack of focus in the area and also due to unavailability of skilled career guidance and counselling. In support Agro (2014) and WHO (1990) assert that our dreams, ideas and wants form our aspirations, and while both the deaf and hearing youth may have unrealistic aspirations these become better adjusted with time and experience. Shield (2006) and Agro (2014) reveal that both subjects may make unrealistic hopes and aspirations toward employment but it is worse with deaf adolescents. Shield (2006) and Punch *et al.* (2004) posit that deaf individual's aspirations always have to be adjusted just like anyone else's. Punch *et al.* (2006) note that vocational education for deaf students needs to move from the stage of awareness to that of implementation, though currently the mood of economic austerity has adverse effects on vocational selection for deaf students. That then, means that, by virtue of impairment deaf students continue to drown in unrealistic job expectations. But WHO (1990) highlights that even after achieving adjustments on self-actualisation, deaf students might still find themselves facing societal rejection where their capabilities are unnoticed. That is likely to reduce their level of aspiration and cause frustration and performance gaps.

Agro (2014) and Luckner and Muir (2001) propose that deaf students can adjust when guided about their shortfalls in jobs such as sales, medicine, pilot and so on and that every child deserves the right to perform to their best abilities. According to the Ministry of Education, Sports and Culture (1989), deaf students should follow the regular curricula tailor-made for the ordinary schools. Curriculum is the content to be taught. The system encourages deaf students to learn all subjects indicated in the syllabus. In other words, Zimbabwe secondary educational inclusive systems exposed individuals to what the school or particular stream offered. If this is a regulated condition, why then does the same system discriminate against students with disabilities, such as those who are deaf, during career exposure presentations as related by the expressed realities? Agro (2014) argues that the main difference between hearing and deaf students is the way they are taught rather than the subjects they are taught. Shield (2006) further argues that deaf students are mostly as physically and mentally fit as their hearing counterparts since their main difficulties are in hearing and communication, which can impose arbitrary limitations on modes of communication. Despite noted challenges, the majority of participants considered deaf students to be capable of undertaking any other jobs pursued by hearing counterparts. Thus, career guidance counselling is regarded necessary in shaping vocational choices of both deaf and hearing students in Zimbabwe and in keeping pace with vocational demands and current technological changes.

The findings imply that an individualised curriculum should be designed which pays great concern to academic achievement against needs created by an impairment and its limiting factors and mitigations. The practice of placing deaf students in vocational classes, as indicated in Table 15.1, needs to be taught in such a way that the consumers benefit and are enabled to make realistic advanced improvements that are market driven and not demanded for the sake of it.

The majority of secondary school teachers noted that deaf individuals in inclusive programmes had impoverished vocational information as compared to hearing counterparts. Most participants suggested that the Zimbabwean educational systems needed to make sure that it engaged in gainful career days. They further suggested that systems needed to give insufficient attention to career guidance to both hearing and deaf students. This is the reason why the chapter recommends that the CRPD should revisit its goals to make career guidance counsellors more instrumental in enhancing vocational choice preparation for people with disabilities to give them lifelong learning and assist in harmonising their aspirations.

The interviewees suggested that some parents' ignorance, family background and/or socio-economic factors contributed to unrealistic job aspirations made by deaf students. The majority of teachers who participated in this study revealed that children from low backgrounds have a tendency to make either too low or too high vocational choices, not matching their competencies or limitations. Another tendency was that girls and boys, respectively, made choices similar to their mother's or father's occupational status which in most instances mismatched their academic pursuits resulting in indexing that as a socio-economic status marking their vocational pursuits.

The interviewees reported that most vocational choices of both hearing and deaf students exiting secondary education were more influenced by their family's job preference trends than from annual district career days in Zimbabwe. Interviewees accepted the yearly career days as a noble commitment though they criticised the system for not specifically involving deaf students. They further proposed that the system needed to recommend each child exiting secondary education to the Ministry of Labour offices for further guidance. The existing yearly career day exposures were further criticised by the majority of teachers in in the study, for giving less focus on individual vocational preparation and for being biased toward hearing students as exemplified by running career days that excluded deaf students by not engaging Sign Language interpreters to meet their linguistic gaps. They further proposed that both primary and secondary school teacher education should produce teachers skilled in managing inclusive practices as a cornerstone enhancing their vocational choices.

The empirical findings imply that Zimbabwe needs to develop robust policies which mandate the education sectors to create fully funded positions for career guidance counsellors. Such actions are likely to help produce not only deaf students but a country workforce with realistic postsecondary vocational choices which promote fulfilling livelihoods and produce workforces matching ongoing technological changes. This would address reasons for schools for all and pave the way for national developments where workforces possess realistic vocational jobs that feed into a sustainable economy, not only in Zimbabwe but globally. It implies that education is the stepping stone for every human being where successful life career needs have been met or enhanced through well-planned focuses on career education for all students. Career guidance can help leverage the talents of not only deaf students but all in Zimbabwe. With such systems in place one might be justified to conclusively suggest that use of career guidance counsellors skilled in Special Needs Education is likely to enhance the ability of people with disabilities to make realistic or meaningful vocational choices in Zimbabwe. The result is likely to enhance fulfilling livelihoods that will sustain meaningful education and economic development in Zimbabwe.

Conclusion

This chapter revealed that the impetus of guidance and counselling in empowering deaf people to make realistic hopes and aspirations was necessary, since most of them were reported to mismatch subjects they were pursuing with their desired vocational interests. The implication is that deaf people need guidance and counselling to enable them to gain the same opportunities as their hearing peers in selecting career paths that match their capabilities and interests. Also, the use of Sign Language or using Sign Language interpreters to make up for the linguistic deprivation caused by hearing loss is necessary in allowing deaf people to make informed decisions about their career paths. The findings also propose that Zimbabwe's Ministry of Education of Primary and Secondary Education needs to engage skilled counsellors if the produced scholars are to meaningfully contribute to the socio-economic developments of the country. Thus, this chapter recommends the use of visual guidance such as Becker's (1988) Reading-Free Vocational Interest Inventory, where deaf individuals identify their vocational choices using pictures from an informed background through counselling interventions. Such procedures are likely to empower all people in selecting their career paths and produce a marketable workforce for Africa where everyone is included in sustainable socio-economic development matters.

Reflective questions

1   Based on the issues emerging from this chapter, examine challenges being faced by deaf students in career preparation and suggest how these can be addressed.
2   How can the teacher training institutions and universities focusing on disability-related courses ensure that their programmes are compatible with inclusive practices?
3   How can educational reforms and legislation in your country be improved in order to assist deaf students to have realistic hopes and aspirations in their vocational choices?

References

Agro, N. (2014). *Public education for deaf and hard of hearing students. USA: American Sign Language (ASL) University lifeprint.* Retrieved from www.lifeprint.com/asl101/topics/public-education-for-deaf-and-hard-of-hearing-students.htm on 10 November 2016.

Becker, R. L. (1988). *Reading-Free Vocational Interest Inventory, Manual.* Columbus: Elburn Pub.

Carnevale, A., Smith, N. & Strohl, J. (2010). *Help wanted: projections of jobs and education requirements through 2018.* Georgetown University of Education and the Workforce, Washington DC. Retrieved from https://cew.georgetown.edu/wp-content/uploads/2014/12/HelpWanted.ExecutiveSummary.pdf on 14 October 2016.

Donaldson, J., Hinton, R. & Nelson, L. (2006). *Preparing students for life: the school-to-work reform movement, issue challenges.* Horizon Site. Retrieved from www.horizon.unc.ed/project/issues/papers/school_to_work.html on 12 October 2016.

Inter-Agency Commission (UNDO, UNESCO, UNICEF, and World Bank) (1990). *Meeting Basic Learning Needs: A Vision for the 1990s: World Conference on Education for All.* New York: UNICEF House Three United Nations Plaza. Retrieved from www.unesco.org/education/pdf/11_92.pdf on 10 November 2016.

Javaraza, R. (2014). *Zimbabwe for Homeless World Cup.* Harare: Zimpapers Ltd. Retrieved from www.b-metro.co.zw/zimbabwe-for-homeless-world-cup/ on 12 October 2016.

Kintrea, K., St Clair, R. & Houston, M. (2011). *The Influence of Parents, Places and Poverty on Educational Attitudes and Aspirations.* London: Joseph Rowntree Foundation.

Lorenzo, T. (ed.) (2011). *Disability Catalyst Africa.* Cape Town: Disability Innovations Africa, School of Health and Rehabilitation Sciences, University of Cape Town.

Luckner, J. L. & Muir, M. (2001). Successful students who are deaf in general education settings. *American Annuals of the Deaf* **146**(5), 450–461.

Madzivanzira, A. (2015). *Include Sign Language in education curriculum.* The Patriot. Retrieved from www.thepatriot.co.zw/old_posts/include-sign-language-in-education-curriculum/ on 10 October 2016.

McMahon, M. & Patton, W. (2002). Using qualitative assessment in career counselling. *International Journal for Educational and Vocational Guidance* **2**, 51–66.

Ministry of Education, Sports and Culture (1987). *Zimbabwe Education Act.* Harare: Government Printers.

Ministry of Education, Sports and Culture (1989). *Circular No. 3 Curricula to Be Followed in Special Educational Institutions.* Harare: Government Printers.

Ministry of Education, Sports and Culture (1991). *Education for Living: 'O' Level Syllabus.* Harare: Government Printers.

Ministry of Education, Sports and Culture (1993). *Education for Living: 'O' Level Syllabus.* Harare: Government Printers.

Mutswanga, P. (2016). *An exploration of personal experiences of deaf people in accessing, participating and completing higher education in Zimbabwe.* Thesis submitted in fulfilment of the requirements for Doctor of Philosophy in Special Needs Education. Harare: Zimbabwe Open University.

Mutswanga, P. & Chakuchichi, D. (2014). A critical analysis of experiences of street vendors in Harare urban: a case of females who are deaf. *The International Journal of Humanities and Social Studies* **2**(9), 331–340.

Punch, R., Hyde, M. & Creed, P. A. (2004). Issues in the school-to-work transition of hard of hearing adolescents. *American Annuals of the Deaf* **149**(1), 28–38.

Rehabilitation International (1990). International Statements on Disability Policy. *Rehabilitation International,* 87–100.

Shield, B. (2006). *Evaluation of the social and economic costs of hearing impairment. A report for HEAR-IT.* Retrieved from www.hear-it.org/sites/default/files/multimedia/documents/Hear_It_Report_ October_2006.pdf on 10 November 2016

United Nations (2006). *Convention on the Rights of People with Disabilities and Optional Protocol.* Retrieved from www.un.org/development/desa/disabilities/convention-on-the-rights-of-persons-with-disabilities. html on 11 September 2016 (pp. 1–5).

United Nations (2012). *Report of the United Nations Conference on Sustainable Development.* United Nations, Rio Janeiro. Retrieved from www.or2d.org/or2d/ressources_files/rapport%20rio%20+%2020.pdf on 10 November 2016.

Warnock, H. M. (1978). *Special Education Needs.* London: Her Majesty's Stationery Office **41**(6), 94–100.

Wolanin, T. R. & Steele, P. E. (2004). *Higher Education Opportunities for Students with Disabilities: A Primer for Policy Makers.* Washington, DC: The Institute for Higher Education Policy.

World Health Organization (1990). *International Classifications of Impairments, Disabilities and Handicaps.* Geneva: WHO.

World Health Organization and World Bank (2011). *Summary World Report on Disability.* Geneva: WHO.

Wyse, S. E. (2012). *Benefits of using cross tabulations in survey analysis.* Retrieved from www.snapsurveys. com/blog/benefits-cross-tabulations-survey-analysis/ on 13 October 2016.

PART V

Religion, gender and parenthood

In Part V, religion, gender and parenthood are discussed to illustrate how they intersect with disability. This results in the exclusion of disabled people, thus highlighting the importance of promoting inclusive sustainable development.

16

THE 'UNHOLY TRINITY' AGAINST DISABLED PEOPLE IN ZIMBABWE

Religion, culture and the Bible

Francis Machingura

Introduction

The negative attitude toward disabled people manifests in the intersections of religion, culture/ tradition and scriptures (the Bible); hence the unholy trinity. Historically, disabled people have experienced discrimination and poverty. Societal interpretation of scriptures in Judaism, Christianity and Islam disabled women, widows, migrants, children and disabled people. Most of the global debates focus on the need to give respect and dignity to disabled people, hence their right to exist. The debates fail to consider the religious dynamics that feed into the stereotypes faced by disabled people. The stereotypes are inextricably bound to culture and different religious traditions. This chapter explores how the interpretation of Judaeo-Christian and African Traditional religio-cultural traditions impact on the wellbeing of disabled people in Zimbabwe. It also advocates for a liberative approach to indigenous traditions, biblical traditions, biblical texts, beliefs and practices on disability. The chapter also engages and interrogates cultural beliefs that fuel the negative beliefs and practices toward disabled people. As a result, all human rights initiatives come to note if men and women of God or religious practitioners in their 'holy talk, spaces, places, platforms and scriptures', do not interrogate certain cultural, religious beliefs, practices and teachings where disability is taken as a sign of sin, curses, disobedience, evil spirits, demons and witchcraft (Chataika, 2013).

African traditional religion and disability in Zimbabwe

The United Nations on the Convention of Rights of Persons with Disabilities (CRPD) defines disability as a socially constructed phenomenon, with a link to human rights and development dimension (United Nations, 2006; Chataika *et al.*, 2012). However, religious traditions, cultures, beliefs/practices as an unholy trinity construct meanings on disability. Some of the religious beliefs, practices, values and norms are part of the constructive forces that create attitudes of either acceptance or rejection and pity toward disabled people. Van Riper and Emerick (1984) note that the cultural and religious assumptions that used to consider disabled people as intolerable nuisances are no longer as prevalent in many societies today as in the past. However, some societies in Africa still look at disabled people with scorn and shame. Perceptions on disability have varied considerably from one society to another (Chimininge, 2016). In African Traditional Religion (ATR), disability is a highly spiritualised reality. It is important to note that ATR is broadly understood and is difficult to define. The discourses and definitions of terms such as African tradition and religion cannot be exhausted in this chapter, though there are general beliefs and practices against disabled people. Disability is generally perceived as a symbol of anomalous relations between the living and the spiritual realm (Magesa, 1997). Each clan or ethnic group in Africa differently maintains its natural cultural, traditional and religious norms that usually assign disabled people to a sub-human status, which is discriminatory. It has become difficult to remove traditional negative myths about disabled people from the followers of ATR (Chimininge, 2016). Several religious and cultural explanations on disability are imbedded in negative myths and beliefs such as the general myths on the causes of disability as resulting from:

- witchcraft;
- a jealous rival who wants the husband of an expectant mother bewitching the child;
- punishment from God;
- curse from ancestors;
- gift from God;
- family trying to get rich but failing to follow the prescribed rituals;
- women ascribing children to men who are not their fathers;
- pregnant woman having sex with a man who is not the father of the baby;
- having sex with disabled people, especially the blind, cures AIDS; and
- women having sex with white men or ghosts.

(Braathen & Ingstaad, 2006; Haihambo & Lightfoot, 2010;
Chataika, 2013; Machingura, 2013)

Critics have argued and associated most negative attitudes and responses to disability as being rooted in beliefs and traditions predominantly attributed to cultural, spiritual or supernatural sources (Claassens, 2013).

Most of the definitions, descriptions and explanations given on disability tend to take away the full humanity of disabled persons. For Biri, Zimunya and Gwara (2016), disabled people are portrayed as tragic victims of an unfortunate accident, disease or as abnormal persons who need urgent help to reverse the disability. Such stereotypes hinder disabled people from freely choosing the lifestyles and careers they wish to enjoy. In fact, societies create or construct attitudes against disabled people. Masolo (2010) argues that all personhood is socially generated. Thus, society defines and characterises all socialisation and participation of all persons and it also plays the environing role. Disability is explained usually by association with witchcraft manifestation of evil and morality challenges (Biri *et al.*, 2016). Witchcraft beliefs are pervasive in ATR. Witches are considered to be sources of evil that make use of extraordinary powers to afflict others (Bourdillon, 1990; Magesa, 1997; Westerlund, 2006). The possibility of witchcraft is always considered when a disabled person is born. Although some afflictions caused by witches are reversible, impairments are culturally considered irreversible and concerned family members must take corrective steps to avoid their recurrence. As such, it can be surmised that attitudes of shame, fear, revulsion, hopelessness and helplessness directed toward disabled people emanate from the irreversibility of impairment.

Rusinga (2012) notes that in ATR, disability is further explained in terms of contravening avoidance rules, traditions and taboos resulting in bad omens. Disability is normally considered a bad omen to the immediate family and the community at large. The bad omen usually results from an avenging spirit (*ngozi*), which for the Shona (Karanga) is another cause of impairments. The word *ngozi* for Aschwanden (1982) is derived from the Karanga word *njodzi*, meaning danger, sorrow or misfortune. For Chimininge (2016), *ngozi* is the spirit of a murdered person seeking reparations, such that a family affected by the *ngozi* spirit experiences various forms of impairments. It is not surprising that any form of impairment is linked to familial shame, curses, social disorder, drought, rejection, disease and famine. The stereotyping of disabled people has resulted in too great a contempt for our fellow brothers and sisters (Addison, 1986). The disability discourse is also associated with sexuality.

In traditional religion, sex is not just a physiological activity but also a religious phenomenon sanctioned and witnessed by the ancestors (Shoko, 2012). Sexual purity and faithfulness are, therefore, practised in honour of not only the living, but also the living dead. Infidelity and engaging in other social ills angers the ancestors because it pollutes family and kinship lineages, leading to experiences of having impairments. Parents of a disabled child are expected to confess their social ills in order for the child to be restored or healed from the impairment. For traditional practitioners, sexual taboos are sacred and any breach of these taboos calls for supernatural vengeance. This explains why the birth of a disabled child is usually blamed on the mother. The suspicion is that the mother could have been unfaithful particularly during pregnancy. Several media reports of men who divorce their wives for giving birth to a disabled child need to be understood in this context. The disabled child is taken as a punishment from God. Yet separations and divorces worsen the economic, moral and social stability of the family. Divorces traumatise the whole family, let alone children. Thus, the disabled child is likely to lose respect, love and joy as s/he grows into adulthood. Hence, it is likely to put women on the receiving end and in a desperate situation such as killing their children for them to be accepted in society. However, there are women who are prepared to be scorned rather than disowning their disabled children.

Barnatt (1992) posits social boundaries that separate the normal from the abnormal pressurise expectant mothers to desist from interacting with disabled people. In Zimbabwe's traditional societies, it is a cultural norm for pregnant women to avoid looking at disabled persons. Disability is believed to emanate from spiritual displeasure; it is generally considered taboo to dare to interact sexually with disabled people. In some cases, some traditional religious practitioners encourage those living with HIV and AIDS to have sex with disabled people in order to be healed. Though, disabled people who are placed on the margins are usually regarded as ritually unclean and defiling and therefore unfit to be married (Douglas, 1988). Hence, they end up earning a conspicuous social stigma that impedes progress in their social development. Whenever people talk about HIV and AIDS, few ever think of disabled people because of the unconscious assumption they are 'asexual'. This practice is hinged on the cultural belief about the transferability of curses. Disability is culturally believed to be a contagious contamination and if an expectant mother comes into contact with a disabled person, she risks contaminating the unborn child. In Zimbabwe, derogatory Shona and Ndebele words are used to describe disabled people, such as *chirema* and *isilima* which have been used, respectively, to imply 'inability to function' and stupidity (Phiri, 2016). The implication is that they are useless people who always wait for help from other people in order to survive.

However, to claim that disabled people are completely rejected in ATR would be an overstatement. Shona society, on the other hand, is generally sympathetic toward disabled people, for example when people are forbidden to mock or laugh at disabled people as evidenced by the Shona idiom *seka urema wafa* (laugh at disability after you are dead) (Machingura, 2013). This idiom implies that there is a high probability for anyone to become disabled, give birth to a disabled child or have any form of impairment in the family. The idiom provides moral sanctions that shape human behaviour and attitudes toward impairment and disabled people. It is considered immoral to laugh at, ridicule or condemn disabled people. Negative remarks are discouraged as the Shona people regard disability as not the property of anybody, but a social construct. There are also many African proverbs that invoke kindness, love, care and protection toward disabled people. Some proverbs even prescribe measures against those who ridicule disabled people. ATR is guided by the philosophy of *ubuntu*, which is an African humanist and ethical world view where a human being is a human being through (*the otherness of*) other human beings (Chataika, 2013). Thus, at the heart of *ubuntu* is respect for diversity of what it means to be human (Eze, 2008). This implies that disabled people are part of a common humanity and embracing diversity is what makes us human.

The African values stand for the values of personhood, hospitality, respect, unity, peace, dignity and worthiness of all human beings, including disabled people. From an African perspective, any denigration and discrimination against disabled people is discrimination against one's own dignity. African values and norms are against the inhumane treatment of others. *Ubuntu* would take any dehumanisation and inhumane treatment of other people as militating against the very nature of the spirit world, which fosters the qualities of cooperation, interconnectedness, partnership, participation, peace, joy, collective identity and reconciliation (Phiri, 2016). Exploitation and dehumanisation of other people based on one's physical condition, disintegrates human dignity, the whole meaning of life and co-existence. African traditions, beliefs, cultures and religions have both positives and negatives when it comes to disability issues. Something that needs to be related or compared with the Bible as the Bible represents the different cultures behind and inside the texts.

The Bible and disability

There are 46 incidents in the Bible where disabled people are portrayed negatively (Bryan, 2006). Some interpretations of the scripture passages in the Old Testament associate disability with impurity or defilement found incompatible with God's holiness. It is not surprising that disabled people are being left to their condition away from the public sphere, thus having any form of impairment becomes a personal tragedy. Visible physical perfection was heavily emphasised over and above the intelligence and moral soundness of the priests (Lev. 21:16–24). In Leviticus, chapter 19, verse 14, we are taught, 'You shall not insult the deaf, or place a stumbling block before the blind.' And in the first chapter of Genesis, we read that each of us is created in the image of God. So there is a tension here in how these chapters of the Bible are interpreted. The reasoning for exclusion is that people judge by looks not by what is within so even then there was awareness of how judgemental society could be. The New Testament includes 'Judge not, that ye be not judged'.

[1] Judge not, that ye be not judged.

[2] For with what judgment ye judge, ye shall be judged: and with what measure ye mete, it shall be measured to you again.

(Matthew 7:1–3 King James Version (KJV))

Judgement causes us to see the other not as a person, but as a thing – as less human and therefore less valuable. And once we do that to a person, or a group of people, it opens the door to all kinds of terrible evil-segregation, injustice, abuse, even genocide. Jesus in Matthew 7:1–3 warns us about excluding anyone, or seeing ourselves or our group as inherently better than any other.

We may disagree and discern another person or group to be wrong – but when that discernment causes us to value another person or group less, then we have crossed the line into judgement, condemnation and exclusion.

For Cochran (2011) and Schofield (2003), the sanctuary was fenced off against pollution, barring priests who were blind, had physical impairments, injured or any kind of blemish from coming close to the altar. The prohibitions emanated from the cultural perceptions and interpretations of purity, ritual stability, morality and holiness (Lev. 19:2; 20:26; 22:32; Ex. 19:6). The early rabbinic readings of Leviticus show that the prohibition to perform priestly duties was originally meant to prevent worshippers from being distracted by the priest's impairment. This was used to draw some connection between soundness of the body and one's spirituality. According to Wenham (1981) and Melcher (1998), one's quality of holiness was measured by one's physical expression of being disabled. Any impairment was deemed as a sign of the person's sin and punishment from God. Any talk on perfection is a human construct that is stigmatising, discriminatory and oppressive to many as well as those labelled as disabled. The issue of social constructionism from the outset has a bearing on everything that is interpreted in life. So different authors have failed to identify that most of the interpretations have come from a particular time period and are linked to cultural ways of thinking. This leaves disabled people exposed to the different territories of the dangers of cultural relativism. Yet disabled people are disabled through social, economic, psychological isolation or exclusion, which underlies the point that disability is a social construct (WHO & World Bank, 2011).

Man was created in the image of God but it is man who denotes perfection. Religious beliefs, traditions and culture as an 'unholy trinity' portray disabled people as not valued by God. It is such traditions, cultures, beliefs and practices that prejudice and disable certain sections of people from participating in the mainstream society. The position of associating sin with disability could have been the understanding by most communities of the time, hence a social construct. Thus, disabled people experience social exclusion and oppression by socially constructed unholy traditions, cultures and religious beliefs. Haihambo and Lightfoot (2010) are right to say that disability is a social construct where each society has its own understanding of disability informed by its cultural beliefs. The Bible also testifies about the different traditions, cultures, religious beliefs and practices that characterise different societies. Eiesland (1994, pp. 73–74) identifies three disabling biblical or theological positions across the major religions that have created obstacles for disabled people where:

- disability is taken as a result of sin;
- disability is taken as suffering that must be endured in order to purify the righteous;
- disabled people are portrayed as cases of charity.

Eiesland's works challenge the above three types of interpretations as being based on societal constructs. She argues that a liberation theology of disability is one that advocates inclusion of disabled people and that much of the disablement experienced by disabled people is socially constructed and therefore open to the possibility of transformation. Disability is biblically viewed as a disease that needs spiritual healing, yet it is supposed to be equated to barriers disabled people face in society (social constructs), which include attitudinal, environmental (physical and communication) and institutional (policies and programmes) barriers (Chataika & McKenzie, 2016). Hence, the need to focus more on the disability (socially constructed barriers) that can be removed with political will, instead of the impairment, which is the loss of or malfunction of a body part (WHO & World Bank, 2011). It matters when disability and sin are conflated when in fact it is society that has imposed these interpretations, not the scriptures. The most common impairments mentioned in the Bible are blindness, deafness, dumbness (*sic*), leprosy, and paralysis.

The general view of the Old Testament writers is that God brings impairments as punishment for transgressions for sin or spiritual disfavour, hence an expression of God's wrath for people's disobedience (Lev. 21:17–21, 26:16). The Hebrew word *mum*, usually translated as 'blemish', refers to many various forms of impairments, such as blindness, deafness or physical impairment (usually referred to in the Bible as lameness, which is derogatory) (Lev. 21:16–23). The blemish is put on the disabled person as well as their immediate family members. Jaeger and Bowman (2005) add that both the Old and New Testaments equate disability with divine punishment for immoral behaviour or sin. Disability is seen as a curse that results from unbelief, disobedience and ignorance (Jewish Encyclopaedia, 1920; The Talmud of Jerusalem, 1956; Encyclopaedia Judaica, 1972; Otieno, 2009). This is the author's interpretation and bound up with cultural assumptions. It is probably worth remembering that when we engage with biblical sources from the past we are touching the very pulse of a society's life. Yet the sources of Oral Law in the Talmud are shaped in a human society and are intimately bound both to the norms of that society and to changes in those norms. The Old Testament takes disability as a religious or theological issue that needs a divine explanation (Gen. 16:2; 20:18; 25:21; 29:31; Ex. 4:11; 23:26; Deut. 7:14; Judges 13:2–3; 1 Sam. 1:5; 2 Chron. 16:22). The curses seem to suggest that any disobedience by any of the children of Israel would result in some form of impairment. Deuteronomy 27 portrays God as admonishing people to obey all His commandments or He will inflict them with blindness. It is not clear whether it is spiritual or physical blindness. We do not know what was meant at the time and this is the issue. We have incidences of Samson who is purported to have sinned against the Lord being punished through his eyes (Judges 14:2; Proverbs 30:17). Hull (2000) points out that the image of God in the Bible is thought of as a perfect body image (Lev. 21:16–23). But what is a 'perfect' body? In the Talmud, a Godly body does not exist because God has no body but instead an essential nature that is divine, an associate in the creation and advancement of the world. Man created in God's image is not God – he is 'a little less' (Ps. 8:6). This is what brings us to the absolute knowledge that all of us are people with disabilities. There is a lot of rabbinical discussion around these points and they do not agree with previous interpretations of disability as a punishment.

Leviticus 13–15 gives detailed instructions for priests when examining a variety of skin diseases. According to Nyamidzi and Mujaho (2016), the prohibitions did not address these skin diseases as medical issues needing treatment but skin diseases as relevant to the larger community religiously and morally. The religious entity influenced and determined the economic, political and social mood of the whole community. Society evaluates the depth of religious belief based on social constructs of bodily perfection and imperfection. The biblical texts show other writers have reified negative definitions of disability because they had failed to reflect. It is assumed that if one is 'right' with the Lord, there is no excuse for having physical flaws in light of any form of impairment (Wenham, 1981). Disabled people are expected to be permanently trapped in the tragedy of their fate. Accordingly, the impression given is that, the God of the Bible is the God of the non-disabled and not of disabled people.

Wilkes (1980, p. 21) notes that the doctrine of the imputation of wholeness and righteousness has brought problems for disabled people, stemming from the belief that strength of faith, or lack of it, has to do with being disabled. Wilkes might claim this but faulty theorising which conflates sin and disability fails to explore where these perceptions and interpretations arise from. Lack of knowledge of what it means to have impairments is the main problem in the broader Zimbabwean communities. This results in fears, for example, of witchcraft, sorcery, *juju* (a spiritual belief system incorporating objects such as amulets, and spells used in religious practice, as part of witchcraft) that might cause expecting mothers having disabled children (Machingura & Masengwe, 2014; Machingura, 2013). Thus, having a disabled child continues to be seen in Zimbabwe as a misfortune and expressions such as, 'Who did wrong that this happened?' or 'Everyone gets what he/she deserves', can still be heard from some people (Wilkes, 1980). The linking of disability to the 'perfect body image' that is found in the Bible has caused disabled people to be viewed and treated negatively even on sexuality issues.

The Hebraic law, Torah and Jewish rituals also classified disabled with legal uncleanness and diseases. According to Stiker (1999, p. 4):

> The disabled had the status of prostitutes or of women whom menstruation made unclean. The Encyclopaedia Judaica develops this concept in the article 'Blemish' by enumerating the impairments that includes: blindness and certain eye diseases, injuries to the thigh, a deformed nose, lameness, a humped back, skin diseases even if not precisely identified, the loss of a testicle.

Blemish may have had different meanings at the time, though we are interpreting it with modern notions around the word. Some of the meanings got changed to suit the meanings as well as serving the interests of men and not women. We will not forget that many words were from Aramaic and old Hebrew. Many of the teachings were passed down through oral traditions and cultures. Translation might have changed the meaning of the word. Women generally in the Old Testament are seen as second-class and impure. It was a patriarchal society and women generally had second-class status, they were often used as bargaining tools to forge dynasties or appease oppressors. This worsened the stigma generated or attached to disabled women. The negative attitude results in a skewed world, first, as physical impairment, second, as an economic impairment (Mark 10:46–52) (Brueggemann, 2008).

However, the Old Testament has texts that talk positively about the total human being and his originality, such as the creation narratives. This helps us to appreciate the multiple voices and diversity in the Bible though we must emphasise those texts that focus on unity, respect, peace and freedom. For Oostrom (1990), everything is good in the hands of the creator God: 'God saw it was good – it was very good.' According to Longchar and Cowan (2014), disabled people are part of the humanity that made the first creation good, as every human being is made in God's image and likeness (*Imago Dei*). This goodness can be understood for its appropriateness for the purposes of God that are there to support all human life in all its forms, find meaning and purpose for being and enhances all human experience. All humanity is the same despite the classification that people give disabled people as 'other'. The *Imago Dei* challenges the notion that considers disabled people as less human, and the unproved perspective that their impairments make them not resemble God. As a result, society negatively interpreted the scriptures and placed its own meaning on them. Vengei (2016) argues that the monarchy initiated discrimination against people in key positions within Israelite society such as politicians, priests, prophets and legislators on the basis of tribal affiliation, gender and disability. Vengei (2016, p. 26) takes true Yahwism as not having been discriminatory against anybody in terms of one's gender, impairment, economic status and tribal background:

> Biblical texts that discriminate against people with disabilities were created during the monarchy to legitimate certain people by discriminating against others. Otherwise, the will, nature and attitude of God toward disability is non-discriminatory.

Though the Bible is a holy book, it has some parts or texts that are violent, abusive and hence not holy. This is important because it underlines a social constructionist perspective of disability and highlights negative attitudes and perceptions. Disabled people deserve respect, love, compassion, protection and dignity just like anybody. The immortality of the soul constitutes the spiritual status of all people in taking the image of God regardless of form and appearance. King David realised the importance of inclusivity by showing great compassion and care to Mephibosheth, son of Jonathan, who was unable to walk (1 Sam. 4:4). For David, Mephibosheth was human like him. David showed great kindness by restoring Mephibosheth's wealth; a sign that justice must be accorded to all people. David did not look at Mephibosheth's physical impairment. David's compassion is crucial today in cultivating societal inclusiveness of all people by fighting off unholy traditions, cultures, biblical texts, religious beliefs and practices that disable and disempower disabled people. Old Testament texts cited against disabled people contradict the Old Testament texts that celebrate diversity. For example, God bestowed the leadership role onto Moses who stuttered, but he still became the chosen national leader of the Israelite nation. People find Moses as the model of liberation but they do not talk about his impairment that did not prevent him from performing his duties as saviour of the people. Our interpretation of the Bible must be influenced by the Bible from its disability context though there is need for a disability hermeneutics that considers current and contextualised theological understanding. Disabled people, too, were created in the image of God as shown by the teachings in the Talmud:

> It happened upon a man who was extremely ugly. The man said, 'Shalom to you, Rabbi!' Rabbi Simeon did not reply. Instead he exclaimed, 'Idiot! How ugly that man is! Could it be that all the people of your city are as ugly as you?' The man said, 'I do not know, why not go to the Artisan who made me, and tell Him, "How ugly that vessel is that You made!"' When Rabbi Simeon realized that he had done wrong, he dismounted from his donkey and fell down at the man's feet, saying, 'I fully accept – please forgive me.' 'I will not forgive you,' said the man, 'until you go to that Artist who made me and tell him, "How ugly that vessel is that You made."'
>
> *(Ta'anit 20a–20b)*

This reinforces that God made man and shames the rabbi for making judgements. This will remove unholy beliefs, practices, myths and teachings that take impairments as a curse. The problems we face in the Old Testament are the same challenges faced when reading the New Testament on disability issues.

In the New Testament, disabled people are also linked to sin and viewed as possessed by evil or cursed. This link is well illustrated in John 9:1–3, when the disciples of Jesus asked him saying: 'Rabbi, who sinned, this man or his parents that he was born blind?' The disciples' questions are evident to the prevailing unholy attitude, beliefs and practices of the time that took impairments as caused by sin. For Nsengiyumwa (2016), this is in accordance with the Old Testament Deuteronomistic doctrine that considers God to be a moral person who rewards people who do right and punishes those who do wrong. Yet the disciples fuelled the pain of the visually impaired man by asking Jesus to explain to the general public what has caused what the disciples took for misfortune. The negative views toward disability as societal constructs are reified by writers who fail to reflect on the historical reasons for these constructions. Contemporary African peoples, like the disciples of Jesus, erroneously take disability as a punishment from God (or the gods). What complicates the whole discourse is that when Jesus healed the physically impaired man who lay by the pool of Bethesda, He said to him: 'See, you are well again. Stop sinning or something worse will happen to you' (John 5:14). When Jesus healed the man with paralysis who was lowered through the roof (Mark 2:1–12), Jesus once again said to him: 'Son, your sins are forgiven' (vs 5), and then continued with the physical healing of the man. In Matthew 9:2, Jesus said to the man with cerebral palsy, 'My son, your sins are forgiven'. Were these unholy words coming from Jesus? No! I do not think so. It might not be Jesus. The position of associating sin with disability could have been the understanding or construct by most communities of the time. We find the same societal construction or understanding of disability among the Jewish religious groups such as the Pharisees, Sadducees, Essenes and Zealots generally excluded disabled people of all kinds.

Instead of Jesus being applauded for the miraculous healing of the blind man; the Pharisees accused him of breaking the Sabbath on the counts:

- healing of the blind man on the Sabbath, which was only permissible if life was in danger,
- kneading the mud on the Sabbath, which was specifically forbidden, and
- anointing the man's eyes on the Sabbath.

The Pharisees could not count the visually impaired man as part of them, as they later threw him out on the streets for arguing against them (John 9:1–34). The biblical texts expose the worlds behind, inside and in front of the texts, that they were written within a context. We, however, need to be aware that the Bible has historically been used to foster intolerance and justify some people's absolute interpretation against those of others such as disabled people, homosexuals, women and children (Kabue, 2016). According to Grant (1997, p. 45), the healing stories of Jesus 'have also been used to serve as proof of the moral imperfection of people with disabilities'. The conflation between sin and impairment confirms unholy cultural models of disability, which views disability as a punishment inflicted upon an individual or family by God as a result of sin. It is proof by man who has interpreted the sayings with a negative intent. Consequently, the presence of impairment stigmatises not only the individual but the whole family. The implication is the exclusion of disabled people from the social, economic, political and spiritual spheres of society. In John 9:41, Jesus responds to the continued questioning of the Pharisees with regard to the healing of a visually impaired person as follows: 'If you were blind, you would not be guilty of sin.' According to Hull (2000), Jesus uses the expression 'blind' as a term of abuse in the Gospel of Matthew. When Jesus attacks certain groups of people, he describes them as 'blind guides' (Matt. 23: 16, 24), 'blind fools' (v.17), and 'you blind Pharisees' (v.26). The metaphoric use of impairment as a symbol of sin, unbelief and ignorance, further highlights the concept of disability as one that is viewed from a moral perspective.

For Kabue (2012), Jesus must be understood in the context of his ministry where Jesus reinterprets his role with regard to disabled people and showing that the fundamental teaching of the Bible is love. Christ announced his mission in the synagogue in Nazareth as follows:

> The spirit of the Lord . . . anointed me to preach the good news to the poor. He sent me to proclaim freedom for the prisoners, and the recovery of sight for the blind, to release the oppressed, to proclaim the year of the Lord's favour.
>
> *(Luke 4: 18–19)*

As people we interpret blindness as physical impairment, but I do not think it is also blindness to the ways of God. It is people who create a culture that negatively regard disability and not God doing it. The four gospels show Jesus spending much time with the 'least' privileged in society, and displaying great compassion for disabled people. The gospel healing stories are seen not as merely cure of the body but more of the individual's restoration in and into the society, hence making them human and part of the broader community. When the blind Bartimeus' sight is restored (Mark 10:46–52), he immediately joins in the procession with the others and is transformed from the beggar on the roadside to a member of the crowd that followed with Jesus (Kabue, 2016). It does not mean that for one to be whole or accepted, he/she has to be healed first before being accepted in the broader community. Healing must not be taken as a conditionality that makes one complete. If we think about the time the book of John was written, people lived in an agrarian society and sight was important in order to till the land, plant seed, cut crops, tend sheep, etc. If we think about how people lived then being able to support yourself when there was no welfare from the state was key to survival, otherwise the disabled people were reliant on begging. Healing is not the only facet that will bring acceptance and inclusivity of all people, including disabled people. People's attitudes must be changed. People were made in God's image, meaning disabled people were also made in God's image. Eiesland (1994) argues that in encountering the Disabled God, if we are all made in His image, it also includes those who are blind, deaf and otherwise disabled, meaning that he is also a disabled God just like his creation. For Jesus, there was no distinction between social restoration and physical healing, hence the holistic theological interpretation and attention to disability. Jesus found it easy to interact and embrace women, the poor, refugees, disabled people and children. Paul makes it clear that Christ came as a perfect sacrifice for all (Rom. 10:4) since all people are sinners who fell short of the glory of God (Rom. 3:23). The New Testament Jesus breaks all forms of discrimination and purity taboos by associating with all people who had been marginalised. Unfortunately, the Bible is intermingled with texts that have been interpreted in oppressive ways and together these continue to reinforce the marginalisation, discrimination and exclusion of disabled people in the social, economic, political and religious life of the society. Contemporary interpreters of the gospels give a wrong impression on the miracles of Jesus as a result of erroneous social constructs, for example portraying him as having healed all disabled people that he met. Yet some were healed and many were not.

Jarvis and Johnson (2015) add that John 5:7 shows that there is the human inaction due to social constructs that implicates human beings in the suffering of others. For example, when the man with impairment said to Jesus, 'Sir, I have no man to put me into the pool when the water is troubled, and while I am going another steps down before me', the man implicates the cruelty of society in abandoning the marginalised sick and disabled people. Interpreters of scripture need to be acutely and sensitively aware of the implications of certain biblical texts that tend to stereotype disabled people (Gillibrand, 2010). The texts tend to give the unholy impression that any form of impairment is a sign of uncleanness, incompetency, flawedness, weakness or the intrusion of demons or Satan. The end result is that all disabled people are relegated to the margins. Yet the New Testament Jesus breaks all forms of discrimination and purity taboos by associating with everybody, including those excluded by the different cultures.

Biblical texts, just like African traditions, beliefs and cultures, must never be taken for granted when it comes to how they shape attitudes, values, beliefs and practices toward disabled people. Biblical texts feed from beliefs found in Judaism and Christianity just like ATR on disabled people, hence 'an unholy trinity'. I am still wondering what makes such an unholy trinity, given the trinity is the Father, Son and Holy Ghost; and they are one and the same thing – implying that God is one. Cultures and religions must help create a tolerant and inclusive society that creates opportunities for all the people. The theological engagement of the Bible must help challenge our theological understandings and misunderstandings of disability. Because of the deeper theological awareness on disability due to societal pressure, religions are now moving toward a new sense of acceptance of disabled people. However, the best pastoral care begins by listening intently to the person's story, for example, their struggles, hopes and fears. Religious beliefs, practices, values, traditions and culture that demean the status of disabled people must be reinterpreted in order to rightly hear their voices. We need to introspect ourselves as a society as to: how do our attitudes become negative and patronising to disabled people? Wouldn't our societies become real homes to all members if negative dispositions are challenged in order to transform the societal thinking?

Conclusion

The broader mainstream society must be conscientised on the beauty and strength that nations have the moment there is an inclusive society that is built on honesty, trust and respect of all members including disabled people. Religions, civic organisations and government must create an inclusive environment that gives hope to the excluded, vulnerable, disfranchised, disabled people and women. Religions, traditions, beliefs, history and culture are always changing because they are dynamic; the changes must also influence the way we look at and understand disability. As people, we live with limitations and there are no superhumans. Culture, tradition and religion must help bring respect, inclusiveness, equality and dignity to all people. All unholy biblical texts must be avoided and ignored in any discourses about disability.

References

Addison, J. (1986). *Handicapped People in Zimbabwe*. Harare: NASCOH.

Aschwanden, H. (1982). *Symbols of Life: An Analysis of the Consciousness of the Karanga*. Gweru: Mambo Press.

Barnatt, N. (1992). Policy issues in disability and rehabilitation in developing countries. *Journal of Disability Policy Studies* **4**, 45–65.

Biri, K., Zimunya, C. T. & Gwara, J. (2016). Personhood and disability in Zimbabwe: a philosophical analysis. In S. Kabue, J. Amanze & C. Landman (eds) *A Resource Book for Theology and Religious Studies* (pp. 387–398). Nairobi: Action Publishers.

Bourdillon, M. F. C. (1990). *Religion and Society: A Text for Africa*. Gweru: Mambo Press.

Braathen, S. H. & Ingstaad, B. (2006). Albinism in Malawi: knowledge and beliefs from an African setting. *Disability and Society* **21**(6), 599–611.

Brueggemann, W. (2008). *Great Prayers of the Old Testament*. Louisville, KY: Westminister John Knox Press.

Bryan, W. V. (2006). *In Search of Freedom: How Persons Living with Disabilities Have Been Disenfranchised from the Mainstream of American Society and How the Search for Freedom Continues*. Springfield, IL: Charles C. Thomas Publisher Ltd.

Chataika, T. (2013). Cultural and religious explanations of disability and promoting inclusive communities. In J. M. Claassen, L. Swartz & L. Hansen (eds) *Search for Dignity: Conversations on Human Dignity, Theology and Disability* (pp. 117–128). Cape Town: African Sun Media (Stellenbosch University).

Chataika, T. & McKenzie, J. A. (2016). Global institutions and their engagement with disability mainstreaming in the South: development and (dis)connections. In S. Grech & K. Soldatic (eds) *Disability in the Global South: The Critical Handbook* (pp. 423–436). Geneva: Springer International Publishing.

Chataika, T., McKenzie, J. A., Swart, E. & Lyner-Cleophas, M. (2012). Access to education in Africa: responding to the United Nations Convention on the Rights of Persons with Disabilities. *Disability & Society* **27**(3), 385–398.

Chimininge, V. (2016). Attitudes of traditional Karanga Society towards people with speech disorder. In S. Kabue, J. Amanze & C. Landman (eds) *Disability in Africa: A Resource Book for Theology and Religious Studies* (pp. 29–41). Nairobi: Action Publishers.

Claassens, J. (2013). Job, theology and disability: moving towards a new kind of speech. *Search for Dignity: Conversations on Human Dignity, Theology and Disability* (pp. 55–66). Cape Town: African Sun Media (Stellenbosch University).

Cochran, E. A. (2011). *Dictionary of Scripture and Ethics*. Grand Rapids, MI: Baker Academy Publishing Company.

Douglas, M. (1988). *Purity and Danger: An Analysis of the Concepts of Pollution and Taboo*. London: Ark Paperbacks.

Eiesland, N. L. (1994). *The Disabled God: Toward a Liberatory Theology of Disability*. Nashville: Abingdon Press.

Eze, M. O. (2008). What is African communitarianism? Against consensus as a regulative ideal. *South African Journal of Philosophy* **27**(4), 386–399. Retrieved from http://dx.doi. org/10.4314/sajpem. v27i4.31526 on 9 April 2017.

Gillibrand, J. (2010). *Disabled Church-Disabled Society: The Implications of Autism for Philosophy, Theology and Politics*. London: Jessica Kingsley Publishers.

Grant, C. (1997). Reinterpreting the healing narratives. In N. Eiesland & D. Saliers (eds) *Human Disability and the Service of God: Reassessing Religious Practice* (pp. 72–87). Nashville: Abingdon.

Haihambo, C. & Lightfoot, E. (2010). Cultural beliefs regarding people with disabilities in Namibia: implications for the inclusion of people with disabilities. *International Journal of Special Education* **25**(3), 76–87.

Hull, J. (2000). *Blindness and the face of God*. Unpublished manuscript.

Jaeger, P. T. & Bowman, C. A. (2005). *Understanding Disability: Inclusion, Access, Diversity and Civil Rights*. New York: Greenwood Publishing Group.

Jarvis, C. A. & Johnson, E. E. (2015). *Feasting on the Gospels: A Feasting on the Word Commentary*. Louisville, KY: Westminster John Knox Press.

Kabue, S. (ed.) (2012). *Disability, Society and Theology: Voices from Africa*. Kijabe: Kijabe Printing Press.

Kabue, S. (2016). Disability: post-modernity challenges to the theology. In S. Kabue, J. Amanze & C. Landman (eds) *Disability in Africa: A Resource Book for Theology and Religious Studies* (pp. 213–230). Nairobi: Action Publishers.

Longchar, W. & Cowan, G. (eds) (2014). *Doing Theology from Disability Perspective*. Manica: The Association for Theological Education in South East Asia.

Machingura, F. (2013). The rights of people with disability from a third world perspective: the Zimbabwean context. In S. S. Bagchi & A. Das (eds) *Human Rights and the Third World: Issues and Discourses* (pp. 287–308). London: Lexington Books.

Machingura, F. & Masengwe, G. (2014). *Dealing with Stereotypes against Persons Living and Working with Disabilities in Zimbabwe*. Williamstown, MA: Piraeus Books.

Magesa, L. (1997). *African Religion: The Moral Traditions of Abundant Life*. Nairobi: Paulus Publications Africa.

Masolo, D. (2010). *Self and Community in a Changing World*. Bloomington: Indiana University Press.

Melcher, S. J. (1998). Visualising the perfect cult. In N. Eiseland & D. Saliers (eds) *Human Disability and the Service of God: Reassessing Religious Practice* (pp. 55–71). Nashville: Abingdon Press.

Nsengiyumwa, F. (2016). Jesus and his healing miracles: insights for people with disabilities. In S. Kabue, J. Amanze & C. Landman (eds) *Disability in Africa: A Resource Book for Theology and Religious Studies* (pp. 111–124). Nairobi: Action Publishers..

Nyamidzi, K. & Mujaho, Z. (2016). Disability and the beauty of creation: an analysis of the Old Testament perception on disability. In S. Kabue, J. Amanze & C. Landman (eds) *Disability in Africa: A Resource Book for Theology and Religious Studies* (pp. 77–96). Nairobi: Action Publishers.

Oostrom, W. F. (1990). *The Message of the Old Testament*. Nairobi: St Paul Communications.

Otieno, P. A. (2009). Biblical and theological perspectives on disability: implications on the rights of persons with disability in Kenya. *Disability Quarterly Studies* **29**(4), 988–1164. Retrieved from http://dsq-sds.org/article/view/988/1164 on 15 July 2016.

Phiri, M. (2016). Constructing an African theology of disability: conceptual imperatives. In S. Kabue, J. Amanze & C. Landman (eds) *Disability in Africa: A Resource Book for Theology and Religious Studies* (pp. 267–287). Nairobi: Action Publishers.

Rusinga, O. (2012). Perceptions of deaf youth about their vulnerability to sexual and reproductive health problems in Masvingo district, Zimbabwe. *African Journal of Reproductive Health* **16**(2), 271–283.

Schofield, R. (2003). *Mystery or Magic: Biblical Replies to the Heterodox*. Blantyre: Kachere Series.

Shoko, T. (2012). Karanga men, culture and HIV in Zimbabwe. In E. Chitando & S. Chirongoma (eds) *Redemptive Masculinities: Men, HIV and Religion* (pp. 91–112). Geneva: World Council of Churches Publications.

Stiker, H. J. (1999). *A History of Disability*. Ann Arbor, MI: University of Michigan.

United Nations (2006). *Convention on the Rights of Persons with Disabilities.* Retrieved from www.un.org/development/desa/disabilities/convention-on-the-rights-of-persons-with-disabilities.html on 18 March 2017.

Van Riper, C. & Emerick, L. (1984). *Speech Correction: An Introduction to Speech Pathology and Audiology.* Englewood Cliffs, NJ: Prentice-Hall.

Vengei, O. (2016). The interpretation of biblical texts on disability: then and now. In S. Kabue, J. Amanze & C. Landman (eds) *Disability in Africa: A Resource Book for Theology and Religious Studies* (pp. 136–164). Nairobi: Action Publishers.

Wenham, G. (1981). *The Book of Leviticus.* Grand Rapids, MI: Eerdmans.

Westerlund, D. (2006). *African Indigenous Religions and Disease Causation: From Spiritual Beings to Living Humans.* Leiden/Boston: Brill.

Wilkes, H. (1980). *Creating a Caring Congregation: Guidelines for Ministry with the Handicapped.* Nashville: Abingdon.

World Health Organization and World Bank (2011). *World Report on Disability.* WHO & World Bank.

17

ADDRESSING DISABILITY AND GENDER IN EDUCATION DEVELOPMENT

Global policies, local strategies

Elina Lehtomäki, Mari-Anne Okkolin
and Magreth Matonya

Introduction

In this chapter, we examine the global approaches and (policy) frameworks on disability and gender, focusing on similarities and differences over decades, their extent and intersection. Key to this chapter are issues of differences in the approaches to gender and disability in education development, as well as the interface of disability and gender, with reference to inclusion, equality and equity. The global frameworks related to disability and gender are studied though a country case, Tanzania, and its strategies for achieving equality and equity in education. By comparing the ways in which disability and gender have been addressed in education development, we analyse what the differences in approaches disclose. Our main argument is that analysing *disability and gender together* provides information both for global policies as well as local strategies about inclusive education as well as requirements for sustainable approaches in broader social changes.

Global policy frameworks for education development

Several global policy frameworks for education development based on universal human rights have aimed to ensure gender equality and equity in education. In 1990, the World Declaration on Education For All (EFA) and in 2000, the Dakar Framework for Action and the Millennium Development Goals (MDGs) set universal primary education and gender equality on the global development agenda. While there has been clear progress in reaching gender parity in lower levels of education, including persons with disabilities in education and ensuring their equality and equity in participating in learning seems seriously more challenging to education systems. The 2006 United Nations Convention on the Rights of Persons with Disabilities (CRPD) has assured the universal right to inclusive education systems without discrimination based on one's impairment. It also states that schools are to be enabling environments for all (United Nations, 2006). Furthermore, the CRPD has called attention to the particularly vulnerable situation of girls and women with disabilities. Reflecting on the impact of the CRPD, Shakespeare (2015, p. 318) has noted that in general, 'there is a huge gap between having a Treaty and achieving human rights'. Also in Africa, global engagements such as the CRPD have little influence in practice, if not combined with local strategies (Chataika *et al.*, 2012). Yet, approaches to reach gender equality in education have contributed to progress over decades, while the process to include students with disabilities has been clearly slower. Are there ways to accelerate it?

In 2015, the United Nations fourth Sustainable Development Goal (SDG) confirmed inclusion, equality and equity as the key factors in quality education. *Inclusion* is to ensure that all learners participate successfully, reaching a minimum standard of knowledge and skills, such as reading, writing and doing basic mathematics. *Equality* refers to equal opportunities to access and attend education and participate in learning processes. *Equity* builds on two fundamental principles, fairness and inclusion in education, meaning that personal characteristics and social circumstances, such as gender, socio-economic status or ethnic origin do not represent obstacles in education (United Nations, 2017). Fair and inclusive education is one of the most powerful levers available to make society more equitable (Morley & Croft, 2011; Ainscow *et al.*, 2012; Unterhalter, 2012).

The SDG 4 specific target 4.5 on gender parity mentions also disability:

> By 2030, eliminate gender disparities in education and ensure equal access to all levels of education and vocational training for the vulnerable, including persons with disabilities, indigenous peoples and children in vulnerable situations with parity indices including disability.
>
> *(United Nations, 2015)*

The parity indices for monitoring progress toward this target (4.5.1) require disaggregated data in terms of female/male, rural/urban, bottom/top wealth quintile and disability status, indigenous peoples and conflict-affected (ibid.). Disaggregated data have, indeed, been invaluable in monitoring gender parity (Subrahmanian, 2005; Unterhalter, 2012), thus providing important information about the changes in education. For monitoring progress toward inclusive education, disaggregated data are necessary at three distinct levels, instructional, school or education system and community or society level (Dyson, 1999). These three levels characterise also the main discourses around inclusive education (ibid.; Kiuppis & Haustätter, 2014). Different from gender parity information, disaggregated data on students with disabilities are mostly missing in education development reports, which suggests that, in the case of persons with disabilities, the progress toward equality and equity in education is not monitored.

In the following sections, we discuss the processes for, and achievements in, gender parity and equality, and compare these with the approaches addressing inclusion of persons with disabilities in education. In addition to the global processes, also changes in Tanzania are analysed. The reason is that Tanzania is one of the sub-Saharan countries that has reached gender parity in primary education and shown promising changes in secondary level education (Okkolin, Lehtomäki & Bhalalusesa, 2010). Furthermore, the Tanzanian government is committed to inclusive education in the broad term, confirming the right to education as universal regardless of gender, ethnicity, language, disability and socio-economic background. The government has also signed and ratified the CRPD and reported on enrolments of students with disabilities (Lehtomäki, Tuomi & Matonya, 2014).

Globally, there have been important steps in creating access to education and reaching parity, i.e. enrolments in education, while the intersection of gender and disability, the case of girls and women with disabilities, reveals how the progress toward quality education for all, equality, equity and inclusion in education requires nuanced consideration of the combination of various factors. In Tanzania, as in most sub-Saharan countries, *being female and with disability* multiplies the risk of facing marginalisation, discrimination and exclusion in education (Meekosha & Soldatic, 2011; Morley & Croft, 2012; Croft, 2012; Matonya, 2016; Chataika & McKenzie, 2016). Therefore, the efforts addressing the gender gap in education need new or, as Groce *et al.* (2011) suggest *more nuanced* understanding to the specific situation of girls and women with disabilities in education and approaches that better bridge policy and practice. Consequently, our core questions are how the approaches addressing gender and those addressing disability in education differ and what these approaches might learn from the intersection of gender and disability.

Addressing the gender gap

The global frameworks have influenced regional and national education strategies and plans to different extent in each country context. Against the broader discussion and research on gender and education, how has gender equality and equity been addressed and assessed in the mainstream development narratives historically? Gross- and Net-Enrolment-Rates (GER and NER) and gender parity have been, and still are, the most widely used indicators that the national bodies and international agencies apply to monitor and evaluate educational advancement.[1] These indicators are, however, static 'snapshots', because neither the GER nor NER can monitor, for instance, how regularly the children actually attend school; neither do they capture the aspects of the quality of teaching and learning. Furthermore, as noted by Unterhalter and Brighouse (2007) and Subrahmanian (2005) *gender parity* in 'access to' and 'participation in' education is neither synonymous with, nor an index for, *gender equality*, nor does it capture the complexity of intersecting and relational dimensions of *gender inequality*.

It is evident that different understandings of *gender, equality* and quality of education generate different approaches with which to *pursue* gender equality in education; different ways by which to *assess* development and change; and finally different *portrayals* of gender equality in education globally and within each country context. In this section, different understandings and approaches regarding gender equality are presented. We will follow the three categories defined by Unterhalter (2005, 2007) and discuss the distributive equality, equality of condition and equality of capabilities (interchangeable in here with the substantive equality) from a historical angle.

Distributive equality approach

To begin with, gender can be understood as a descriptive characteristic of a person based ontologically on biology, 'meaning no more than having short hair or a birthday in September' (Unterhalter, 2005; 2007, p. 98). As per this understanding, equality in education is connected first and foremost to distribution, such as to the availability of schools (for all) and an equal number of years of schooling. This understanding dominates and guides the ways in which governments collect and present statistical data, and international organisations such as UNESCO and the OECD make comparisons (Unterhalter, 2005; Okkolin & Lehtomäki, 2005). According to Subrahmanian (2005, p. 397), this is not, however, gender equality, but gender *parity*, offering only the 'first-stage' measure of progress toward gender *equality*. Unterhalter (2007) has termed this understanding as for a *distributive equality*, having its undertones significantly in the 'women in development' approach that emerged in the 1970s.[2]

The main targets for the first wave of feminism in development and 'women in development' (WID) advocates were to make women a recognised constituency, a visible and distinctive category in development policy and discourse, in response to the denial of the voice and agency of women (see e.g. Kabeer, 1994; Fennel & Arnot, 2009). It became clear that this recognition was rather categorical and symbolic, that it was unsupported by material resources or political commitment, and this paved the way for the shift from 'women' to 'gender relations' as the focus of analysis (Kabeer, 1994, p. xii). The implication of relying categorically on 'women' only, was that the 'problem' too, for instance, to achieve gender equality in education, like the solution, concerned women only, and put aside the very essence of the 'problem', that is, the relational and hierarchical nature of it. For this reason, the gender and development (GAD) approach, having a more structuralist perspective with which to re-examine similar kinds of 'problems' that the WID had sought to address, took root in the development discourse and agenda. As remarked on by Kabeer (1994, p. xiii), just as a class analysis can be used to understand and address the problems of the poor, so too a gender analysis can be used to understand and address the problems of women's subordination. Thus, having its undertone in Marxist thinking, but moving well beyond the tradition, the analyses moved toward structured and socially constructed disadvantages that women face relative to men, drawing attention to positions constituted by social relations.

Equality of conditions approach

The GAD approach resonates with the *second* understanding of gender equality in education, defined as the *equality of conditions* by Unterhalter (2007), and deriving from structuralist and quite different post-structuralist approaches (associated ideas drawing from critical theory and post-colonialism). Evidently, and in contrast to the value-neutral first meaning with regard to 'having a birthday in September', the *equality of conditions* approach is packed with structural inequalities and discriminatory processes, practices and meanings, on which grounds gender is ontologically constituted and constructed. Hence, gender equality means the removal of structural barriers and institutionalised discriminatory values, norms, procedures and rules (Unterhalter, 2005), the post-structuralist discourse tends to place more emphasis on multiplicity and the prospect for *difference* rather than for equality, and thus to complex forms of negotiations exercised by the excluded groups, such as women.

The key point and methodological challenge in here is that gender equality is not just about counting numbers, nor is it about an equal amount of education, equality of outcomes or achievements; rather, it is about creating equal empowerment and enabling conditions for people, which, in turn, require creating an understanding about the complex array of social relations and arrangements embedded in the girls' and women's education and schooling. In other words, within the *equality of conditions* approach, gender resonates with deeply imbued social relationships and positions, while equality refers to equalised conditions in school, and education in its broadest sense (interlinked with other areas of social policy); alike, it refers to 'equal regard', influenced by an appreciation of considerable difference (Unterhalter, 2007). As remarked on by Unterhalter (ibid.), the vision of equality in here is enormously important as a goal to be aimed at, yet it might be too overwhelming a policy challenge for governments.

Substantive equality/equality of capabilities approach

Kabeer (1999, in Subrahmanian, 2005) has made a statement according to which the achievement of *substantive equality* requires the recognition of the difference between capacities of women and men based on biology, *and* in terms of social constructed disadvantagement. To continue with this idea, Subrahmanian (2005) has proposed that to achieve substantive equality depends on two further processes to reveal *how* it has been reached. She (ibid.) suggests focusing on the socially constructed pathway(s) to equality, referring at first to the *quality of experience* (access *to* education, participating *in* it and benefiting *from* it), presuming that there is equality of treatment and equality of opportunity, and second, to a *commitment* to non-discrimination. Yet, assessing gender equality reaches beyond the aspects of treatment and opportunity and involves the elements of agency and autonomy. In other words, for Subrahmanian (ibid.), to achieve and to assess substantive equality, and for the process to be meaningful from the perspective of gender, it depends profoundly on the equal distribution, equal opportunities *and* the recognition of the fundamental freedoms.

What Subrahmanian (2005) asserts, corresponds with the *third* meaning of gender equality in Unterhalter's (2005) definition arguing that gender implies both socially constructed constraints on women's *capabilities* (well-being freedoms) and the negotiation processes dependent on women's *agency* (achievements and freedoms) (e.g. Sen, 1992, 1993, 1999; Robeyns, 2005, 2006). The key here is the possibility for change, referring to the attributes of the person, on the one hand, and to social relations, on the other. For instance, girls from different families and broader social and societal contexts might 'do gender' differently at different moments in their own lives, sometimes because of the demands of the structures, but sometimes because of negotiations and contestations; this meaning of gender acknowledges the power of macro-level social relations, yet analogously to gendered micro-identities, comprehends the gendered educational hierarchies and institutions to be challengeable and changeable (Unterhalter, 2007).

Unterhalter relates the third understanding of gender equality to the concept of representational justice, referring to the work of Nancy Fraser, who locates the dimensions of *process* and *difference* at the core of equality assessment by comparing (1) whether women participate in terms of parity with men in the decision-making and (2) whether the languages and routes to power they have are equal. Thus, when framed within the discussion and assessment of gender equality in education, the focus is on the micro-level pathways and processes, and on the macro-level commitments to non-discriminatory policies in education, acknowledging that different groups of people, such as female students, might need different kinds of initiatives to advance. Obviously, this understanding of gender equality in education overlaps with the second definition, and elsewhere, too, the conceptual boundaries and the approaches per se cross over.

Reflecting Tanzanian approaches

The Government of Tanzania has defined education as a national priority and is committed to equity and non-discrimination policies in education. Over the last decades the government has initiated a series of reforms to ensure equal access to primary education of good quality for all children, to expand secondary education, and also to promote education and empowerment of girls. Since 1975 universal primary education has been the goal in Tanzania. The Education Act of 1978 made primary education compulsory, though not free.

In practice, reflecting the commitments formulated by the global development community, gender equality has been recognised as a development goal per se and moreover, as a cross-cutting issue in sustainable social development and the poverty-reduction process in Tanzania. Tanzanian educational reforms entail both gender parity and gender equality objectives, which are quantitative and qualitative goals, respectively. Presumably, gender inequalities cannot be addressed by any single approach to gender or equality, but various initiatives, such as all three approaches discussed above, are needed to 'overlap' and complement each other to enhance policy and practice. Yet the focus in Tanzania, for example, is notably on the realisation of distributive equality, some notions are given to, and strategic priorities and practices linked with the equality of condition approach, with very little focus on the equality of capabilities.

Presumably, as remarked on by Subrahmanian (2005), both kinds of assessment are needed to monitor and evaluate progress toward both numerical and qualitative goals. However, as she points out, it is somewhat disconcerting that the Dakar Framework of Action, for instance, did not actually define the concept of gender equality; hence, making the measurement of progress toward EFA goals hard, if not impossible, and a subject of contestation and dispute (ibid.). Similar criticism was pointed out at the time of the global consultations to debate and define the post-MDGs development agenda and SDGs (see e.g. Fukuda-Parr, 2012; Unterhalter, 2014).

Distributive equality is the mainstream approach to assess progression in Tanzania, through monitoring the rates and parity in the 'access to' and 'participation in' education. In the national statistical data in Tanzania, some of the educational indicators, such as enrolment, performance and completion rates, were monitored and presented according to gender, although unsystematically. On the grounds of this understanding and approach, where gender equality signifies an equal number of girls and boys enrolled in school, attending classes, performing and completing in examinations, Tanzania is doing well in primary education.

As stated by Moser (2007, p. 10), to decide what to assess is a political process; yet, in practice, assessment depends on objectives and goals; it also depends on the identification of the changes that are required to achieve these goals; and finally, it depends on the decision regarding aspects and indicators that enable the measurement of the progress toward the desired changes. Consequently, in practice, referring to Moser's notions and the previous discussion on different kinds of understandings of gender equality in education, it is somewhat clear that it is much easier to assess development when it is understood as a change in numbers and amounts, and in contrast, it is more complicated if the change is targeted toward the less explicitly defined goal of equality.

Addressing the disability gap

While gender parity and distributive equality have clearly become strategic goals in education development in many sub-Saharan African countries, disability has seldom been addressed in terms of parity or distributive equality but it is either expected that inclusive education approaches cover also education of persons with disabilities or, that special education settings provide for students with disabilities. Bines and Lei (2011) state, however, that disability often means the biggest challenge or the last priority for inclusion efforts. One evident reason is lack of reliable statistics, though recently census data for demographics have included items aiming to identify prevalence of disability in populations also in sub-Saharan Africa (Eide & Loeb, 2016). Still, in low-income countries the prevalence rate of disability in populations is low, only 2–5%, while in industrialised countries it is 12–15% or higher (Mont, 2007; Loeb, 2013). In low-income countries, the causes for the lack of reliable disability statistics are manifold, related to unclear definitions, lack of systematic identification of impairments and persons with disabilities, limited health and social services, traditional beliefs attached to impairments and lack of policies to guide data collection (Eide & Loeb, 2016).

Where information about persons with disabilities exists, usually it is health or social services that have collected the data, and education systems or schools do not use or refer to it. Due to the lack of reliable demographic data that include disability status, education statistics that report on numbers of students seldom provide more information or indicators, such as proportion of persons with disabilities in relation to age-level student population, parity and distributive equality (see Mont, 2007; Croft, 2012; Loeb, 2013; Lehtomäki, Tuomi & Matonya, 2014; Eide & Loeb, 2016). What education statistics do inform is that where educational opportunities exist, boys have priority, and thus regarding literacy among adults, men with disabilities outnumber women with disabilities (Eide & Loeb, 2016; Groce *et al.*, 2011).

On the one hand, lack of education opportunities increases marginalisation and social isolation of persons with disabilities, which, in turn, contributes to limited or inaccurate data. To end this vicious circle, education has the potential and task to intervene. Croft (2012) has suggested that an ethically appropriate way of collecting data on disability in low-income countries would be through developing and improving provision of basic services, such as health and education. Thereby, inclusion in education would mean an important way to develop both data collection as well as education services. This is in line with the critical realists' theorisation that education of persons with disabilities represents a challenge to education systems world-wide due to the underlying theoretical and ontological assumptions that tend to reduce 'disability' and 'being with disability' to simple models (Bhaskar & Danermark, 2006; Danermark, 2002). Their argument is that disability is a complex phenomenon that requires multidisciplinary knowledge and multidimensional understanding of the combination of genetic, psychological, psycho-social, economic, political and cultural factors (ibid.). But could such a complexity be addressed in global policy frameworks and local education strategies, especially in low-income countries? Yet, addressing gender seemed just as impossible a challenge some decades ago and it has taken several phases and still various types of approaches are necessary to ensure *equality of conditions*, the third type of addressing gender in education (Unterhalter, 2007). In this, the key question is how addressing gender in education may inform disability-inclusive development in education. In what aspects do the efforts to address the gender gap and disability gap in education differ in Tanzania?

Efforts to address the disability gap in Tanzania

The global EFA process and, in particular, the CRPD have laid a favourable policy foundation for the inclusive education provision for persons with disabilities. In practice, however, in many countries, including countries in sub-Saharan Africa, there is a huge gap between the international commitments and their implementation. Tanzania, for instance, ratified the CRPD in 2009 (United Nations, 2018). The government has also launched a strategy for inclusive education and collected annual statistics on students with disabilities. Regardless of these efforts, the number of persons with disabilities in formal education has remained very small; according to the recent estimates below 1% (HakiElimu, 2008).

In Tanzania, the critical points in education are transitions from primary to secondary education and to upper grades in secondary school. While gender parity in primary education has been achieved and girls continue to secondary school, the inequality persists in upper secondary school, where boys still outnumber girls. About students with disabilities in secondary school, there is little information. In total, 18 secondary schools have enrolled students with disabilities, but less than 9% of students with disabilities continued from primary school to secondary education – and most of them were boys (United Republic of Tanzania, 2014). Problems students with disabilities have reported are unfriendly and inaccessible learning environments, inadequacy of teachers and learning/teaching materials, fees and payments, and irrelevance of training programmes to the future lives of the students. Inappropriate school construction and infrastructures still seem serious barriers to learning and participation in secondary education (DOLASED, 2005; Matonya, 2016; Morley & Croft, 2012; Mwaipopo, Lihamba & Njewele, 2011).The students' views show that there is no equality of conditions.

In Tanzania, the involvement of girls and women in the efforts to reach gender equality has been of utmost importance. In this vein, the development of education services for persons with disabilities requires involving all education stakeholders and, in particular, including children, students and adults with disabilities in planning education, designing teaching and learning practices (Croft, 2012). A review of studies and reports on education of persons with disabilities in Tanzania supports this view but also provides evidence of the lack of information and data (Lehtomäki, Tuomi & Matonya, 2014). Therefore, Croft's (2012) suggestion to combine service development with data collection, reaching across health and education, deserves attention. Without reliable data it is impossible to verify progress toward the globally and nationally set goals for inclusive education.

Data on gender parity are not sufficient, as Unterhalter (2012, 2014) has underlined, to inform about social changes. In the same line, Terzi (2005, 2008) has applied the capability approach and suggested that inclusion requires an understanding of the socially constructed notions of disability and special needs, and education as other social institutions contributes to these constructions. Also Vehmas and Watson (2014) have stated the importance of the global policy frameworks, such as CRPD, influencing local strategies but emphasised the need for tools to measure the desired social changes. In their view, the capability approach provides a multidimensional perspective to disability in society while promoting also the agency of persons with disabilities (ibid.). Participation of persons with disabilities is, according to Meekosha and Soldatic (2011), a prerequisite for responding to the necessary social change to end the marginalisation and exclusion of persons with disabilities. In Tanzania, there are clear signs of growing agency among persons with disabilities, contributing to policy and practice, and claiming equality of conditions, and advocating for social change (Macha, 2002; Mwaipopo *et al.*, 2011; Matonya, 2016). The situation of girls and women still requires specific attention.

The voice of girls and women with disabilities: education for agency

Over 20 years ago, the World Education Forum issued the Salamanca Statement and Framework for Action, which made a specific point about the significant vulnerability of girls and young women with disabilities (Lehtomäki & Hukkanen, 2015; Lehtomäki *et al.*, 2014). Yet, there are hardly any reports on measures taken to improve their participation in education. Furthermore, the challenging situation of girls and women with disabilities has been researched in relation to health, poverty, livelihoods and marginalisation in society but the social meaning of education for girls and women with disabilities, in terms of their *capabilities*, values, freedom of choice and *agency*, is a new theme in education (Beauchamp-Pryor, 2012; Gable, 2014; Tuomi, Lehtomäki & Matonya, 2015; Chataika & McKenzie, 2016).

In Tanzania, Matonya (2016) interviewed 22 women with disabilities, who studied at the University of Dar es Salaam, that is, all she could identify. These women talked about their experiences of being girls and women with disabilities in education and in the Tanzanian society. They emphasised their own goals, reasons for education and efforts, as this one quote shows: 'I am putting my efforts into my studies so that I can get a good job and manage my life as a woman with disability without depending on anybody' (Analisa in Matonya, 2016, p. 126).

The women wanted to end the prevailing stereotypes against women with disabilities, change the attitudes in society and overcome the challenges related to disability, marriage and dependence. Furthermore, they wanted to assist their counterparts, influence and encourage parents and families to ensure their daughters with disabilities received education (Matonya, 2016). The women explained how they had accepted themselves as women and with their impairments. Psychologically, this acceptance helped them to reduce stress, tension and depression, and increased their self-confidence, resilience and determination to meet their goals. These women emphasised the importance of the encouragement of their parents, families and communities. Therefore, they wanted to become role models for others and contribute to broader social change (ibid.), as these two examples depict:

> The love, intimacy and kindness of my family members are the key to my success; they appreciated my education and helped to raise me as a woman with disability.
>
> *(Upendano in Matonya, 2016, p. 135)*

> The parents and community members use me as an example to other children. Their parents would always remind them that their blind sister performed so well that she has progressed to university now, so why shouldn't they, considering that they were not blind, yet were not performing well.
>
> *(Suzana in Matonya, 2016, p. 130)*

Matonya's (2016) findings show that women with disabilities perceived families to be essential in creating conditions for education and (higher) education as a significant instrument for social change. The key factors were the agency of the women themselves and their families, as they can inform education development with knowledge and experience concerning the combination of being a woman and with disability. Until now, the importance of agency and the motivation of women with disabilities have been largely ignored in efforts aiming to include girls and women in education in sub-Saharan African countries. Disability-inclusive and gender-inclusive developments combined can reveal the gaps in both approaches but, moreover, they mean a move toward engaged approaches, respecting those targeted by policies, giving them voice.

At the same time, the combined approach suggests complementing current forms of evidence or data collection based on parity and distributive equality toward more equality of conditions, and addressing disability as a social construction, i.e. engaging educational and social stakeholders, including families and persons with disabilities in service development and data collection. Thus, as Croft (2012) points out, engagement of the stakeholders seems to be the key to developing what Unterhalter (2007) calls, *equality of conditions*. Our observation has been that education monitoring reports and even research have had too little room for the voices of those targeted by equality and equity policies and strategies. The evidence-informed policy making and research-guided policies only may ignore whose voice, lived experience and stories are of relevance and heard, and how voices are represented and listened to. There are mechanisms and tools for listening to women's voices and meaningfully engaging them in education development processes concerning their experiences, and ways to integrate their 'voice' in educational development from planning and management to implementation and evaluation. We argue for engaging women with disabilities in research, policy and practice, thus considering 'not only the global benchmarks, but also, and most importantly, the situation on the ground' (Lehtomäki *et al.*, 2014, p. 142). Inclusive development requires active engagement as well as local interpretations of the global policies and national strategies.

In Tanzania, those women who Matonya (2016) interviewed were ready to get involved and contribute to broader social changes. These women with disabilities had used (higher) education to develop their agency. Considering that the Tanzanian government is serious with its global and national commitments to gender equality, equity and inclusion, the highly educated women with disabilities are committed to support these efforts with their knowledge and experience, as those who have overcome challenges in society. Further research that engages girls and women with disabilities in processes aiming to transform society is needed. A comparative perspective could highlight how involvement of stakeholders contributes to social changes across sub-Saharan Africa.

Conclusion

Both gender-inclusive and disability-inclusive developments call for engaged approaches, while the interface of gender and disability seriously challenges education development. Parity indices used in monitoring of progress toward the globally agreed SDGs by 2030, including gender equality in education, provide only the first step of evidence which is insufficient for confirming equality. To observe and confirm that quality education is provided for all requires multiple types of evidence and perspectives of all stakeholders, such as families, persons with disabilities, and ensuring that views of both men and women are heard. The stakeholders' participation both in service development as well as data collection is essential for ensuring equality of conditions, equality of experience (having the experience of access, participation and equal treatment) and institutions' commitment to non-discrimination. Through engagement in the development processes and evidence production the stakeholders use their capabilities and freedoms to grow agency that is needed for sustainability of equality, equity and inclusion in education.

Reflective questions

1   What kind of information do parity indices, distributive equality and equality of conditions provide for education development?
2   What is your understanding of the education of girls and women with disabilities in your context (e.g. country, district, education institution or school)?
3   How can equality of conditions be ensured in your context?
4   Examine the equality of experiences of persons with disabilities in your context.

Notes

1   The gross-enrolment rate indicates the number of children attending school (in a census) regardless of their age, for which reason the rate is often above 100% due to a large number of under-aged and over-aged children. The net-enrolment rate, in turn, is adjusted to the official school age, being for example 7–13 for primary education in Tanzania.
2   The emergence and evolution of gendered thinking and discourse in the development agenda is discussed comprehensively by Kabeer (1994), Kabeer and Subrahmanian (1996) and Moser (1993). See also the comparison between UNESCO and the World Bank understandings and approaches concerning girls' and women's education by Vaughan (2010).

References

Ainscow, M., Dyson, A., Goldrick, S. & West, M. (2012). *Developing Equitable Education Systems*. London: Routledge.

Beauchamp-Pryor, K. (2012). From absent to active voices: securing disability equality within higher education. *International Journal of Inclusive Education* 16(3), 283–295.

Bhaskar, R. & Danermark, B. (2006). Metatheory, interdisciplinarity and disability research: a critical realist perspective. *Scandinavian Journal of Disability Research* 8(4), 278–297.

Bines, H. & Lei, P. (2011). Disability and education: the longest road to inclusion. *International Journal of Educational Development* 31(5), 419–424.

Chataika, T. & McKenzie, J. A. (2016). Global institutions and their engagement with disability mainstreaming in the south: development and (dis)connections. In S. Grech & K. Soldatic (eds) *Disability in the Global South: The Critical Handbook* (pp. 423–436). Switzerland: Springer International Publishing.

Chataika, T., McKenzie, J. A., Swart, E. & Lyner-Cleophas, M. (2012). Access to education in Africa: responding to the United Nations Convention on the Rights of Persons with Disabilities. *Disability & Society* **27**(3), 385–398.

Croft, A. (2012). Promoting access to education for disabled children in low-income countries: do we need to know how many disabled children there are? *International Journal of Educational Development* **33**(3), 233–243.

Danermark, B. (2002). Interdisciplinary research and critical realism: the example of disability research. *Journal of Critical Realism* **5**, 56–64.

DOLASED (Disabled Organisation for Legal Affairs and Social Economic Development). (2005). *The Research in the Status of Disabled Children's Rights in Tanzania: Access to Education Perspective.* Dar es Salaam: DOLASED.

Dyson, A. (1999). Inclusion and inclusions: theories and discourses in inclusive education. In H. Daniels & P. Garner (eds) *World Yearbook on Education 1999: Inclusive Education* (pp. 36–53). London: Routledge.

Eide, A. H. & Loeb, M. (2016). Counting disabled people: historical perspectives and the challenges of disability statistics. In S. Grech & K. Soldatic (eds) *Disability in the Global South: The Critical Handbook* (pp. 51–68). Switzerland: Springer International Publishing.

Fennel, S. & Arnot, M. (2009). *Decentring Hegemonic Gender Theory: The Implications for Educational Research.* Vol. 21 of Working Paper. London: DFID.

Fukuda-Parr, S. (2012). *Recapturing the Narrative of International Development.* Geneva: UNRISID.

Gable, A. S. (2014). Disability theorising and real-world educational practice: a framework for understanding. *Disability & Society* **29**(1), 86–100.

Groce, N., Kett, M., Lang, R. & Trani, J. F. (2011). Disability and poverty: the need for a more nuanced understanding of implications for development policy and practice. *Third World Quarterly* **32**(8), 1493–1513.

HakiElimu (2008). *Do Children with Disabilities Have Equal Access to Education? A Research Report on Accessibility to Education for Children with Disabilities in Tanzania Schools.* HakiElimu: Dar Es Salaam.

Kabeer, N. (1994). *Reversed Realities: Gender Hierarchies in Development Thought.* London and New York: Verso.

Kabeer, N. & Subrahmanian, R. (1996). *Institutions, Relations and Outcomes: Framework and Tools for Gender-Aware Planning.* No. 357 of Discussion Paper. Brighton: Institute of Development Studies.

Kiuppis, F. & Hausstätter, R. S. (2014). *Inclusive Education Twenty Years after Salamanca.* New York: Peter Lang.

Lehtomäki, E. & Hukkanen, S. (2015). Girls and women with [dis]abilities in Tanzania claim their right to education. In F. Kiuppis & R. S. Hausstätter (eds) *Inclusive Education: Twenty Years with Salamanca* (pp. 231–249). New York: Peter Lang.

Lehtomäki, E., Tuomi, M. & Matonya, M. (2014). Educational research from Tanzania 1998–2008 concerning persons with disabilities: what can we learn? *International Journal of Educational Research* **64**(2), 32–39.

Loeb, M. (2013). Disability statistics: an integral but missing (and misunderstood) component of development work. *Nordic Journal of Human Rights* **31**(3), 306–324.

Macha, E. (2002). *Gender, Disabilities and Access to Education in Tanzania.* PhD Thesis. University of Leeds. Retrieved from http://etheses.whiterose.ac.uk/282/ on 27 April 2018.

Matonya, M. (2016). Accessibility and participation in higher education from the perspectives of women with disabilities. *Jyväskylä Studies in Education, Psychology and Social Science*, 568. Jyväskylä: University of Jyväskylä.

Meekosha, H. & Soldatic, K. (2011). Human rights and the global south: the case of disability. *Third World Quarterly* **32**(8), 1383–1397.

Mont, D. (2007). Measuring disability prevalence. *The World Bank Social Protection. Discussion Paper, No. 0706.* Washington, DC: The World Bank.

Morley, L. & Croft, A. (2012). Agency and advocacy: disabled students in higher education in Ghana and Tanzania. *Research in Comparative and International Education* **6**(4), 383–399.

Moser, A. (2007). *Gender and Indicator: Overview Report.* Brighton: Institute of Development Studies.

Moser, C. O. N. (1993). *Gender Planning and Development: Theory, Practice & Training.* New York: Routledge.

Mwaipopo, R. N., Lihamba, A. & Njewele, D. C. (2011). Equity and equality in access to higher education: the experiences of students with disabilities in Tanzania. Special issue on African higher education: researching absences, equalities and aspirations. *Research in Comparative and International Education* **6**(4), 415–429.

Okkolin, M. A. & Lehtomäki, E. (2005). Gender and disability: challenges of education sector develop-ment in Tanzania. In O. Hietanen (ed.) *University Partnerships for International Development, Finnish Development Knowledge (FFRC-publications)* (pp. 204–216). Finland: Turku School of Economics and Business Administration.

Okkolin, M. A., Lehtomäki, E. & Bhalalusesa, E. (2010). Successes and challenges in the education sector development in Tanzania: focus on gender and inclusive education. *Gender and Education* **22**(1), 63–71.

Robeyns, I. (2005). The capability approach: a theoretical survey. *Journal of Human Development* **6**(1), 93–114.

Robeyns, I. (2006). The capability approach in practice. *Journal of Political Philosophy* **14**(3), 351–376.

Sen, A. (1992). *Inequality Re-examined*. Oxford: Oxford University Press.

Sen, A. (1993). Capability and well-being. In M. Nussbaum & A. Sen (eds) *The Quality of Life: Studies in Development Economics* (pp. 30–53). Oxford: Oxford University Press.

Sen, A. (1999). *Development as Freedom*. Oxford; Oxford University Press.

Shakespeare, T. (2015). Human rights and disability advocacy. *Disability & Society* **30**(2), 316–318.

Terzi, L. (2005). A capability perspective on impairment, disability and special needs: towards social justice in education. *Theory and Research in Education* **3**(2), 197–223.

Terzi, L. (2008). *Justice and Equality in Education: A Capability Perspective on Disability and Special Educational Needs*. London: Continuum.

Tuomi, M., Lehtomäki, E. & Matonya, M. (2015). 'As capable as other students': Tanzanian women with disabilities in higher education. *Disability, Development and Education* **62**(2), 202–214.

Subrahmanian, R. (2005). Gender equality in education: definitions and measurements. *International Journal of Educational Development* **25**, 395–407.

United Nations (2006). *Convention on the Rights of Persons with Disabilities (CRPD)*. Retrieved from www. un.org/development/desa/disabilities/convention-on-the-rights-of-persons-with-disabilities.html on 25 April 2018.

United Nations (2015). *Sustainable Development Knowledge Platform*. Retrieved from https://sustainable development.un.org/sdg4 on 9 November 2016.

United Nations (2017). *Sustainable Development Report 2017*. United Nations. Retrieved from https://unstats. un.org/sdgs/files/report/2017/TheSustainableDevelopmentGoalsReport2017.pdf on 22 August 2017.

United Nations (2018). *United Nations Treaty Collection, Chapter IV, Human Rights, 15*. Convention on the Rights of Persons with Disabilities (Signatures and ratifications by states). Retrieved from www. un.org/development/desa/disabilities/convention-on-the-rights-of-persons-with-disabilities.html on 25 April 2018.

United Republic of Tanzania (2014). *Education for All (EFA) Report for Tanzania Mainland*. Dar es Salaam: Ministry of Education and Vocational Training.

Unterhalter, E. (2005). *Gender Equality and Education in South Africa: Measurements, Scores and Strategies Gender Equality in South African Education 1994–2004: Perspectives from Research, Governments and Unions*. Cape Town: Human Sciences Research Council Press.

Unterhalter, E. (2007). Gender, equality, education and the capability approach. In M. Walker & E. Unterhalter (eds) *Amartya Sen's Capability Approach and Social Justice in Education* (pp. 87–107). New York: Palgrave Macmillan.

Unterhalter, E. (2012). Inequalities, capabilities and poverty in four African countries: girls' voice, schooling, and strategies for institutional change. *Cambridge Journal of Education* **42**, 307–325.

Unterhalter, E. (2014). Walking backwards into the future: a comparative perspective on education and a post-2015 framework. *Compare* **44**(6), 852–873.

Unterhalter, E. & Brighouse, H. (2007). Distribution of what for social justice in education. In M. Walker & E. Unterhalter (eds) *Amartya Sen's Capability Approach and Social Justice in Education* (pp. 67–86). New York: Palgrave Macmillan.

Vaughan, R. (2010). Girls' and women's education within UNESCO and World Bank, 1945–2000. *Compare: A Journal of Comparative and International Education* **40**(4), 405–423.

Vehmas, S. & Watson, N. (2014). Moral wrongs, disadvantages, and disability: a critique of critical disability studies. *Disability & Society* **29**(4), 638–650.

World Health Organization and the World Bank (2011). *World Report on Disability*. Retrieved from www. who.int/disabilities/world_report/ on 23 September 2016.

18

SOCIO-ECONOMIC BARRIERS FACED BY WOMEN WITH DISABILITIES IN ZIMBABWE

Tafadzwa Rugoho and France Maphosa

Introduction and background

Research reveals that women with disabilities in Zimbabwe have endured widespread violations of their rights for a long time. Museva (2012) observed that the oppression and suppression of women with disabilities have not been well-documented; hence, little is known about the challenges they face. While Zimbabwe has been judged as being on the right track in the promotion of the rights of women in general (Southern African Development Community [SADC], 2013), there has not been specific policy focus by the government to uplift women with disabilities from poverty and the general violation of their rights. Non-governmental organisations (NGOs) and donors have also made little effort to improve the plight of women with disabilities. Issues that affect women with disabilities in Zimbabwe have therefore largely remained at the periphery of policy making and intervention. Zimbabwe does not yet have any legislation and policy on the empowerment of women with disabilities. Consequently, women with disabilities in Zimbabwe have become victims of multi-layered discrimination (Rugoho & Siziba, 2014). They experience discrimination on the basis of their sex and impairment (Grobbelaar-du Plessis, 2007).

The levels of poverty experienced by women with disabilities, relative to those experienced by women without disabilities is a vivid example of their marginalisation. The government of Zimbabwe has generally failed to enunciate policies that help on the reduction of poverty. United Nations Development Programme 2014, Human Development Index ranked Zimbabwe number 156 out of the 187 countries, which demonstrates that it is struggling in supporting its population. This indicates that Zimbabwe has one of the highest prevalences of poverty and is not able to provide basic necessities to its populace. This finding is further supported by Government of Zimbabwe (2015), which noted an average poverty prevalence rate of 70%. The poverty rates are even as high as 83% in some rural areas of Zimbabwe. This paints a poor picture considering the fact that the majority of women with disabilities in Zimbabwe reside in the rural areas. The Ministry of Health and Child Welfare (2013) also confirmed that people with disabilities, especially women, are heavily burdened by poverty. Unemployment has risen to unprecedented levels of around 90% (Zimbabwe Independent, 2012). Unemployment levels are even higher among people with disabilities, especially women. Agriculture, which used to be the backbone of the Zimbabwean economy and largest employer, has collapsed. The higher poverty rates among women with disabilities than among other groups is a result of an intricate combination of factors such as cultural and religious practices toward women with disabilities and lack of policies and interventions intended to address the marginalisation of women with disabilities. These factors present barriers for women with disabilities to employment, education and political participation.

Many women with disabilities in Zimbabwe are from poor families (Mitra, Posarac & Vick 2011). As a result, they are disadvantaged at an early age. Throughout their lives, they endure prejudices and injustices from their families, community and the government (Mokomane, 2012). History is replete with accounts of women with disabilities being neglected and mis-treated. The media in Zimbabwe and organisations of people with disabilities have reported horrific stories of children with disabilities who have been kept in confinement by their families for several years. Some parents are so ashamed of their children with disabilities that they keep them isolated from the rest of society. This isolation has adverse impacts on their socialisation as well as their mental development.

Zimbabwe is a patriarchal society in which women are generally disadvantaged. Historically women were not accorded the same opportunities as those enjoyed by their male counterparts (Rutoro, 2012). The generality of women have struggled to access education and the means of production. As a result of sustained advocacy and lobbying, significant strides have been made toward giving women without disabilities access to those opportunities they had been previously denied. However, women with disabilities have not benefited much from these developments. They still experience stigmatisation and discrimination even by other women. Women with disabilities are at the bottom of the social hierarchy. The experiences of marginalisation and discrimination have had serious psychological and mental ramifications (Green *et al.*, 2005); for example, impacting on the women with disabilities' confidence to fight for their rights.

Models of disability and the empowerment of women with disabilities in Zimbabwe

The management of disability issues in Zimbabwe and other southern African countries has historically been influenced by two models; namely, the medical and the charity models. The medical perspective looks at disabled people as sick people who require the attention of medi-cal specialists. The charity model requires that community sympathise with disabled people by assisting them with food handouts and other things, which makes their life comfortable (Kachaje *et al.*, 2014). Despite increasing calls to adopt a rights-based approach, these two models still influence the manner in which disability issues are managed in the country. The medical and charity models, which date back to the colonial era, were adopted by the post-colonial government which has failed to transform its approach to disability management. This is despite a global shift in disability programming and management toward a rights-based approach. The country has failed to embrace the rights-based approach. The disability models adopted by any country have a strong bearing on the protection and promotion of the rights of people with disabilities. They are an indicator of how the government is committed to the promotion of disability rights.

Buntinx and Schalock (2010) argue that disability models have implications on how disabil-ity issues are promoted and programmed. Countries that still adhere to the medical and charity models of disability, struggle to promote the rights of people with disabilities. A comparison between Zimbabwe and Uganda will illustrate this point. Uganda has largely adopted a rights-based approach to disability (Nyende, 2012). This is provided for in the Constitution of Uganda.

The adoption of a rights-based approach to disability management and programming in Uganda has seen a number of persons with disabilities occupying key decision-making positions in the private and public sectors of the country. A third model, the spiritual model has also been gaining some prominence due to the mushrooming of churches that emphasise spiritual healing and researchers are beginning to pay serious attention to it.

While Zimbabwe was the first country to adopt a disability law in Africa (Manatsa, 2015), the continued influence of the medical and charity models of disability has stiffed the promotion of disability rights. The government and its development partners seem to be fixated on the medical and charity models. Mtetwa (2014) notes that even the tone of the new Constitution has charity connotations when referring to the rights of persons with disabilities. The use of the word 'assist' in the Constitution on disability issues clearly shows that the State is still entangled in the welfare approach (Mtetwa, 2014). Although the new Constitution provides for some rights for people with disabilities, the enjoyment of such rights is limited by the insufficient resources provided by the State toward disability issues. For example, Section 83 of the Constitution, which deals with the rights of persons with disabilities, hinges the fulfilment of disability rights on the availability of resources. This demonstrates that the government is yet to fully commit to the promotion of the rights of people with disabilities as they seem to enjoy the least protection by the Constitution when compared to other social groups such as women, war veterans and political detainees.

The Government of Zimbabwe has left non-governmental and faith-based organisations to deal with disability issues and welfare. It considers that non-governmental and faith-based organisations having the capacity to deal with the social and economic issues that affect women with disabilities. Most of the self-empowerment projects and activities that are done for women with disabilities have been driven by non-state actors (Rugoho & Maphosa, 2017). In most cases, such activities do not focus on the improvement of the legal environment when dealing with issues affecting women with disabilities. They are short-term interventions that are embedded in the charity model; mainly, donations of food and assistive devices. These activities contribute to the marginalisation of women with disabilities as they only mitigate the problems faced by women with disabilities and do not address the conditions that bring about those problems.

Zimbabwe is witnessing an unprecedented growth of the Pentecostal movement, which believes in miracle healing (Biri, 2013). People with disabilities are often invited to such churches so that miracles can be performed on them. Women with disabilities are among those who have attended these churches in large numbers expecting to be healed of their impairments. The spiritual approach focuses on physical healing and overlooks the socio-economic marginalisation of people with disabilities. It therefore does not seek to provide ways to empower people with disabilities. By viewing them as objects of pity rather than people with the capabilities to engage in productive activity, the church is perpetuating the charity model; thus it is also perpetuating the marginalisation of women with disabilities.

Barriers to political participation

Political participation by women has been regarded as the engine for their emancipation. It gives them a voice and enables them to ascend to strategic positions. Political participation also offers leverage on economic inclusion. Due to the efforts of the women's movement in Zimbabwe, a number of women have become active in politics, at least by taking up active membership of political parties. However, women with disabilities still face enormous challenges in their quest for political participation (Chabaya, Rembe & Wadesango, 2009). While the Constitution of

Zimbabwe reserves a quota of the seats in parliament for women, women with disabilities still have no representation in parliament. No disabled woman was elected by the parties in the current parliament to occupy those seats reserved for women. Only one seat in the upper house of parliament among the lower house seats reserved for women is occupied by a disabled woman. The factors that inhibit the political participation of disabled women in Zimbabwe include poverty, low educational attainment and systematic discrimination (Rugoho, 2017). The virtual absence of women with disabilities in decision-making bodies limits democracy and hinders inclusive economic development. If non-disabled men and women continue to monopolise the democratic and political processes in Zimbabwe, the interests of disabled women will not be taken into consideration (Chataika, 2013a).

The political environment also is generally not accommodating to disabled women who aspire to enter into politics. Zimbabwean politics, particularly in the period between 2000 and 2013, has been characterised by pre-election violence. This environment discourages the participation of women with disabilities because of their multiple vulnerabilities as women and people with disabilities. Rugoho and Maphosa (2017) observed that political parties generally prefer non-disabled men as their candidates for election while women are often treated as voters. While disabled women have been considered, their selection in political office is rare, implying that disabled women are not acceptable in the political sphere. The political manifestos of some of the major political parties in Zimbabwe, such as the Zimbabwe African National Union Patriotic Front (ZANU PF, 2015), Movement for Democratic Change (MDC, 2011) and Mavambo show that these parties do not have any agenda for facilitating women with disabilities to stand as candidates for elections (Rugoho & Maphosa, 2017). Women with disabilities generally occupy peripheral positions in these political parties.

Rugoho and Maphosa (2017) observed that women with disabilities are mainly found in the low levels of political structures. While there are some women with disabilities from the lowest to the provincial levels, their presence at the national level is very rare. Gaidzanwa (2006) observed that in Zimbabwe, for one to succeed in politics s/he requires skills and wealth to distribute to his/her followers. Women with disabilities generally do not have the wealth to distribute to followers. With low levels of educational attainment and without skills, women with disabilities often face challenges in shaping and articulating their development agenda. Rugoho and Maphosa (2017) noted that women's organisations such as Women's Trust, Women's Coalition and Disabled Women's Organisation are working toward capacitating women with skills that would enable them to participate in the socio-economic transformation of the country. Women with disabilities, many of whom are dependent on family members and well-wishers are often unable to travel long distances to access this training, due to both physical limitations and lack of transport money. Rugoho and Maphosa (2015) noted that in some cases, in the rural areas of Zimbabwe, families do not allow their female disabled members to travel. They are confined to their homes mainly out of the fear that they might be abused if they venture outside their homes. This curtailment of the movement of women with disabilities is one of the factors contributing to their socio-economic marginalisation, including lack of political participation.

Cultural barriers

Certain cultural practices have resulted in barriers to the socio-economic participation of women with disabilities. There are still a lot of myths that continue to reinforce and perpetuate the isolation of women with disabilities in Zimbabwe. The government and its development partners have made little effort to help demystify these myths. Lang and Charowa (2007) found that there are some communities in Zimbabwe where there is still a strong belief that there is a strong relationship between witchcraft and disability. The belief is that disability is a curse cast upon the children for their parents' transgressions, especially witchcraft (Chataika, 2013b). Thus, people acquire impairments as a result of curses by the gods and ancestors angered by their parents' involvement in witchcraft. This perception endangers the lives of women with disabilities because it results in them being discriminated against and ill-treated. Negative cultural beliefs toward disability affect the socio-economic inclusion of women with disabilities, because they cause them to be relegated to objects of pity and ridicule (Rugoho & Maphosa, 2017).

Legislative and policy environment

Zimbabwe is a signatory to a number of international treaties and laws, which seek to improve the status of women. These include the Convention on Economic, Social and Cultural Rights; the Convention on Civil and Political Rights; the Convention on the Elimination of All Forms of Discrimination against Women (CEDAW); the Beijing Declaration and Platform for Action; the Universal Declaration of Human Rights; the 1997 SADC Declaration on Gender and Development with its addendum on the Prevention and the Eradication of Violence against Women and Children; the SADC Protocol on Gender and Development; as well as the Protocol to the African Charter on Human and People's Rights on the Rights of Women. Recently, it signed the Convention on the Rights of Persons with Disabilities. However, the convention has not yet been domesticated to become part of the country's laws. Women with disabilities are yet to benefit from all these international agreements. This demonstrates a non-committal attitude by the Zimbabwean government in improving the welfare of women with disabilities.

Zimbabwe was once regarded as a progressive country with regard to promoting the rights of persons with disabilities. It was one of the first countries in Africa to enact a disability Act in 1992 (Manatsa, 2015). The Disabled Persons Act was enacted by the Parliament of Zimbabwe to promote the rights of people with disabilities. However, Choruma (2007) notes that the Act was rarely implemented, resulting in people with disabilities not benefiting from it. The Act called for the appointment of a director of the National Disability Board. It was envisaged that the director would be responsible for promoting disability-related issues within the government ministries and departments. The Zimbabwe Disabled Persons Act also called for the provision of access to public premises, services and amenities accessible to people with disabilities. It outlawed discrimination against disabled persons in employment. However, there is no Employment Equity Act, Social Assistance Act, Skills Development Act and Skills Development Levy Act designed specifically for people with disabilities. All these Acts are mentioned in passing in the Disabled Persons Act. As a result, the Disabled Persons Act has remained insignificant in addressing the challenges faced by people with disabilities because it was only partially implemented (Manatsa, 2015).

In 1992, a National Disability Board was formed in Zimbabwe by the then Ministry of Public Service, Labour and Social Welfare (now Ministry of Labour and Social Services) whose mandate was to act as a watchdog to ensure fair treatment and accessibility to the country's facilities, services and resources by people with disabilities. Further, it was supposed to help the government in formulating progressive policies on disability. Lack of resolve has disabled the Board and compromised its ability to execute its responsibilities. While membership of the Board includes women with disabilities, yet constituency has not yet benefited from its establishment. There is nothing tangible to show for its existence in the socio-economic empowerment of women with disabilities.

In 2013, Zimbabwe adopted a new Constitution. During the Constitution-making process, a number of submissions were made by organisations of disabled people. Women with disabilities made a number of representations, which were allegedly ignored by the drafters of the Constitution. The new Constitution clearly spells out the political rights of women. It calls for the representation of women in all democratic processes. However, the political rights of women with disabilities are not clearly spelled out. The Constitution provides for women with disabilities to be represented by only one senator. The Senate is the upper house of the bicameral parliament of Zimbabwe. The Senate is not responsible for introducing new laws. Hence, the concerns of women with disabilities are likely to be overlooked.

An official of the Disability Agenda Forum of Zimbabwe (an organisation representing people with disabilities) was quoted by *Radio Dialogue*:

> The draft constitution has got nothing really new to offer the disabled [people], it is far short of the demands of persons with disabilities, and it leaves these people at the mercy of the state powers. The draft constitution speaks on issues of the welfare of persons with disabilities without empowering them. . . . while the draft constitution makes provisions for a gender commission for the purposes of women empowerment, it is silent on the formation of a disability commission. It gives proportions about representation of women in parliament or in government institutions but there is no proportion of representation for people with disabilities in these offices elected or appointed meaning that for there to be representation of disabled people, it will be at the mercy of the incumbent president, it will not be a constitutional right.

The statement provides evidence that while people with disabilities in Zimbabwe had made representations on issues they wanted included in the new Constitution, their voices were ignored. Hence, Mtetwa (2014) observes that the new Constitution of Zimbabwe has not promoted the rights of people with disabilities.

Education and women with disabilities

The educational attainment for women with disabilities remains very low. Many of them seem not to complete primary school education (Mangwaya, 2015). Women with disabilities in the rural areas face more challenges than their urban counterparts in accessing education. The failure of women with disabilities to access education is caused by their general neglect by both the government and the communities they live in. An analysis of national budgets for the period 1980 to 2016 clearly shows that the funds committed to a more inclusive education were negligible. Peresuh and Barcham (1998) note that between 1980 to 2000 the Zimbabwean government invested substantial amounts of money in the expansion of access to education, a strategy that resulted in the country attaining higher levels of literacy than many other African countries. However, the benefits of this expanded access to education did not accrue to people with disabilities as their education was mostly left to non-state actors. Peresuh and Barcham (1998) further asserted that the Government of Zimbabwe inherited, from the colonial government, a system that was unjust toward black people with disabilities. Up to now, the country does not have an inclusive education policy (Chataika, 2016), which is contrary to Article 24 (inclusive education) of the CRPD, which Zimbabwe ratified in 2013 (United Nations, 2006). Peresuh and Barcham (1998) observed that, prior to 1998, the provision of education to people with disabilities was only a moral and religious obligation rather than a right. However, without an inclusive education policy, it implies that the situation has not changed much.

The role of gender activism in addressing marginalisation of women with disabilities

Gender activism in Zimbabwe has grown from strength to strength (Maranan, 2007). Having started very small soon after independence, the movement gradually gathered momentum to a point where government could not ignore it. It addressed issues that affected women in both the private and public spheres. Its impact has been felt in economic, social, health and political sectors of the Zimbabwean society, grappling with issues such as livelihoods, access to education, land ownership, inheritance and many others. Kurebwa (2014) observed that the women's movement in Zimbabwe has been able to deal with a wide range of issues and won many struggles. For example, the women's movement has been pivotal in the enhancement of women's participation in democratic processes. This makes it well-placed to deal with issues of gender inequalities.

In 1999, the Women's Coalition was established. The organisation became a force to reckon with by confronting issues that inhibited the political participation of women. Among other things, it lobbied political parties to include women among their lists of candidates for elections. It also conducted a series of training workshops in which women were instructed on how to be involved in democratic processes including elections (Research and Advocacy Unit, 2010). The organisation has structures in all the ten provinces of Zimbabwe. With a membership that included some very powerful and influential women from various fields, the Women's Coalition started working with the women's leagues of several political parties in an effort to influence the structures of those parties (Reeler, 2014). Its emphasis was on the need for those political parties to create an enabling environment for women to participate in democratic processes. With the media on their side, they gradually influenced policy changes by the government and political parties toward the inclusion of women. The Women's Coalition has been credited for the appointment of Joyce Mujuru as the first female vice-president of Zimbabwe.

The women's movement also established various organisations in the business sector also in an effort to ensure that their concerns are addressed (Manatsa, 2015). Organisations such as the Indigenous Business Women's Organisation (IBWO) and Women in Business (WIB) were established with the aim of mainstreaming women's issues in business. Zimbabwe Young Women in Business (ZYMB) was also formed to deal with issues that affect young women in business or intending to venture into business. These organisations have facilitated a number of training sessions and arranged for loan facilities to their constituency (Viriri & Makurumidze, 2014). This has enabled a number of women to venture into business areas which had previously been male-dominated. These organisations have, however, not benefited women with disabilities. They have no strategies in place to attract women with disabilities to join them or to help address the specific challenges faced by women with disabilities or intending to venture into business.

The women's movement has successfully lobbied for women's inclusion in national bodies such as the Gender Commission, Media Commission, and Human Rights Commission among many others. It demanded a 50–50 gender representation in these bodies and these demands have generally been accepted as reflected in the new Constitution. However, it is not clear how the concerns of women with disabilities are incorporated into the structures and functions of these commissions. Several factors have contributed to this state of affairs and these include disabled people's low educational attainments, prevailing prejudices against them and lack of political will to address their issues on the part of government, especially those for disabled women.

Women with disabilities' economic empowerment initiatives

A study carried out by Museva (2012) on the level of participation of women with disabilities in economic empowerment programmes portrayed a bleak picture. She noted that these programmes gave little attention to women with disabilities and that they were rarely consulted when such programmes were designed to address their challenges to economic participation. Economic planners seem to regard them as charity cases who would not make any meaningful contribution to the development of economic empowerment programmes. Museva (2012) concludes that there are numerous cultural, social, physical and psychological barriers to the participation of women with disabilities in economic activities. Rugoho and Siziba (2014) noted that because of limited opportunities for women with disabilities in the formal economy, women with disabilities are resorting to begging and vending as their livelihood.

As observed by Viriri and Makurumidze (2014), attempts by women with disabilities to operate formal small-scale businesses experience major challenges, the major one being the bureaucratic and costly process of registering a company in Zimbabwe. As a result of their generally low levels of educational attainment and economic status, women with disabilities often find it difficult to negotiate the bureaucracy associated with the process of registering a business and also often lack the means to pay for the process. Hence, they end up resorting to street begging.

Viriri and Makurumidze (2014) further noted that because of the informal nature of most of the businesses owned by women with disabilities, it is difficult for them to operate from fixed and designated spaces. As a result, they are unable to erect proper business structures. They also do not benefit from the existing business support infrastructure. The issue of lack of infrastructure was also raised by Museva (2012) as a major obstacle against the participation of women with disabilities in economic activities. The government has allocated vending places in a number of towns and cities; an initiative supported by local authorities. Women cross-border traders have been the major beneficiaries of this initiative. However, the process of allocating of the operating spaces was marred with corruption and political patronage; hence, women with disabilities did not benefit from this initiative (Museva, 2012).

Women with disabilities have also faced the challenge of accessing financial assistance to start businesses (Viriri & Makurumidze, 2014). Most women with disabilities do not own properties which they can offer as collateral security to the banks. Handicap International (2006) noted the difficulties faced by women with disabilities in low-income countries in accessing financial assistance from banks and microfinance institutions. In support, Bwire, Mersland and Mukasa (2009) argued that microfinance institutions do not include people with disabilities in their mainstream programmes. Banks and microfinance institutions usually do not have lending policies tailor-made for the needs of women with disabilities (Viriri & Makurumidze, 2014). Bank personnel often have prejudices against people with disabilities, which makes it difficult for them to get the same attention given to non-disabled people when they approach the banks for loans (Simanowitz, 2001; Bwire *et al.*, 2009).

The manner in which some of the empowerment initiatives are implemented in Zimbabwe also makes it extremely difficult for women with disabilities to participate. As indicated earlier, projects apparently meant to economically empower women, are often characterised by political patronage.

Nyezwa and M'kumbuzvi (2003) noted that women with disabilities do not have access to information relating to economic empowerment initiatives. Rugoho and Siziba (2014) observed that the majority of people with disabilities spend most of their time at home. This lack of mobility limits their access to sources of information, including social networks that can be facilitated by mobility. Maziriri and Madinga (2016) also observed that lack of education and training, lack of access to finance, inadequate government support and lack of equipment are major challenges that are faced by disabled people in general. The Ministry of Finance and Economic Development (2011) acknowledged that the majority of disabled people, including women with disabilities, are self-employed. However, despite its acknowledgement, there is little planning and resource allocation toward the improvement of the economic participation of women with disabilities (Rugoho & Siziba, 2014).

The Ministry of Women and Gender Affairs in Zimbabwe has rolled out a number of initiatives for the empowerment of women. One of the most outstanding initiatives is the establishment of the Women's Development Fund (WDF). The fund enables women to get access to grants and loans for income generating projects. Tshuma (2012) reported that the WDF has enhanced the livelihoods of the recipients through initiation of income-generating projects. The other programmes that have been initiated by this ministry include community gardens and bee-keeping. However, evidence demonstrates that women with disabilities have not benefited from these initiatives (Museva, 2012). They seem to be excluded from participating in such programmes because of the absence of a national disability policy. The ministry does not have a deliberate policy or programme for economically empowering women with disabilities.

The disability movement and women with disabilities

Majiet and Africa (2015) argue that the role played by women with disabilities is little known because it is undocumented. Traustadottir (1997) also observes that historically, women with disabilities have been neglected by those concerned with disability, including the disability rights movement as well as the feminist movement. Most of the studies on women's disability movements that have been carried out and documented tend to focus mainly on European, American and Asian women (Muthukrishna, Sokoya & Moodley, 2009).

The disability movement has existed in Zimbabwe for the past three decades. Most of the Disabled People's Organisations (DPOs) were for a long time led by men who had been injured during Zimbabwe's liberation struggle (Majiet & Africa, 2015). This absence of women in these organisations deprived them of the ability to articulate the issues that affected women with disabilities. The male leaders of DPOs have come under severe criticism for paying lip-service to gender issues. Consequently, women with disabilities have recently started establishing their own organisations (Majiet & Africa, 2015). The Disabled Women's Support Organisation, whose focus is the empowerment of women with disabilities, has made some strides toward fulfilling its mandate. However, like other DPOs in Zimbabwe, it faces several challenges, including poor funding and lack of organisational capacity. As a result, it has not had a significant impact on the improvement of the socio-economic condition of women with disabilities. The Women's Disability Movement and other DPOs have failed to be vehicles for the empowerment of women with disabilities. They seem to have challenges at collectively lobbying and advocating for disability rights.

Conclusions and recommendations

Women with disabilities in Zimbabwe face myriad challenges to socio-economic participation. A number of factors combine to confine them to the margins of society. Despite being lauded for its efforts to advance the interest of women in general, Zimbabwe has no policy that specifically addresses the concerns of women with disabilities. The country's new Constitution does not have specific provisions for addressing the concerns of women with disabilities. The majority of women with disabilities are trapped in poverty because of many social, economic and political barriers. The approaches to dealing with issues affecting women with disabilities have traditionally been influenced by the medical and charity models. Together with the emerging spiritual model, these models have treated people with disabilities as being in need of help. At best, such approaches merely tinker with the socio-economic marginalisation of women with disabilities; and at worst, they perpetuate it. Government should treat disability issues as human rights issues and not relegate them to charity issues to be dealt with by non-state actors.

In the light of the views expressed above, we make the following recommendations:

- The rights of women with disabilities should be clearly spelt out in the Constitution.
- Government should take a leading role in promoting the rights of women with disabilities.
- Women with disabilities should be given access to the means of production.
- Decision-making bodies should adopt a quota system so as to guarantee the inclusion of women with disabilities in all areas of development, including access to social services.

Reflective questions

1 Why are women's organisations marginalising fellow women with disabilities?
2 How can disabled women's organisations be strengthened to lobby and advocate for their involvement in decision-making at government level?
3 What strategies can be employed by political parties to mainstream women with disabilities in the political spaces?

References

Biri, K. (2013). Religion and emerging technologies in Zimbabwe: contesting for space? *International Open & Distance Learning Journal* **7**(1), 19–27.

Buntinx, W. H. E. & Schalock, R. L. (2010). Models of disabilities: quality of life and individualized supports: implications for professional practice in intellectual disability. *Journal of Policy and Practice in Intellectual Disabilities* **7**(4), 283–294.

Bwire, F. N., Mersland, F. & Mukasa, G. (2009). Access to mainstream microfinance services for persons with disabilities: lessons learned from Uganda Disability Studies. *Disability Studies Quarterly* **29**(1), 7–18.

Chabaya, O., Rembe, S. & Wadesango, N. (2009). The persistence of gender inequality in Zimbabwe: factors that impede the advancement of women into leadership positions in primary schools. *South African Journal of Education* **29**(6), 235–251.

Chataika, T. (2013a). *Gender and Disability Mainstreaming Training Manual: Prepared for Disabled Women in Africa*. Germany: GMZ and GIZ. Retrieved from www.diwa.ws/index.php?option=com_phoca download on 4 September 2017.

Chataika, T. (2013b). Cultural and religious explanations of disability and promoting inclusive communities. In J. M. Claassen, L. Swartz & L. Hansen (eds) *Search for Dignity: Conversations on Human Dignity, Theology and Disability* (pp. 117–128). Cape Town: African Sun Media (Stellenbosch University).

Chataika, T. (2016). African perspectives on Article 24 of the CRPD. In C. O'Mahony & G. Quinn (eds) *Disability Law and Policy: An Analysis of the UN Convention* (pp. 113–135). London: Clarus Press.

Choruma, T. (2007). *The Forgotten Tribe: People with Disabilities in Zimbabwe*. London: Progressio.

Gaidzanwa, R. (2006). *Gender, Women and Electoral Politics in Zimbabwe*. Johannesburg: EISA.

Government of Zimbabwe (2013). *Constitution of Zimbabwe Amendment (No. 20)*. Harare: Government Printers.

Government of Zimbabwe (2015). *Poverty Atlas of Zimbabwe*. Harare: Government Printers.

Green, Sara, Davis, Christine, Karshmer, Elana, Marsh, Pete & Straight, Benjamin (2005). Living stigma: the impact of labeling, stereotyping, separation, status loss, and discrimination in the lives of individuals with disabilities and their families. *Sociological Enquiry* **75**(2), 197–215.

Grobelaar-du Plessis, I. (2007). *African Women with Disabilities: The Victims of Multi-layered Discrimination*. Pretoria: University of Pretoria.

Handicap International (2006). *Good Practices for the Economic Inclusion of Persons with Disabilities in Developing Countries*. Paris: Handicap International.

Kachaje, R., Dube, K., MacLachlan, M. & Mji, G. (2014). The African Network for Evidence-to-Action on Disability: a role player in the realisation of the UNCRPD in Africa. *African Journal of Disability* **3**(2), Art. #86.

Kurebwa, J. (2014). Rural women's representation and participation in local governance in the Masvingo and Mashonaland Central Provinces of Zimbabwe. *IOSR Journal of Humanities and Social Science* **19**(2), 125–132.

Lang, R. & Charowa, G. (2007). *Scoping Study: Disability Issues in Zimbabwe. Final Report.* London: DFID.

Majiet, S. & Africa, A. (2015). Women with disabilities in leadership: the challenges of patriarchy. *Disability & Gender* **29**(2), 101–115.

Manatsa, Proceed (2015). Are disability laws in Zimbabwe compatible with the provisions of the United Nations Convention on the Rights of Persons with Disabilities (CRPD)? *International Journal of Humanities and Social Science Invention* **4**(4), 25–34.

Mangwaya, E. (2015). Challenges faced by learners and teachers in special classes in secondary schools: the case of Dzivaresekwa District in Harare. *The International Journal of Humanities & Social Studies* **3**(9), 151–154.

Maranan, F. (2007). *Reflection and insight on the status and directions of women's political participation: Re-imagining women's movements and struggles in conversations with women: A collaborative project between the women's education development, productivity and research.* Philippines: WEDPRO.

Maziriri, E. T. & Madinga, N. W. (2016). A qualitative study on the challenges faced by entrepreneurs living with physical disabilities within the Sebokeng Township of South Africa. *International Journal of Research in Business Studies and Management* **3**(5), 1–13.

Ministry of Finance and Economic Development (2011). *Zimbabwe National Budget.* Harare: Government Publishers.

Ministry of Health and Child Welfare (2013). *The Living Conditions among Persons with Disability Survey.* Harare: Government Publishers.

Mitra, Sophie, Posarac, Aleksandra & Vick, Brandon (2011). *Disability and Poverty in Developing Countries: A Snapshot from the World.* Health Survey. SP Discussion Paper.

Mokomane, Zitha (2012). *Role of Families in Social and Economic Empowerment of Individuals.* United Nations Expert Group Meeting on 'Promoting Empowerment of People in Achieving Poverty Eradication, Social Integration and Full Employment and Decent Work for All', 10–12 September 2012. New York: United Nations.

Movement for Democratic Change (2011). *Constitution of the Movement for Democratic Change.* Harare: MDC.

Mtetwa, E. (2014). Disability policy and practice in Zimbabwe. In J. Mugumbate (ed.) *Development Policy and Practice: Making Use of Population Census Data in Zimbabwe* (pp. 165–180). Harare: IDA Publishers.

Museva, L. (2012). The level of participation of women with disabilities in economic empowerment programmes in Gweru District. *Journal of Emerging Trends in Educational Research and Policy Studies* **3**(6), 955–963.

Muthukrishna, N., Sokoya, G. & Moodley, S. (2009). Gender and disability: an intersectional analysis of experiences of ten disabled women in Kwazulu-Natal. *Gender & Behaviour* **7**(1), 2264–2282.

Nyende, F. (2012). *Children with Disabilities in Universal Primary Education in Uganda: A Rights-Based Analysis to Inclusive Education.* Unpublished Master's Thesis, The Hague Institute of Social Studies, Netherlands.

Nyezwa, H. & M'kumbuzvi, V. R. P. (2003). Participation in community based rehabilitation programmes in Zimbabwe: where are we? *Asia Pacific Disability Rehabilitation Journal* **6**(3), 56–63.

Peresuh, M. & Barcham, L. (1998). Special education provisions in Zimbabwe. *British Journal of Special Education* **15**(4), 18–23.

Reeler, T. (2014). Women and democracy in Zimbabwe: insights from Afrobarometer. *Afrobarometer Policy Paper* No. 14.

Research and Advocacy Unit (2010). *Women, politics and the Zimbabwe crisis. Report produced by the Institute for Democracy in Africa (IDASA), the International Center for Transitional Justice (ICTJ), the Research and Advocacy Unit (RAU), and the Women's Coalition of Zimbabwe (WCoZ).* Harare: RAU. Retrieved from http://archive.kubatana.net/html/archive/demgg/100526rau.asp?orgcode=RES002&year=2010&range_start=1 on 15 August 2017.

Rugoho, T. (2017). Fishing in deep waters: sex workers with disabilities in Harare, Zimbabwe. *International Journal of Gender Studies in Developing Societies* **2**(3), 227–240.

Rugoho, T. & Maphosa, F. (2015). Gender-based violence amongst women with disabilities: a case study of Mwenezi district, Zimbabwe. *Gender Questions* **6**(13), 12–27.

Rugoho, T. & Maphosa, F. (2017). Challenges faced by women with disabilities in accessing sexual and reproductive health in Zimbabwe: the case of Chitungwiza town. *African Journal of Disability* **6**(0), a252. Retrieved from https://doi.org/10.4102/ajod.v6i0.252 on 17 August 2017.

Rugoho, T. & Siziba, B. (2014). Rejected people: beggars with disabilities in the city of Harare, Zimbabwe. *Developing Country Studies* **4**(26), 51–56.

Rutoro, E. (2012). *An analysis of the impact of socio-cultural factors on the effective implementation of gender sensitive policies in education management*. Unpublished PhD Thesis, Zimbabwe Open University, Zimbabwe.

Southern African Development Community Gender Monitor (2013). *Tracking Progress on Implementation of the SADC Protocol on Gender and Development: Women in Politics and Decision-Making Positions*. Gaborone: Southern African Development Community (SADC) Gender Unit.

Simanowitz, A. (2001). From event to process: current trends in microfinance impact assessment. *Small Enterprise Development* **12**(4), 11–21.

Traustadottir, R. (1997). *Obstacles to Equality: The Double Discrimination of Women with Disabilities*. New York: Center for Human Policy, Syracuse University.

Tshuma, M. C. (2012). A review of the poverty and food security issues in South Africa: is agriculture the solution? *African Journal of Agricultural Research* **7**(28), 4010–4020.

United Nations (2006). *The Convention on the Rights of Persons with Disabilities and Optional Protocol*. New York: United Nations. Retrieved from www.un.org/disabilities/documents/convention/convoptprot-e.pdf on 27 April 2018.

United Nations (2014). *The United Nations Human Development Index*. Geneva: UN.

Viriri, P. & Makurumidze, S. (2014). Engagement of disabled people in entrepreneurship programmes. *Journal of Small Business and Entrepreneurship Development* **2**(1), 1–30.

ZANU PF (2015). *Zimbabwe African National Union Partiotic Front (ZANU PF) Manifesto*. Harare: Jongwe Printers.

Zimbabwe Independent (2012). Workers bear brunt of trade union strife. 3 May, in Business, Politics.

19

DISABILITY, INTIMACY AND PARENTHOOD

Deconstructing 'mutually exclusive' constructs

Joanne Neille

Introduction

Sexuality is often the source of our deepest oppression; it is also often the source of our deepest pain. It is easier for us to talk about and formulate strategies for changing discrimination in employment, education and housing, than to talk about our exclusion from sexuality and reproduction.

(Finger, 1992, p. 9)

Internationally, there has been a move toward a human rights approach to disability. This implies that disabled people are placed in control of making decisions, which affect all aspects of their lives, including decisions about intimate relationships and reproductive health. However, despite the adoption of policies that advocate for the human rights approach, myths and beliefs regarding the ways in which disabled people are expected to behave abound, with disabled people often being viewed as eternal children, asexual, or unable to inhibit their sexual impulses. This chapter aims to explore the experiences of disabled people in the establishment and maintenance of long-term intimate relationships and their experiences of pregnancy and child-rearing. Narrative interviews were conducted in SiSwati with 30 disabled adults with various forms of impairments living in rural South Africa. Data were analysed using thematic analysis. Findings revealed that contextual beliefs pertaining to the cause of impairments, together with stereotypical beliefs regarding the nature of relationships that disabled people should engage in and the behaviours that they should portray serve to have a significant impact on their identities. Furthermore, disabled women reported numerous accounts of psychological violence inflicted on them by healthcare professionals during antenatal check-ups. This was compounded by exposure to sexual violence in the community. These results hold implications for the training of healthcare providers in terms of the way in which they engage with persons with disability, and highlight the need for contextually relevant information that can be made accessible to disabled people to support their right to freedom of choice, while at the same time protecting them from becoming victims of sexual assault. Furthermore, there is a need to evaluate the ways in which human rights policies are put into practice and how these relate to contextual beliefs pertaining to disability, intimacy and parenthood.

Background

One does not need to inspect cultural norms too closely in order to conclude that, for most people, it is a priority to have a significant other with whom to share social and intimate relationships. With few exceptions, the pursuit of these types of interpersonal relationships is fraught with complexity and anxiety. This is particularly true for disabled people who are frequently excluded from social participation in everyday activities for a variety of reasons, including stigma, discrimination, fear, limited access and lack of support. This chapter will explore the experiences of establishing and maintaining intimate relationships, and the experiences of pregnancy and child-rearing among disabled people living in a rural area of South Africa.

Despite the numerous international and local policies set out to protect the rights of disabled people, including the United Nations Convention on the Rights of Persons with Disabilities (United Nations Enable, 2006), the World Programme of Action Concerning Disabled People (United Nations Enable, 1982), the United Nations Rules on the Equalisation of Opportunities for Persons with Disabilities (United Nations Enable, 1993), the White Paper on an Integrated National Disability Strategy (1997), the African Charter on Human and People's Rights (African Commission on Human and Peoples' Rights, 1979), and the Patient Rights Charter (2005), few policies specifically promote the right to healthy intimate and sexual relationships among disabled people. Conversely, desires to engage in intimate relationships among this population are often viewed as symptoms of mental illness needing to be prevented or constrained (Tennille & Wright, 2013). The idea that disabled people have any form of sexuality is often responded to negatively, with society viewing them as asexual or 'other' to the social norm (Wickenden, Nixon & Yoshida, 2013). Disabled adults are frequently viewed as being intensively passive and helpless or are viewed as 'over-sexed' or sexually inappropriate (Rohleder & Swartz, 2012) and are consequently infantilised, prohibited from engaging in sexual activity and marriage, sterilised, and excluded from social and leisure activities (Wickenden *et al.*, 2013). These perceptions violate the individual's sense of liberty and dignity.

Current literature suggests two pivotal areas of concern for disabled people in relation to the establishment and maintenance of intimate relationships. First, disabled people experience discrimination and marginalisation, affecting their abilities to establish and maintain mutual intimate relationships as a consequence of stigma, limited access to potential partners, sexually restrictive environments, reduced physical and emotional defences, communication barriers, and psychosocial challenges to forming relationships (Tennille & Wright, 2013; Neille & Penn, 2015). Second, disabled people are particularly vulnerable to a variety of forms of violence, including sexual exploitation (Plummer & Findley, 2012; Neille & Penn, 2015). This is of particular concern in the context of HIV/AIDS. Despite the emphasis on 'vulnerability' in society's response to the HIV pandemic, the impact of HIV on disabled people has been grossly overlooked (Wickenden *et al.*, 2013). This has magnified the sense of inequality experienced by disabled people, and exacerbated the entrenched sense of denial, blame and stigma against this population (ibid.). The stigma and silence surrounding HIV and disability thus serve as a double form of discrimination.

Research suggests that human sexuality is a product of cultural socialisation (Dune & Mpofu, 2015) and is constructed through the interaction of psychological and social processes within a specific culture (Schooler & Ward, 2006). This is supported by Thornton (2009) who claims that sexual relationships involve a complex combination of emotions, social roles, attitudes, actions and economic exchanges, all of which are embedded within complex social relationships and identities. Thus, in order to understand the complexities associated with intimate relationships and the act of childbearing, it is essential to take into account the complexities of social and cultural structures (Thornton, 2009). Sexual Script Theory (Simon & Gagnon, 1986) suggests that individuals express their sexuality through socially imprinted schemas which outline how they should interact with others, what types of intimate activities are permitted, and when and where these activities may take place. These behavioural dispositions are created through the individual's involvement in cultural, interpersonal and intrapsychic schemas (Dune & Mpofu, 2015).

Three different schemas are combined when creating sexual behaviour scripts. These include public, interpersonal and intrapsychic scripts, all of which influence individual constructions and expressions of sexuality. Public scripts guide the individual within collective life by dictating the requirements needed to fulfil specific roles, including the process by which an individual enters roles and how they should behave within these roles (Ronen, 2010). Interpersonal schemas define people as being both actors of scripts and agents of their formulation, and are characterised by the formulation of interpersonal relationships (Dune & Mpofu, 2015). Through these schemas individuals try to act out what has been culturally scripted (Weeks, 2010). The construct of interpersonal schemas reinforces the relevance of public schemas because people act out their perceptions of appropriate identities and the desired expectations from playing out these roles (Simon & Gagnon, 1986). Intrapsychic schemas involve inner dialogue and influence the ways in which individuals adopt the script of what is sexually desirable and how they fit into that scenario.

Within African culture, marriage is conceptualised as the linking of two families rather than of two people (Kuper, 1963; Niehaus, 2002a). The homestead is fundamental to the family, and it is here that roles are played out in dynamic interpersonal relationships (Maverick, 1966). In control of the homestead is the patriarchal headman whose prestige is enhanced by the size of his family and his number of dependants (Kuper, 1963; Delius, 2007). Thus the notion of childbearing is considered to be essential to the consummation of wifehood (Niehaus, 2002a). Naturally, the act of sexual intercourse is intimately related to the act of childbearing, and has been found to be fundamental to male masculinity in this area (Niehaus, 2002b). Sexual intercourse is believed to ensure a balanced supply of blood within the body, essential to the maintenance of good health, while prolonged periods of celibacy might result in poorly regulated bodily fluids, short temper, recklessness and the inability to think clearly (Niehaus, 2002b). This notion is expanded on by Knox (2008) who adds that in African culture, sexual relationships are valued as an expression of kinship, while childbearing signifies the bonding of both visible and invisible worlds. Thornton (2008) explains how sexuality relates both toward the cultural representation of the body and the flow of substances as gifts between partners during sexual intercourse, and thus disability and illness may originate through the action of sexual intercourse. This implies that individuals are permeable to both physical and spiritual substances of other persons, and suggests that the biological boundaries of the individual are rooted in the cultural concepts of the body (Thornton, 2008).

To date, research into the ways in which disabled people make sense of intimate interpersonal relationships has remained limited, largely due to narrow conceptualisations of sexuality among this population, with limited insight into the diverse factors that shape intimate interpersonal behaviours. This is particularly true for persons living in developing countries (Shuttleworth *et al.*, 2010).

Research setting

The study took place within the Nkomazi East Municipality of the Mpumalanga Province, which is located within the Southern Lowveld area of Mpumalanga, approximately 350 kilometres east of Johannesburg. The Nkomazi East Municipality continues to be one of the poorest municipalities in the Mpumalanga Province (Comprehensive Rural Development Programme, 2013). Approximately 409,000 people live in the area (Nkomazi Integrated Development Plan, 2014–2015), the majority of whom are black SiSwati-speaking residents, with the highest portion of the population falling within the age range of 5–19 years (Nkomazi Integrated Development Plan, 2014–2015). Population growth has slowed significantly in recent years for a number of reasons, including increasing mortality rates, decreasing birth rates, and increases in the working-age population migrating to urban areas in search of work (Nkomazi Integrated Development Plan, 2014–/2015). Currently, no published data exist on the numbers of disabled

Table 19.1 Community profile of the Nkomazi East Municipality

Employment	• 55% of the population fall into the economically active population
	• However, many of these persons are immigrants from Mozambique and Swaziland and do not have the documents required for formal employment
	• Thus, 40% of the economically active population are unemployed. 80% of the employed population work in the informal sector
Dependency ratio	• 1:8
Household density	• 6 persons per household
Population distribution	• 47% population under 19 years old
Water provision	• 14.9% of the population have piped water supply inside their homes
	• 44.4% of the population have piped water within the perimeters of their property
	• 31.4% of the population access piped water at a community tap
	• 9.3% of the population collect water from rivers, dams and rainwater tanks
Sanitation	• 5.6% of the population have flush toilets connected to a sewerage system
	• 1.9% of the population have a flush toilet with a septic tank
	• 39.1% of the population have a chemical toilet
	• 35.8% of the population have a pit latrine with ventilation
	• 17.4% of the population have no sanitation facilities
Waste management	• No organised waste management or disposal sites outside of the urban towns
Electricity	• 44.1% of the population have electrification in their homes
	• 2% of the population use gas
	• 6.1% of the population use paraffin
	• 41.2% of the population use wood
	• 6.4% of the population use coal
	• 0.1% of the population use solar energy
	• 0.2% of the population burn animal dung for energy purposes
Roads	• 80.9% of roads are gravel/sand tracks
	• 40% of villages are roads almost inaccessible by car
Health	• Two 24-hour hospitals functioning at a primary healthcare level
	• One 24-hour clinic
	• 27 day clinics
	• Numerous informal home-based care initiatives
Education	• 49% of the population are illiterate
	• 25% of the population have no formal education
	• 35% of the population have a primary school education, with 16% of the population having completed school

Adapted from the Nkomazi Integrated Development Plan (2014–2015). Retrieved from http://mfma. treasury.gov.za/Documents/01.%20Integrated%20Development%20Plans/2014-15/02%20Local%20 Municipalities/MP324%20Nkomazi/MP324%20Nkomazi%20%20DRAFT%20IDP%202014%20-2015. pdf accessed on 12 April 2018.

people residing in the Nkomazi East Municipality. Current statistics reveal that the Nkomazi East Municipality has an HIV prevalence rate of 47.3% (Comprehensive Rural Development Programme, 2013) as reflected in Table 19.1.

Access to setting

I have a long history with members of the disabled community in the Nkomazi East Municipality. Over the period 1 January–31 December 2003, I was employed at Tonga Hospital as a Community Service Speech-Language Therapist and Audiologist, providing an in- and out-patient speech and hearing therapy service at the hospital, at outreach clinics in the surrounding area, and making home visits for patients who were unable to access the clinics or hospital. This enabled a first-hand experience of the community, its culture, belief systems and practices, and exposed me to many of the frustrations that the local community face, including lack of provision of municipal services, poor conditions of the roads and limited access between the hospital and many of the homes in the community, as well as the frustration of travelling long distances in order to acquire basic products. Considerable time was spent with the local leaders and elders in order to gain access to the community and in order to develop an understanding of the needs of the community so as to deliver a basic rehabilitation service. This experience provided a degree of understanding of the way of life within the community, the beliefs and cultural practices, as well as the support structures and roles of various members of the community.

In 2006–07, I returned to the Nkomazi East Municipality in order to gather material for a study on caregivers' experiences of parenting children with cerebral palsy. This study relied on qualitative methods, including semi-structured interviews and participant observation, and enabled a profoundly powerful snapshot of the link between disability and daily life, the interface between historical, social and demographic factors, and the relationship between the individual and the community (Barratt & Penn, 2009). Based on the findings that emerged from this study, a number of issues were highlighted that required further investigation, in order to develop a better understanding of the lived experience of disability and the needs of disabled people in rural areas. These issues formed the rationale for returning to the area over the period 2010–11 in order to explore the lived experiences of adults with disabilities living in a rural context.

Throughout all of my engagements with the people of the Nkomazi East Municipality, I worked through the community-based rehabilitation worker (CBRW). The CBRW is a local woman with a physical impairment who acquired polio during childhood. She is consequently confined to a wheelchair. The CBRW took on the role of a mediator and was able to put me into contact with a variety of contextual issues that, as an outsider, I would not otherwise have been able to engage in (Angrosino & Rosenberg, 2011). The nature of the research was socially grounded and it was acknowledged that the stories that people consider as most expressive of their lives often remain told within their community only (Frank, 2012). For this reason, together with the fact that I only possess a basic command of SiSwati (local language spoken in Mpumalanga), the mediator served as a cultural broker, assisting me in traversing linguistic, cultural and contextual barriers.

Participants

Participants were sampled from within 12 villages in the Nkomazi East Municipality using a combination of snowball sampling and intensity sampling. Over the period of data collection, 30 participants were interviewed in SiSwati. Participants were visited in their homes on a number of occasions and were asked to 'tell their story'. Table 19.2 provides a summary of the informants who were interviewed.

Table 19.2 Participants' demographics

Age in years	Gender	Nature of impairment					
		Physical	Multiple	Visual	Cognitive	Psychiatric	Total
19–40	Male	6	3	–	–	–	9
	Female	3	1	–	1	1	6
41–60	Male	3	2	1	–	–	6
	Female	4	2	1	–	–	7
61–80	Male	–	–	–	–	–	0
	Female	–	–	–	–	–	0
80+	Male	–	–	–	–	–	0
	Female	1	1	–	–	–	2
Total	30	17	9	2	1	1	30

Narratives on the intersection between disability, intimacy and parenthood

Listening to the narratives through a Sexual Script Theory lens appeared to provide a useful means for understanding the ways in which adults with disabilities living in a rural area make sense of attempts to develop and sustain intimate interpersonal relationships and to negotiate the complexities of pregnancy and childbearing. The process of data collection and data analysis is reflected in Figure 19.1.

Substantial evidence emerged to suggest that despite the challenges associated with maintaining interpersonal relationships, the majority of adults with disabilities attempted to align themselves with existing socio-cultural scripts. However, a number of the informants positioned themselves in contrast to extant scripts, thereby redefining their positions as adults with disabilities. The complexities and pluralities that emerged within the narratives are discussed below in relation to Sexual Script Theory.

Public scripts

Interactional constructions of sexuality are reinforced through socio-cultural attitudes within communities, and these interpretations influence who can engage in sexual activity with whom (Simon & Gagnon, 2003). The construction of normative public scripts frequently excludes adults with disabilities, and as a result their experiences of intimacy are poorly understood.

Three dominant public scripts emerged in the current study which appeared to challenge the ways in which adults with disabilities were able to make independent and supported decisions to engage in long-term interpersonal relationships.

Impact of impairment on intimate partners

In a number of cases, participants with acquired impairments reported that their intimate and social relationships had broken down, for numerous reasons including interpersonal collapse and death, and that these had led to the onset of disability. Examples of this emerged when Participant 22 said, 'They [family] said she [wife] is a witch and she caused me to be injured' and when Participant 12 said, 'I became disabled because my father died before he finished paying *lobola* or dowry'.

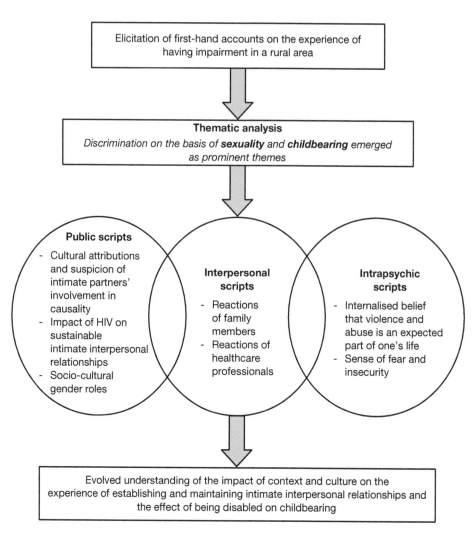

Figure 19.1 Process of elicitation of narratives and management of data

Given the clear and important kinship ties existing in SiSwati culture, threats to interpersonal relationships have far-reaching effects in both the community and for the individual. The ubiquitous presence of death within the community appeared to create a sense of uncertainty among informants, and place limitations on the nature of relationships which were deemed 'safe' to engage in. This served to magnify the sense of isolation, social exclusion, and barriers to accessibility of potential partners, and social support. This is evident where Participant 22 lamented: 'So now it is difficult for me. It is like I have no one who I can trust and I would like to meet a lady and marry her but what can I do? Because it was my wife who caused me to be like this.'

These examples highlight the ways in which relationships are drawn between context, death, disability and interpersonal relationships, suggesting that cultural attributions have the potential to manipulate the psychosocial needs of individuals and influence the ways in which individuals engage in intimate interpersonal relationships.

Effects of HIV to sustainable intimate interpersonal relationships

Over the last three decades, sexual scripts have been increasingly influenced by the HIV pandemic (Ross-Bailey *et al.*, 2014). South Africa continues to have the highest rate of HIV infection in the world, with current statistics suggesting that there are over six million people living with HIV, giving rise to an overall prevalence of between 11 and 12% (Statistics South Africa, 2015). The highest rate of infection is in the age group 15–49 years, with over three million deaths due to AIDS, and over two million children orphaned as a result of the pandemic (UNAIDS, 2015). Despite the vast coverage that HIV has received, the impact of the disease is believed to be much deeper than that of other conditions since '*these merely kill*' (Thornton, 2008, p. 32), while HIV challenges the fundamental values of individuals and society (ibid.).

Current public scripts surrounding HIV/AIDS promote safe sex, monogamy, and the need to test regularly for the presence of the virus in the blood. However, the enactment of these scripts can be challenging for disabled people who might be disempowered from negotiating safe sexual relationships, and who might not have access to information regarding the nature and transmission of HIV, or access to condoms. Evidence of this emerged in the narratives as follows:

> It is difficult for me to say to my husband that we can't have sex. You see we are two wives with one husband, and I know that one of his girlfriends died because of AIDS. So they say we must use condoms but for me it is difficult to get to the clinic to get them and the man, he doesn't like to use them. So for me, I just hope that I am not infected.
>
> *(Participant 3)*

> My husband says he doesn't believe in this thing called HIV, even though you can see he used to have a big tummy and now he is very skinny and sick all the time. Even the neighbours are saying he has HIV. So for me, I am just happy when he is working in Johannesburg, then I know I am safe.
>
> *(Participant 6)*

> Yes, I think about illnesses like HIV. Like if I propose to someone and they refuse, I quickly say 'Ah, I'm safe'. If I get sick it will be a problem for me. Who will give me money to go to hospital?
>
> *(Participant 9)*

Of particular concern was the anecdotal evidence that emerged suggesting that having sex with a disabled person could cure an infected person from HIV. This concurs with findings by Rohleder (2017) and is not unlike the myths that sex with an infant or young child can cure HIV (Mahlalela & Kang'ethe, 2015). This places all vulnerable persons at risk for sexual violence and transmission of HIV. Participant 30 provided insight into the fear that these types of myths evoke among the disabled population:

> So for people like us who are disabled, we are very scared because some, they say, if they are HIV positive and they have sex with you, they will be cured. So for us, we are not safe anywhere, even in our houses, we are scared they will come and rape us.

These narratives highlight the ways in which HIV challenges traditional public scripts on safe sex and consequently impacts on the ways in which adults with disabilities explore and negotiate ways of engaging in intimate interpersonal relationships. Significantly, it appears that, despite a desire to engage in intimate interpersonal relationships, in the context of HIV these decisions are governed by fear.

Socio-cultural gender roles and the exclusion of disabled people

Great value and importance are associated with marriage and childbearing in SiSwati culture. Thus, in order to understand the complexities associated with sexual relationships and the act of childbearing, it is essential to take into account the complexities of social and cultural roles and structures (Thornton, 2009).

Many of the participants in the sample positioned themselves according to whether or not they were parents. Given that the majority of the sample fell within the childbearing age range, this is not surprising and is consistent with the culturally expected norms for the community (Knox, 2008; Thornton, 2008). Kuper (1963) states that within the Swazi culture, childbearing is essential to the consummation of wifehood, and should a married woman be unable to bear children, her family might be requested to return the cattle that were paid for her hand in marriage. However, bearing of children is not only a core aspect of identity for women, but also for men, since a man's prosperity and importance in the community is measured by his number of dependants (Kuper, 1963). Similarly, both Caldwell and Caldwell (1996) and Thornton (2008) describe the significance that fertility carries within African cultures in relation to kinship, property regimes and the exchanges in networks and relations. This is expanded on by Knox (2008), who states that, particularly within the Afro-centric worldview, the prospect of being unable to bear children is a source of great distress, raising the question as to who will remember the individual after their death. This leads to the shame of '*cosmological insignificance*' (Knox, 2008, p. 175) given the potential of not having a future in the next life. In addition to this, Niehaus (2007) found that bachelors living in the Lowveld area of Mpumalanga were considered suspiciously, with prolonged celibacy being considered to be abnormal, distrustful and linked to witchcraft. Thus, the lack of opportunity to bear children has the potential to impact significantly on the ways in which family and community members respond to individuals, and consequently on the individual's interpretation of experiences.

Within the current study, some of the most common areas where participants revealed conflict and distress were in relation to establishing resilient identities as partners, providers and homemakers. The source of this conflict appeared to be from a combination of both inter- and intra-personal turmoil, as evidenced where Participant 1 said, 'People are always wondering like can I have sex like a normal person, and will I be able to look after them like a husband or will they just have to care for me.' Participant 3 also agreed with Participant 2: 'The neighbours are always talking behind my back, saying things like, how can I sleep with a man if I can't even clean my own house.'

Many of the female participants reported that their family and neighbours were upset or angry when they found out that they (the participants) were pregnant. Consequently, participants experienced negative reactions from the community during pregnancy, yet their narrative positioning as mothers and caregivers provides evidence of defying the community's definitions and responses to disability. These perceptions are further confounded by the cultural associations with childbearing. Given the traditional beliefs regarding the onset of disability as a consequence of *umuti*, it is possible that family and community members might be concerned about the transmission of evil spirits or misfortune through sexual encounters. *Umuti* here refers to the onset of impairment in cases where the family (usually the parents) have not heeded cultural norms and processes, such as planting crops or family obligations, or in cases where the male head of the household has more than one wife.

Masculinity was also defined in terms of whether male participants had children or not, which implies that taking on the role of a parent is not only a priority for females. For example, Participant 2 defines himself by saying, 'I am a father of four children, and I have supported them up until now.' Also Participant 23, a 39-year-old man with a physical impairment, who is married to a woman with a hearing impairment, had this to say:

> My wife had four children from before, and we have three children together, so all together we have seven children. My wife's family were not happy when we had children, but I will not allow them to rule my life. I am supporting all the children – even those from another man.

This highlights the importance assigned to being able to portray oneself as a provider and a parent.

The positioning of the self in relation to being a partner and provider was thus a prominent theme among both male and female participants. These identity constructions are important because they do not only reflect a sense of agency and independence, but also a sense of kinship. Similarly, in each of these quotations the notion of cultural and gendered norms of childbearing and child-rearing is reflected. This implies that parenthood and the notion of being a partner and provider serves as a marker of success and contribution among disabled adults. Following this, it can also be understood that the inability to form intimate relationships and limited opportunities to bear children has the potential to affect the participants' sense of self. This is evident where participants made comments such as, 'I want to have children, because that is the will of God' and 'I want to have children and things that belong to me'. These narratives suggest that the enactment of socio-cultural and gendered scripts for disabled people living in the context of poverty not only places significant physical and emotional demands on the individual, but questions the individual's identity in relation to basic human elements such as the value placed on sex and childbearing.

Interpersonal scripts

Interpersonal scripts are based on the ways in which individuals view existential conditions within their environments, and how they negotiate interpersonal relationships and interpret other people's intentions, purposes, assumptions and points of view (Kimmel, 2007).

Within the realm of interpersonal scripts, narratives of the ways in which adults with disabilities established relationships with members of their communities and the ways in which they interpreted community members' reactions to them emerged. The most common sources of interpersonal scripts emerged in relation to the reactions and responses of family members, community members and healthcare professionals in relation to the notion of intimacy and parenthood among disabled people.

Reactions of family members

For the majority of participants, the experience of developing close interpersonal relationships and the act of childbearing were fraught with anxiety and the sense of disapproval from others. The lack of support and stigmatisation surrounding disability served to marginalise and disempower the adults in this study, resulting in a fragmented sense of self. Adults with disabilities reported isolation and abandonment secondary to the onset of disability, as well as strained inter-personal relationships at home causing stress. Participants confirmed these sentiments:

> My wife is gone because I'm no longer working. I wasn't able to maintain her any-more so she met another man and he took her.
>
> *(Participant 9)*

> (My girlfriend's family) said, 'This one is disabled. What is he going to be able to give you? He doesn't have money'.
>
> *(Participant 20)*

> At home they accepted me but my wife left me. I was still in hospital when she left me.
>
> *(Participant 22)*

> My parents were angry (when I was pregnant) and didn't want me to go and stay with my husband.
>
> *(Participant 24)*

The quotations above highlight the ways in which family members stigmatise adults with disabilities, displaying the ways in which deeply ingrained myths and stereotypes regarding disability, and beliefs regarding the ways in which disabled people should act and behave, come to the fore. These perceptions appeared to weaken the individuals' resilience, lead-ing to narrative incoherence. This in turn seemed to affect disabled adults' abilities to align themselves with socially and culturally acceptable roles, leading to further isolation, margin-alisation and insecurity, and detracting from the ability to reveal a sense of independence within the community.

Reactions of healthcare professionals, specifically nurses

Women with disabilities appeared to have faced significant forms of overt discrimination during their pregnancies from the wider community as well as from healthcare professionals, reflecting exposure to psychological violence. Historical attitudes, together with limited mobility, lack of accessibility and social isolation appear to contribute significantly to this form of marginalisation and oppression. These attitudes are dehumanising and devaluing, and as a consequence serve to strengthen the negative cycle of psychological violence to which disabled people are exposed.

An example of psychological violence inflicted during pregnancy was reported by Participant 3:

> It was embarrassing for me to be pregnant. I was afraid of myself, the way I was, and the nurses were saying, 'Who did this to you?' Like as a disabled person you are not supposed to sleep with a man, like you are an animal. The other women at the clinic were pointing fingers at me, talking a lot, saying, 'If I were you, I would not do that' or 'Stop this and don't do it again! Look at you!' like I have done something wrong, like I am not supposed to have feelings for a man.

Similarly Participant 11 reported, 'I had my first child when I was 24 years old. People in my area were not happy about it. They were saying someone was abusing me and that it was a sin to be sleeping with a disabled person'. Participant 30 indicated that, 'People are thinking that if you have a boyfriend, then you are a prostitute'. These reports of psychological violence and overt discrimination are in direct defiance of Chapter 2 (section nine) of the South African Bill of Rights (Constitution of the Republic of South Africa, 1996) which ensures the right to freedom from discrimination, including discrimination on the grounds of pregnancy and disability. These findings have the potential to significantly impact on the development of a coherent sense of self, as well as on the individuals' abilities to position themselves in culturally and gender-appropriate positions, and concur with the findings of Kulick (2012) who laments that for disabled people in search of safe and equitable intimate relationships, the obstacles in the way feel frighteningly large.

Intrapsychic scripts

Intrapsychic scripts refer to the ways in which individuals make sense of and act upon wishes and desires that originate in the deepest recesses of the self (Simon & Gagnon, 1986). Simon and Gagnon (1986) further suggest that these desires are not necessarily related to a desire for a person or object, but rather reflect what an individual might expect to experience through another person or object, and mirror in part the process of creation of the self.

The majority of participants in this study reflect that despite attempts to align with mainstream socio-cultural scripts, the experience of repeated exposure to a variety of forms of violence and discrimination appear to result in the internalised belief that violence and abuse is an expected part of one's life. This reflects a sense of fear and insecurity, as evidenced when Participant 24 commented, 'I met a guy who fell in love with me but I was afraid to sleep with him because of my disability'. Participant 30 lamented, 'I didn't want to love anyone. I didn't think that me, I could have a boyfriend, I was always thinking it was not for me, it was only for normal people to love each other'. These experiences can be explained by Jeffreys (2008) who suggests that society's focus on biological flaws serves to position blame on the individual, and in so doing, disabled people continue to be exposed to increasing and complex forms of violence. These experiences continue to negatively affect disabled people as seen when Participant 21 commented, 'I was always feeling afraid, like I was not a human being'. Similarly, Participant 3 recalls her response to the sexual abuse she endured, coupled with the nurses' responses to her when she was pregnant, 'I was always afraid of myself, the way I was'.

Conclusion

The inaction of cultural, interpersonal and intrapsychic sexual scripts by disabled people reflects a complex intersection along the axes of biology, history and power dynamics. Limited research into this field has resulted in narrow understandings of the challenges and experiences of disabled people in establishing resilient identities where they are able to enjoy rights to freedom and equality in all spheres of life. Conversely, by refraining from engaging in discussions relating to sexual health and equality we are all complicit in perpetuating negative stereotypes. Significantly, the absence of first-hand experiences of disabled people in research inhibits the development of policies and practices that take into consideration the impact of context and cultural safety for all.

The experiences of disabled people in their attempts to establish intimate interpersonal relationships discussed in this chapter extend beyond the current literature on the topic. Incorporating these issues into research serves to acknowledge and validate the reality of living with a disability in a rural area. Despite the negative physical and emotional effects that violence has on the individual, these narratives allow individuals to reveal their vulnerabilities, and in so doing, to bear witness by transforming memory into language. This serves to crystallise their experiences within history. Through exposing their vulnerabilities, disabled people reveal the possibility of constructing new realities of the lived experience of disability or impairments.

Reflective questions

1   How can current attitudes toward the intimate interpersonal relationships of adults with disabilities be addressed in ways that promote freedom of expression and equality?
2   In what way does the interplay between violence, marginalisation and disability affect the opportunities adults with disabilities have when engaging in intimate interpersonal relationships?
3   How can sexual rights be incorporated into current policy in a way that promotes cultural safety for all?
4   Consider how healthcare professionals working in rural areas can improve models of practice through prioritising the needs of disabled people.

References

African Commission on Human and Peoples' Rights (1979). *African Charter on Human and Peoples' Rights*. Retrieved from www.achpr.org/instruments/achpr/ on 13 June 2010.

Angrosino, M. & Rosenberg, J. (2011). Observations on observation: continuities and challenges. In N. K. Denzin & Y. S. Lincoln (eds) *The SAGE Book of Qualitative Research*, 4th edn. (pp. 467–478). Thousand Oaks, CA: SAGE Publications, Inc.

Barratt, J. & Penn, C. (2009). Listening to the voices of disability: experiences of caring for children with cerebral palsy in a rural South African setting. In L. Swartz (ed.) *Disability and Development* (pp. 191–212). New York: Springer.

Caldwell, J. & Caldwell, P. (1996). The African AIDS epidemic. *Scientific American* **274**(3), 62–68.

Comprehensive Rural Development Programme (2013). *Selected Socio-Economic Indicators of the 7 Municipal Areas in Mpumalanga – December 2013*. Retrieved from www.ruraldevelopment.gov.za/publications/evaluation-reports/file/3500-implementation-evaluation-of-the-comprehensive-rural-development-programme-crdp-2013 accessed on 12 April 2018.

Constitution of the Republic of South Africa (1996). Retrieved from www.info.gov.za/documents/constitution/ on 15 July 2010.

Delius, P (ed.) (2007). *Mpumalanga: History and Heritage*. Scottsville: University of Kwazulu Natal Press.

Dune, T. & Mpofu, E. (2015). Allowing yourself to sexual freedom: making sense of sexual spontaneity with disability. *Advances in Social Sciences Research Journal* **2**(11), 36–47.

Finger, A. (1992). Forbidden fruit. *New Internationalist* **233**, 8–10.

Frank, A. (2012). Practicing dialogical narrative analysis. In J. Holstein & J. Gubrium (eds) *Varieties of Narrative Analysis* (pp. 33–52). Los Angeles, CA: SAGE Publications.

Jeffreys, S. (2008). Disability and the male sex right. *Women's Studies International Forum* **31**(5), 327–335.

Kimmel, M. (2007). *The Sexual Self: The Construction of Sexual Scripts*. Nashville, TN: Vanderbilt University Press.

Knox, P. (2008). *AIDS, Ancestors, and Salvation: Local Beliefs in Christian Ministry to the Sick*. Nairobi: Paulines Publications Africa.

Kulick, D. (2012). A stale and lamentable view of people: men, sex and disability. In R. Jönsson & L. Forsberg (eds) *Other Men (Andra Män)* (pp. 25–44). Stockholm: Gleerups.

Kuper, H. (1963). *The Swazi: A South African Kingdom*. New York: Holt, Rinehart and Winston.

Mahlalela, V. & Kang'ethe, S. (2015). Dimensions and manifestations of sexual risk taking behaviours in the era of STIs and HIV/AIDS in South Africa. *Journal of Human Ecology* **49**(3), 255–262.

Maverick, B. (1966). *The Swazi: An Ethnographic Account of the Natives of the Swaziland Protectorate*. London: Frank Cass.

Neille, J. & Penn, C. (2015). The interface between violence, disability, and poverty: stories from a developing country. *Journal of Interpersonal Violence* **32**(18), 2837–2861.

Niehaus, I. (2002a). Renegotiating masculinity in the South African Lowveld: narratives of male-male sex in labour compounds and prisons. *African Studies* **61**, 77–97.

Niehaus, I. (2002b). Perversion of power: witchcraft and the sexuality of evil in the South African Lowveld. *Journal of Religion in Africa* **32**(3), 269–299.

Niehaus, I. (2007). Death before dying: understanding AIDS stigma in the South African Lowveld. *Journal of Southern African Studies* **33**(4), 845–860.

Nkomazi Integrated Development Plan (2014–2015). Retrieved from http://mfma.treasury.gov.za/Documents/01.%20Integrated%20Development%20Plans/2014-15/02%20Local%20Municipalities/MP324%20Nkomazi/MP324%20Nkomazi%20%20DRAFT%20IDP%202014%20-2015.pdf accessed on 12 April 2018.

Plummer, S. & Findley, P. (2012). Women with disabilities' experience with physical and sexual abuse: a review of the literature and implications for the field. *Trauma, Violence, & Abuse* **13**(1), 15–29.

Rohleder, P. (2017). Disability and HIV in Africa: breaking the barriers to sexual health care. *Journal of Health Psychology* **22**(11), 1404–1414.

Rohleder, P. & Swartz, L. (2012). Disability, sexuality and sexual health. In P. Aggleton (ed.) *Understanding Global Sexualities: New Frontiers* (pp. 138–152). London: Routledge.

Ronen, S. (2010). Grinding on the dance floor: gendered scripts and sexualized dancing at college parties. *Gender & Society* **24**(3), 355–377.

Ross-Bailey, L., Moring, J., Angiola, J. & Bowen, A. (2014). The influence of sexual scripts and the 'better than average effect' on condom responsibility. *Journal of College Student Development* **55**(4), 408–412.

Schooler, D. & Ward, M. (2006). Average Joes: men's relationships with media, real bodies, and sexuality. *Psychology of Men & Masculinity* **7**(1), 27–41.

Shuttleworth, R., Russell, C., Weerakoon, P. & Dune, T. (2010). Sexuality in residential aged care: a survey of perceptions and policies in Australian nursing homes. *Sexuality and Disability* **28**(3), 187–194.

Simon, W. & Gagnon, J. (1986). Sexual scripts: permanence and change. *Archives of Sexual Behaviour* **15**(2), 97–120.

Simon, W. & Gagnon, J. (2003). Sexual scripts: origins, influences and changes. *Qualitative Sociology* **26**(4), 491–497.

Statistics South Africa (2015). *Mid-year Population Estimates*. Retrieved from https://www.statssa.gov.za/publications/P0302/P03022015.pdf on 2 August 2016.

Tennille, J. & Wright, E. (2013). Addressing the intimacy interests of people with mental health conditions: acknowledging consumer desires, provider discomforts, and system denial. *Temple University collaborative on community inclusion of individuals with psychiatric disability*, 1–22.

Thornton, R. (2009). Sexual networks and social capital: multiple and concurrent sexual partnerships as a rational response to unstable social networks. *African Journal of AIDS Research* **8**(4), 413–421.

Thornton, R. (2008). *Unimagined Community: Sex, Networks, and AIDS in Uganda and South Africa*. Berkley: University of California Press.

UNAIDS (2015). *HIV and AIDS Estimates 2015*. Retrieved from www.unaids.org/en/regionscountries/countries/southafrica on 10 August 2016.

United Nations Enable (1982). *World Programme of Action Concerning Disabled People*. Retrieved from www.un.org/documents/ga/res/37/a37r052.htm on 15 August 2010.

United Nations Enable (1993). *Rules on the Equalisation of Opportunities for Persons with Disabilities*. Retrieved from www.un.org/development/desa/disabilities/standard-rules-on-the-equalization-of-opportunities-for-persons-with-disabilities.html accessed on 12 April 2018.

United Nations Enable (2006). *Convention on the Rights of Persons with Disabilities*. Retrieved from www.un.org/disabilities/documents/convention/convoptprot-e.pdf accessed on 12 April 2018.

Weeks, J. (2010). Making the human gesture: history, sexuality and social justice. *History Workshop Journal* **70**(1), 5–20.

White Paper on an Integrated National Disability Strategy (1997). Retrieved from www.info.gov.za/whitepapers/199/disability.htm on 14 October 2008.

Wickenden, A., Nixon, S. & Yoshida, K. (2013). Disabling sexualities: exploring the impact of the intersection of HIV, disability and gender on the sexualities of women in Zambia. *African Journal of Disability* **2**(1), 1–8.

PART VI

Tourism, sports and accessibility

In Part VI, authors challenge discrimination of disabled people in tourism and sports and suggest ways of increasing accessibility for them to participate in recreational activities.

20

DISABILITY AND TOURISM IN SOUTHERN AFRICA

A policy analysis

Oliver Chikuta and Forbes Kabote

Introduction

Disability as a tourism study area, has not been adequately addressed in most southern African countries, with few studies having been done (Dube, 2005; Chikuta, 2015). However, there are abundant studies on disability in African countries (Eide & Ingstad, 2013; McKenzie *et al.*, 2014; M'kumbuzi *et al.*, 2015a, 2015b) and tourism (Snyman, 2012; Fabricius *et al.*, 2013) as independent subjects. This chapter interrogates disability policy issues as applied in the southern African region's tourism industry. The two concepts *disability* and *tourism* are discussed in unison. The chapter identifies the legal frameworks (or lack thereof) that increase disabled people's opportunities and allow them to participate in tourism and recreational activities. This is done by analysing government documents for Botswana, Zambia, Zimbabwe and South Africa. Disability advocates might want the following questions answered: what legal frameworks exist in these countries to promote tourism access by disabled people? How inclusive are these policies especially looking at the diversity of disabilities? This chapter attempts to answer these questions, among other things. This is important as the World Health Organization and World Bank (2011) reported that disabled people constitute about 15% of the world's population. By December 2016, southern Africa had a total population of 63.2 million people. Thus, assuming the 15% rate, the region has approximately 9.48 million disabled people. This is a significant niche for the region's tourism industry if they are recognised and tapped for sustainable tourism development.

The recognition of disabled people within southern African countries contributes to pursuing sustainable development goals as tourism is key in sustainable development (Pegas *et al.*, 2015). Thus, by addressing disability in the tourism context, southern African countries are likely to address sustainable development within the region. The benefits derived from approaching tourism using a disability lens are likely to benefit disabled people from local and international markets visiting these countries as tourists. Yet, the challenge has been that disability and tourism concepts have not been considered in relation to one another. This has emanated from the way the two concepts are conceptualised and operationalised by various stakeholders within the disability and tourism fields, thus undermining the fact that disability is a cross-cutting issue; an aspect emphasised within the social model of disability.

Models of disability

Before discussing the models of disability, it is important to understand what the term disability means. The United Nations (2006) defines persons with disabilities as people with long-term physical, mental, intellectual or sensory impairments, which in interaction with various barriers, can hinder a person's full and effective participation in society on an equal basis with others. Disabled people constitute a diverse community with various needs. Hence, several models of disability have been developed to conceptualise disability, with implications for policy and practice (Oliver, 1990, p. 7). In this chapter, three models of disability are discussed, which are: (1) the traditional model, (2) the medical model, and (3) the social model (Samaha, 2007; Darcy, 2002; Oliver, 1990). However, the chapter is informed by the social model of disability, which rides on the notion that disability is a social construct, not an individual problem (Oliver, 1990, 1996; Darcy, 2002). It does not victimise the person with impairment but blames the environment for the state of affairs. The model emphasises that society should put supportive mechanisms in place in order to remove barriers to social, physical and recreational participation (Buhalis & Darcy, 2011; Aitchison, 2003). It is out of the social model that a rather more recent approach is born called the *Human Rights-Based Model*. This approach advocates for the recognition of human dignity regardless of their social, political and economic status. Humans are to be valued simply because of their inherent self-worth. This therefore implies that disability is not a basis for discrimination and everyone has a right to everything that humans are entitled to. This chapter adopts the social model of disability.

Understanding tourism

With the joint efforts of UNWTO and UNSTAT, the definition of tourism was approved, with universal acceptance in 1994 as the activities of persons travelling to and staying in places outside their usual environment for not more than a year, for any main purpose (leisure, business or other personal purpose) other than to be employed by a resident entity in the country or place visited (Candela & Figini, 2012). This definition hinges around three main aspects on which tourism has to be defined and distinguished from other forms of travel: (1) the movement (where does the tourist travel to?); (2) the time (for how long does the tourist travel?) and (3) the motivation (why does the tourist travel?). However, tourism is conceptualised as mainly a preserve for the rich (Bigano *et al.*, 2006; Scheyvens, 2012). It becomes an exercise embarked on by those who have time, money and ability to be away from their known environment in another unknown environment. Here, travellers are exposed to unknown situations but are confined to use the resources they came with without generating anything within the visited area; a situation that Korstanje (2013) believes demands a lot of physical and mental endurance. Thus, disability and tourism appear to be incompatible. However, these perceptions are a gross misunderstanding motivated by lack of appreciation of both disability and tourism concepts by stakeholders. Globally, some national governments have been affected by the belief that disability and tourism are two separate concepts that can never meet. This is evidenced by the absence of policies that promote tourism among disabled people.

Government policy on disability and tourism

According to Mayaka and Prasad (2012, p. 53), policy formulation and implementation is a political process earmarked to attain certain set objectives. Many governments globally, guided by the UN resolutions in the United Nations Decade of Disabled Persons (1983 to 1992), tried to bring disabled people into mainstream lifestyle including in tourism. African countries ratified the United Nations Convention and Rights of Persons with Disabilities, obligating them to abide by the expectations of the convention and its related protocols. By 1992, Africa had achieved minimal inclusion of disabled people's rights in policies, particularly on tourism participation.

However, to underline their commitment to improving life for disabled people, African governments through the African Union launched The African Decade of Persons with Disabilities (1999 to 2009). This was acknowledgement that there was a need to provide for the disabled people in Africa. Despite coming seven years after the expiry of the United Nations Decade of Disabled Persons in 1992, the document is quite instrumental in the advancement of disabled people's rights in Africa. One of its objectives was to:

> [p]romote more efforts that encourage positive attitudes towards children, youth, women and adults with disabilities, and ensure the implementation of measures to ensure their access to rehabilitation, education, training and employment, as well as to cultural and sports activities and access to the physical environment.
>
> *(Chalklen, Swartz & Watermeyer, 2006, p. 5)*

Tourism is implied through culture and sporting activities and access to the physical environment. Thus, it is from this particular objective that access to tourism by disabled people derives. Equal access entails bringing the disabled people on a par with the non-disabled people when it comes to both physical access and access to opportunities. Examples of physical access include hearing aids for the deaf, Braille for the blind, and wheelchairs and ramps for the physically challenged among other accessibility aids.

It is from these general guidelines given in African Union objectives as set out in The African Decade of Persons with Disabilities (1999 to 2009) that most African governments developed their own disability policies. An analysis of national constitutions, disability policies, tourism policies and other related statutory instruments of selected countries in southern Africa highlighted fundamental issues around disability and tourism.

The southern Africa block has many member states whose approach to disability and tourism may vary. Using convenient sampling, four southern African countries (Zambia, Zimbabwe, Botswana and South Africa) were selected for analysis. The focus of analysis was on inclusivity of disabled people in tourism through various statutory instruments such as constitutions, disability policies and tourism policies among other government directives. Each country is addressed independently, however the common threads are that all are SADC members and signatories to the UN resolutions on disabled people.

Disability and tourism in Botswana

The Botswana Constitution became operational in September, 1966. While it covers a lot of vital sections and is more explicit on essential and non-essential aspects for the people of Botswana, there is no reference whatsoever to disabled people. Section 15 on protection from discrimination, subsection 3 states that:

> Discrimination means affording different treatment to different persons, attributable wholly or mainly to the respective descriptions by race, tribe, place of origin, political opinions, colour or creed.
>
> *(p. 15)*

From the given section, which is the only one in the whole Constitution that points at discrimination, disability is not listed. It can be argued that the Botswana Constitution, which is the supreme law, does not directly address disability issues. However, disability was addressed via other statutes and policy documents.

First is the National Policy on Care for People with Disabilities (Republic of Botswana, 2013). This was adopted on 14 February 1996 almost 30 years after adoption of the operating Constitution. From the title to the contents of the policy, emphasis is placed on caring for disabled persons (sections 1, 2 and 3.3). According to the Cambridge Dictionary, care means the process of protecting someone. This implies that someone is vulnerable and cannot protect themselves; people whose situation can only be improved through intervention by second parties. The focus of such care in Botswana is education, health and other social sectors (section 1.2). According to Maslow's (1943) theory of motivation, the needs highlighted by the policy are more of basic needs that everyone is expected to have in a normal environment. One might conclude that Botswana adopted the traditional model of disability where disabled people are considered as recipients of care and sympathy from the non-disabled (Thomson, 1997). This approach is incommensurate with the much advocated social model which takes disability as a social construct not an innate disposition (Darcy, 2002; Pfeiffer, 2001; Oliver, 1996).

Throughout the National Policy on Care for People with Disabilities, there is no mention of how the government, through its various agencies, is going to help disabled people to participate in tourism. There are implied gestures to tourism, but section 1.3 states that a national response 'which engages all sectors of the society meaningfully in the care for people with disabilities is required' (p. 1). The underlining theme here is care. In caring there are two main aspects considered. First, there is the emotional care, as in the burdensome sense of responsibility that people and organisations in Botswana are expected to have in order to serve disabled people. Second, is the physical care where societal sectors are supposed to take action to ensure physical safety and prosperity of disabled people. These sectors include the tourism industry. Such general recommendations do not mandate any organisation to provide for disabled people. Rather, organisations can do what they feel is enough, such as providing just a ramp on a hotel entrance, and claim to be taking care of disabled people. This is just too small an incentive for disabled people since they require many more personalised services (Darcy, 2010).

Section 4.1 states: 'The purpose of the policy is to guide those parties interested in disability issues, in order to involve them in the process effectively' (p. 4). This policy objective gives stakeholders options to be interested in disability issues in order to be involved. The disabled people's welfare is not protected as stakeholders are not obliged under law to provide for them. This is evidenced by lack of any disability requirements when grading hotels in Botswana. In Chapter 42:09 of 1996 – Tourism: Subsidiary Legislation, Index to Subsidiary Legislation (Government of Botswana, 1996), which lists all the requirements for hotel registration, there is no disability requirement for the hotels to be registered. However, in what appears to be an afterthought, there is a sweeping statement on quality indicators that requires accommodation providers to have a parking bay for disabled people. This bay should be unobstructed, clear and specially marked for easy access by disabled people.

The Department of Tourism Regulations for Licencing (Government of Botswana, 1996), only points to disability issues in brief under minimum requirements for all tourist enterprises. It states that a bedside cabinet or table shall be accessible to all adults. More pointers are given under 'Other requirements for accommodation facilities' as follows:

> There shall be a room with facilities for the disabled with ramps and rails. Parking space for the disabled should be clearly marked and near the entrance of the building. Bath tubs and toilets with rails should be provided in the rooms for the disabled.
>
> *(p. 33)*

Many organisations and countries at large still subscribe to the idea that there should be a paraplegic room in hotels instead of making all rooms accessible to disabled people. This is the reason why the above guidelines prescribe that there should be a room for the disabled. Another misconception even at policy level is thinking that disability issues can be dealt with by simply providing a ramp and rail. This presupposes that all disabilities are of a mobility and physical nature. Even when issues of parking are discussed, only mobility-impaired people are considered in most cases.

The Development Control Code of Botswana 2013, a set of regulations for use of land and the activities on it, also marginally addresses disability issues without necessarily specifically referring to tourism. However, the following areas can be applied to tourism:

> Accessible routes: This shall cater for the handicapped [*sic*]. The ends of all raised walkways . . . shall provide ramps that are accessible, and walkways shall provide direct route to primary building entrances.
>
> *(Government of Botswana, 2013, p. 141)*

The deliberate use of handicapped in the code is a direct violation of the rights of disabled people. It is also a manifestation of the traditional or medical model of disability where the individual is to blame for their disability. Also, no consideration is made for those with forms of impairments other than physical. Accessible parking is also addressed in this section where for every 25 public parking spaces, one accessible parking space is required. The parking spaces are expected to be at least three metres wide and adjacent to an aisle which is at least 1.5 metres wide. These requirements, though not specific to tourism, are applicable to the tourism industry. Botswana developed many statutory instruments between 1996 and 2008 to grade hotels but still failed to capture the interests of disabled people.

Section 2.1 of the Final Draft of the 2010 Botswana Tourism Policy (Government of Botswana, 2010) requires that there should be 'accessible environments' for disabled people. Despite not being explicit on which environment, the government gives the impression that tourism should be accessible to everyone, including disabled people. In making a more bold statement, the policy states in section 3.10 (iv) that 'Government shall initiate a campaign that sensitises the sector, to provide disabled friendly facilities'.

The keyword here is sensitising, which from a psychological perspective mean the process of becoming highly sensitive to specific emotional events or situations. The policy position is sensitisation not enforcement. Thus, the tourism sector can determine on their own how much they would want to give to their disabled customers. This implies that some might choose not to do anything for disabled people.

However, the government offered a platform for the development of disability tourism. For example, section 3.7: Training and Education subsection (iv) states: 'the training levy will be used to improve learners with flair in tourism access'. This long-term policy position presupposes that decisions on accessible tourism become more favourable as tourism professionals with disability knowledge become dominant in the tourism industry.

The Botswana Tourism Organisation (2012) also scarcely acknowledged the need to have disabled people's requirements in its annual report for the year ended 31 March 2012. These are reported as recommendations to enhance the hotel grading system as follows:

> Consider how to recognize and encourage universal access to tourism facilities. Universal access encourages provision of facilities that allow easy accessibility for disabled members of the society in using buildings and facilities. e.g. provision of a ramp for wheelchairs, Braille (in elevators) for the visually impaired and provide hearing aids for the hearing impaired.
>
> *(p. 30)*

Recent developments in Botswana, where concerns for disabled people have been transferred from the Ministry of Health to the President's Office are hoped to increase the recognition of disabled people's rights, including tourism. Meanwhile, although some efforts have been put in place by both government and private organisations in trying to improve accessibility for disabled people to tourism, no specific legislation has been enacted to deal with disability issues in a tourism context. It is therefore recommended that the tourism authorities in Botswana extrapolate from the other legal instruments that deal with disability issues and come up with a tourism-specific set of guidelines on disability.

Disability and tourism in Zambia

Disabled Zambians are among the most vulnerable members of society, with limited access to most social utilities as most buildings, including hotels and other facilities, were never built with disabled persons in mind (OSISA, 2011). Disability in Zambia has been a subject of national laws and policies since colonial times under the Rhodesia Federal Government. To protect disabled people, Zambia enacted the Blind Persons Ordinance in 1961 leading to the establishment of the Northern Rhodesia Council for the Blind. This institution, however, focused only on blind persons, leaving out other disabilities.

In 1968 the government enacted the Handicapped Persons Act. This led to the formation of the Zambia Council for the Handicapped, which aimed at incorporating other impairments other than blindness. Handicapped [*sic*], which is meant to imply people with impairments, in this case, focus on physical deformities that hinder equal participation by disabled people. Thus, this Act directly excludes other disabled people such as those without physical deformities. This was followed by the signing of International Labour Organisation Convention 159 on vocational rehabilitation and employment of persons with disabilities in 1983 which sought to increase employment opportunities, establish medical and rehabilitation centres and educational institutions for disabled people in Zambia.

While all these developments empowered the disabled people there were no specific pointers to tourism. However, literature states that economically empowered and educated disabled people tend to travel more as tourists (Silberberg, 1995; Lück, 2015). Thus, Zambia indirectly opened the door for tourism participation by disabled people. Despite opening up tourism to disabled people, there is still a paucity of data on disabled tourists in Zambia.

In 1996, Zambia enacted the Persons with Disabilities Act No. 33 which replaced the Handicapped Act. Its purpose was to eliminate all forms of discrimination on the grounds of having impairments and regulated programmes targeting persons with disabilities. With the Act, the Zambian Council for the Handicapped (ZCH) was replaced by the Zambian Agency for Persons with Disabilities (ZAPD). One major thrust of this agency was the provision of micro-credit to disabled persons through the National Trust Fund for the Disabled. The facility enabled disabled persons to start projects such as selling crafts that were to economically empower them, with the hope that they would be able to sustain their everyday life and also engage in tourism activities.

While efforts are being put in place to include disabled people in mainstream life, the Zambian Federation of Disability Organisations reports that the tourism industry is still lagging behind with regard to accessible tourism. Challenges range from physical access barriers to actual denial of entry to tourism facilities. This clearly highlights that despite various legislative instruments, government efforts are more general and do not meet the expectations for tourism development and/or participation. The government is perhaps regarding tourism as a luxury which it cannot afford to support, a position consistent with evidence from literature (Park *et al.*, 2010).

In its tourism policy, the Zambian government has 14 aims. These include redistributing 'both the opportunities to participate in tourism growth and access to the benefits from it towards Zambians' (Government of Zambia, 2001, p. 43). This aim clearly spells out the need to participate and benefit from tourism. Participation can be as service providers hence business people who benefit from tourism. Here disabled people are catered for through the micro-credit facility from the National Trust Fund for the Disabled. However, on access to benefits such as participation as tourists, this aim seems too blurred to further the rights of disabled people. More emphasis on how disabled people are to gain access to benefits would clarify more fully their ability to influence sustainable development. However, this aim could be used by disabled people to claim their right to tourism. Once Zambians become active tourists, this becomes a base for international disabled tourists to visit Zambia as they become aware of the accessible tourism in Zambia (Ritchie & Crouch, 1993). Finally, the policy also aims 'to promote domestic tourism, leisure and recreation' (p. 4).

Supported by the Disabled Persons Act No. 33 in which the government aims to eliminate discrimination, this tourism policy aim would help disabled people, both domestic and international, to access tourism as tourism resources are reshaped to accommodate disabled tourists. If not satisfied, disabled people in Zambia can use these two government instruments to fight for their right to tourism as domestic tourists.

Just like Botswana, Zambia has come up with a number of pieces of legislation to alleviate the plight of disabled citizens. The concern of this chapter is however still not addressed adequately. There is a need for tourism authorities in Zambia to formulate policies that address disability issues in the tourism context in order to avail tourism opportunities to disabled people.

Disability and tourism in Zimbabwe

Mandipa (2013, p. 73) believes Zimbabwe still has a long way to go in fulfilling the rights of disabled people, as a lot of misconceptions and myths still surrounding disability are hindering disabled people's emancipation. As such, many disabled people are kept hidden from the public for fear of community stigma. Despite these general conditions, some sections of society now view disability differently, with some parents sending their disabled children to school and some companies employing disabled people (Mizunoya & Mitra, 2013).

The Zimbabwean Constitution had not included disabled persons in its non-discriminatory clauses prior to 2005 (Mandipa, 2013). However, following widespread campaigns by the National Disability Board and other disability activists, the Constitution was amended in 2005. The amendment included people with physical impairments in the non-discrimination list. While this was applauded, there was a problem in that the amendment ignored all forms of impairments other than physical. This meant that a person could still be discriminated against if they were intellectually disabled, yet the Convention on the Rights of Persons with Disabilities (CRPD) is concerned with people with all forms of impairments (United Nations, 2006).

On 22 August 2013, Zimbabwe adopted and operationalised a new Constitution, which contained major improvements relating to disabled people. For example, the inherent dignity of disabled people and their equal worth as human beings is specified (Mandipa, 2013). Furthermore, there is clear mention of the rights of disabled people. Unlike in the old Constitution where disability rights were the duty of the Ministry of Health and Child Welfare and the Department of Social Welfare, the new Constitution mandates all government departments and agencies to recognise the rights of disabled people, especially when it comes to being treated with dignity (Mandipa, 2013). The Constitution also acknowledges Sign Language as one of Zimbabwe's official languages (section 6). In section 22 of the Constitution, subsection 4 states that 'the State must take appropriate measures to ensure that buildings and amenities to which the public has access are accessible to persons with disabilities' (p. 21).

This fits well with Article 9 of the CRPD which promotes equal access to the physical environment and transportation and other facilities so as to enable disabled people to live as independently as possible (United Nations, 2006).

The Disabled Persons Act was passed in 1992 and amended in 1996, falling directly under the Ministry of Health and Child Welfare. It provided for the protection of the rights of disabled persons in Zimbabwe. One could, however, argue that the fact that disability issues were placed under the health ministry gives connotations that policy makers believed that disabled people have a health condition and thereby subscribe to the medical model of disability. In section 8, the Act forbids any form of discrimination on the basis of ability or lack thereof:

> 8. (1) No disabled person shall, on the ground of his disability alone, be denied admission into any premises to which members of the public are ordinarily admitted; or . . . provision of any service or amenity ordinarily provided to members of the public, unless such denial is motivated by a genuine concern for the safety of the disabled person concerned.
>
> (2) . . . proprietor of a premises referred to in paragraph (a) of subsection (1) shall not have the right on the ground of a person's disability alone to reserve right of admission to his premises against such a person.
>
> (3) A disabled person who is denied admission into any premises or the provision of any service or amenity in terms of subsection (1) shall be deemed to have suffered an injury and shall have the right to recover damages in any court of competent jurisdiction
>
> *(p. 2)*

The Act also established the National Disability Board to enforce the aforementioned principles. If this board is satisfied that certain facilities are not accessible to disabled persons, it must issue an adjustment order. It is a criminal offence to fail to comply with an adjustment order or to deny disabled people access to premises that admit members of the public. This is indeed a positive step toward emancipating disabled people (Mandipa, 2013). However, the question is: have there been instances where an inaccessible tourist facility (or any other) was issued with an adjustment order to make their facility accessible? In other words, no orders to make facilities accessible have been made.

In Zimbabwe, the Zimbabwe Tourism Authority (ZTA) is mandated to enforce industry requirements as prescribed in the tourism policy. The Zimbabwe Tourism Policy (Government of Botswana, 2010) has very little to say about disability and accessibility issues. Section 5.10 highlights the 'Role of Physically Handicapped [*sic*]' as follows:

> Government will ensure that all the major tourism destinations/products will be provided with the facilities that are user friendly to persons with disabilities. Government will promote the mainstreaming of people with disabilities to participate in mainstream tourism activities for their 'tourists' socio-economic benefits.

The Zimbabwe Tourism Policy gives these two statements on what is to be done for the disabled tourist. The statements appear to be wishful and only time will tell how much of this will be introduced for the benefit of the disabled tourist in Zimbabwe. The statements also sound vague enough to leave room for escape in the event of litigation by aggrieved disabled people in situations where the policy framework is not implemented or only partially implemented.

Due to the briefness of the tourism policy, the ZTA is guided by Statutory Instrument (SI) 128 of 2005 (Grading and Standards Regulations) and Statutory Instrument 106 of 1996 (Declaration and Requirements for Registration). Section 5 of the 3rd schedule of SI 128 of 2005 provides that accommodation facilities should have ramps to enhance access to all areas of the hotel, lodge, motel or any other accommodation facility. It also provides that all hotels with three-star grading and above must have at least two rooms for disabled people while those with two stars and below should have at least one room for disabled persons.

Statutory Instrument (SI) 106 of 1996 provides that, as a requirement for registration, all accommodation facilities should have at least one properly working and well maintained cubicle toilet to cater for disabled people. While these two statutory instruments might seem pro-disability, a closer examination reveals that SI128 of 2005 is only concerned with people with mobility disabilities, specifically wheelchair users. Nothing is said of the other dimensions of disability. SI 106 of 1996 also has simple requirements when it comes to access for disabled persons. It does not specify what the toilet should contain, in contrast to the Scandic accessibility standard which stipulates the position of the toilet seat, the grab bars and toilet paper. At the end of the day, one can conclude that the provisions in the statutory instruments are too general and many establishments can make superficial changes and get away with it. While hotels are kind of mandated to cater for disabled people, other tourism players such as safari operators, among others, are not mandated in any way to cater for disabled tourists.

While Zimbabwe can be applauded for coming up with a tourism policy after many decades of trying, it is worrying to note that disabled people are barely addressed in the document. When reporting tourist statistics, Zimbabwe does not give any information about disabled tourists as a niche market in the same way they group tourists according to source markets. This shows the extent to which disability rights advocates have to work to educate Zimbabweans from grassroots to policy level on the importance of disabled people, not only as citizens but also as tourists.

Disability and tourism in South Africa

The Republic of South Africa has adopted a number of pieces of legislation that directly and indirectly affect disabled people. The Republic of South Africa's premier law, the Constitution of 1996 section 9 provides for equal protection and benefit of the law and the right of all to non-discrimination. In article 9(3), the *State* is mandated not to discriminate against anyone on the basis of race, gender, sex, pregnancy, marital status, ethnic or social origin, colour, sexual orientation, age, *disability*, religion, conscience, belief, culture, language and birth (Republic of South Africa, 1996). This is a vertical application, i.e., the relationship between the State and the individual.

Likewise, section 9(4) pertains to the horizontal application of the right to non-discrimination. It provides that *no person* may unfairly discriminate directly or indirectly against anyone on one or more grounds including race, sex, pregnancy, marital status, ethnic or social origin, colour, sexual orientation, age, *disability*, religion, conscience, belief, culture, language and birth. These are the only two sections that deal directly with disability. However, the Constitution indirectly addresses the rights of disabled people through its Bill of Rights.

The Bill of Rights provides for the rights of all citizens, not specific to disabled people; therefore, one assumes that since disabled people are citizens, they are also equally covered by the Bill of Rights. These rights include human dignity, life, freedom and security of the person, and freedom of trade, occupation and profession as contained in Sections 10, 11, 12 and 22, respectively, among other rights.

It is sad to note that South Africa does not have a comprehensive disability Act that deals with matters directly relating to disabled people (Ngwena, 2013). However, the country has enacted policies and acts of parliament that mention issues to do with disabilities in passing. These include: Employment Equity Act of 1998, Skills Development Act of 1998, Promotion of Equality and Prevention of Unfair Discrimination Act of 2000, Labour Relations Act of 1998, Mental Health Care Act and Library for the Blind Act, to name but a few (Dube, 2005). These Acts and policies seek to achieve some form of equity or equality in the way people are treated at the workplace, in the development of skills and the general and socio-economic welfare of all citizens. The disabled are included.

Another important document is the Disability Charter of South Africa written by disabled people in South Africa. It clearly spells out what they expect from their government. Through this charter, disabled people demand the following: non-discrimination, self-representation, health and rehabilitation, education, employment, sport and recreation, social security, and housing and transport, among other things (Bokone Bophirima Provincial Government, 2014). Although the charter is not a law, it has informed a number of disability related acts and laws.

One of the policy documents that have their roots in the charter is the Universal Accessibility in Tourism Declaration formulated by the South African Government as it moved toward implementation of the CRPD. The document was guided by the provisions of the Promotion of Equity and Prevention of Unfair Discrimination Act, Act 4 of 2000, which prohibits unfair discrimination on the grounds of disability. It was also informed by the White Paper on an Integrated National Disability Strategy, released by the Presidency in November 1997 which recommends that 'Department of Environmental Affairs and Tourism, in consultation with the National Environmental Accessibility Programme and the South African Tourist Organisations must develop national norms and standards as well as monitoring mechanisms to ensure barrier-free access in the tourism industry' (Department of Tourism, 2018).

The tourism stakeholders also consulted in section 2.2 of the UNWTO Global Code of Ethics for Tourism which states that tourism activities should respect the equity of men or women, and more particularly, the individual rights of the most vulnerable groups, notably children, the elderly, disabled people, ethnic minorities and indigenous people (UNWTO, 2005). Among other provisions, the Declaration on Universal Accessibility in Tourism (Department of Tourism, South Africa, n.d.) mandates tourism service providers to:

- Provide the same choices for all consumers to ensure the full participation of disabled persons, the elderly and parents with young children and ensure the protection of individual rights.
- Ensure that disabled persons have equal rights of access to all tourism infrastructure, products and services, including employment opportunities and benefits offered by the tourism industry.
- Introduce universal accessibility as a criterion in the grading of hotels and restaurants.

The declaration mandates government to undertake the following, among other things:

- Ensure that tourism master plans, policies and programmes incorporate the principles of universal access to tourism infrastructure, products and services;
- Ensure that government and state owned enterprises at all levels conduct access audits of key public facilities on a regular basis and use the findings to enhance policy development and effect immediate action. The findings should be made available to the public in accessible formats.

With proper implementation, no tourism and hospitality facility in South Africa would remain inaccessible to disabled people.

Conclusion

This chapter explored policies related to disability and tourism in four southern African countries: Botswana, Zambia, Zimbabwe and South Africa. The main common element within these countries, as in most developing countries, is lack of an implementation and enforcement framework. Without properly laid down policies and pieces of legislation on disability and tourism, there is no implementation to speak of.

Southern African countries must take disability issues more seriously if the desires of disabled people are to be met. It is evident in these countries investigated that they have disjointed instruments to deal with disability and tourism issues. Only South Africa has what looks like a more tourism-specific document (the Declaration on Universal Accessibility in Tourism (Department of Tourism, South Africa, n.d.). In all the tourism policies discussed, little or no mention is made of disability issues and this is a great concern.

However, looking at the various statutes, acts and policy documents developed in these countries since the 1960s there is hope for disabled tourists. Evidence is abundant that organisations guided by national interests in disabled people are altering their services to meet the minimum requirements ideal for disabled clients. Other organisations have heeded the encouragement to do more for this special market and are offering tailored service just for the disabled customers.

Reflective questions

1 To what extent have southern African governments promoted tourism among disabled people?
2 Discuss the importance of policy in the emancipation of disabled people in southern Africa.
3 Which of the four case countries is doing well in protecting the rights of disabled people?
4 Disability does not mean ability. Discuss in relation to tourism participation.

Acknowledgement

The authors would like to acknowledge the work by Oliver Chikuta in his unpublished PhD Thesis: *The development of a universal accessibility framework for National Parks in South Africa and Zimbabwe*; submitted in fulfilment of the requirements for the degree Doctor of Philosophy in Tourism Management at the Potchefstroom Campus of the North-West University. Much of the information on Zimbabwe and South Africa was taken from it with minor adjustments.

References

Aitchison, C. (2003). From leisure and disability to disability leisure: developing data, definitions and discourses. *Disability & Society* **18**(7), 955–969.

Bigano, A., Hamilton, J. M. & Tol, R. S. (2006). The impact of climate on holiday destination choice. *Climatic Change* **76**(3–4), 389–406.

Bokone Bophirima Provincial Government (2014). *Premier Mahumapelo Content with Tourism and Economic Growth*. Retrieved from www.nwpg.gov.za on 23 July 2017.

Botswana Tourism Organisation (2012). *Botswana Tourism Organisation Annual Report*. Retrieved from www.botswanatourism.co.bw/sites/default/files/publication/bto_annual_report_2012.pdf on 15 July 2017.

Buhalis, D. & Darcy, S. (2011). *Accessible Tourism: Concepts and Issues*. Ontario: Channel View Publications.

Candela, G. & Figini, P. (2012). *The Economics of Tourism*. London: Springer.

Chalklen, S., Swartz, L. & Watermeyer, B. (2006). Establishing the secretariat for the African decade of persons with disabilities. In B. Watermeyer, L. Swartz, T. Lorenzo, M. Schneider & M. Priestly (eds) *Disability and Social Change: A South African Agenda* (pp. 93–98). Cape Town: HSRC Press.

Chikuta, O. (2015). Is there room in the inn? Towards incorporating people with disability in tourism planning. *Review of Disability Studies: An International Journal* **11**(3), 57–69.

Darcy, S. (2002). Marginalised participation: physical disability, high support needs and tourism. *Journal of Hospitality and Tourism Management* **9**(1), 61–73.

Darcy, S. (2010). Inherent complexity: disability, accessible tourism and accommodation information preferences. *Tourism Management* **31**(6), 816–826.

Department of Tourism, South Africa (2018). *Tourism to create jobs around the world*. Retrieved from www.tourism.gov.za/AboutNDT/Ministry/News/Pages/Tourism_to_create_jobs_around_the_world.aspx on 16 April 2018.

Department of Tourism, South Africa (n.d.). *Universal Accessibility in Tourism Declaration*. Retrieved from https://tkp.tourism.gov.za/documents/ua%20declaration.pdf on 17 April 2018.

Dube, A. K. (2005). The role and effectiveness of disability legislation in South Africa. *Samaita Consultancy and Programme Design*, 1–89.

Eide, A. H. & Ingstad, B. (2013). Disability and poverty: reflections on research experiences in Africa and beyond. *African Journal of Disability* **2**(1), 1–7.

Fabricius, C., Koch, E., Turner, S. & Magome, H. (2013). *Rights Resources and Rural Development: Community-based Natural Resource Management in Southern Africa*. London: Routledge.

Government of Botswana (1996). *Chapter 42:09 – Tourism: Subsidiary Legislation Index to Subsidiary Legislation*. Retrieved from http://extwprlegs1.fao.org/docs/pdf/bot91750.pdf on 15 July 2017.

Government of Botswana (2010). *Botswana Tourism Organisation Regulations* (Chapter 42:10). Retrieved from www.ecolex.org/details/legislation/botswana-tourism-organisation-regulations-chapter-4210-lex-faoc115294/ on 12 March 2017.

Government of Botswana (2013). *The Development Control Code of Botswana 2013*. Retrieved from www.gov.bw/en/Ministries--Authorities/Ministries/Ministry-of-Lands-and-Housing/About-MOA/Reports-and-Publications/DEVELOPMENT-CONTROL-CODE-OF-2013/ on 16 June 2017.

Government of Zambia (2001). Action programme for the development of Zambia 2001–2010. *Paper presented at the Third United Nations Conference on the Least Developed Countries*, 12–20 May 2001, Brussels, Belgium. Retrieved from unctad.org/en/docs/aconf191cp9zam.en.pdf on 18 June 2018.

Korstanje, M. E. (2013). The darker side of travel: the theory and practice of dark tourism. *International Journal of Contemporary Hospitality Management* **24**(1), 160–162.

Lück, M. (2015). Education on marine mammal tours: but what do tourists want to learn? *Ocean & Coastal Management* **103**, 25–33.

Mandipa, E. (2013). Critical analysis of the legal and institutional frameworks for the realisation of the rights of persons with disabilities in Zimbabwe. *African Disability Rights Yearbook Journal 2013* 1, 73–96.

Maslow, A. H. (1943). A theory of human motivation. *Psychological Review* 50(4), 370.

Mayaka, M. A. & Prasad, H. (2012). Tourism in Kenya: an analysis of strategic issues and challenges. *Tourism Management Perspectives* 1, 48–56.

McKenzie, J., Mji, G. & Gcaza, S. (2014). With or without us? An audit of disability research in the southern African region. *African Journal of Disability* 3(2), 1–6.

Mizunoya, S. & Mitra, S. (2013). Is there a disability gap in employment rates in developing countries? *World Development* 42, 28–43.

M'kumbuzi, V., Myezwa, H. & Desmond, N. (2015a). Adaptation of global frameworks for community based rehabilitation in southern Africa. *Physiotherapy* 101, 1019–1020.

M'kumbuzi, V. R. P., Myezwa, H., Shumba, T. & Namanja, A. (2015b). Disability in southern Africa: insights into its magnitude and nature. In T. Halvorsen, H. Ibsen & V. R. P. M'kumbuzi (eds) *Knowledge for a Sustainable World: A Southern African-Nordic Contribution* (pp. 31–55). Cape Town: African Minds & Southern African-Nordic Centre.

Ngwena, C. (2013). *Western Cape Forum for Intellectual Disability v. Government of the Republic of South Africa*: a case study of contradictions in inclusive education. *African Disability Rights Yearbook* 1, 139–164.

Oliver, M. (1990). *Disability Definitions: The Politics of Meaning – the Politics of Disablement*. London: Springer.

Oliver, M. (1996). *The Social Model in Context: Understanding Disability*. London: Springer.

OSISA (2011). *OSISA in Zambia*. Retrieved from www.osisa.org/banda/osisa-zambia on 19 August 2017.

Park, K. S., Reisinger, Y. & Noh, E. H. (2010). Luxury shopping in tourism. *International Journal of Tourism Research* 12(2), 164–178.

Pegas, F. D. V., Weaver, D. & Castley, G. (2015). Domestic tourism and sustainability in an emerging economy: Brazil's littoral pleasure periphery. *Journal of Sustainable Tourism* 23(5), 748–769.

Pfeiffer, D. (2001). The conceptualization of disability. *Research in Social Science and Disability* 2, 29–52.

Republic of Botswana (2013). *National Policy on Care for People with Disabilities*. Retrieved from http://www.gov.bw/en/PrintingVersion/?printid=2827 on 17 April 2018.

Republic of South Africa (2006). *Constitution of the Republic of South Africa*. Retrieved from www.acts.co.za/constitution-of-the-republic-of-south-africa-act-1996/ on 27 April 2018.

Ritchie, J. R. B. & Crouch, G. (1993). *Competitiveness in International Tourism: A Framework for Understanding and Analysis*. Calgary: World Tourism Education and Research Centre, University of Calgary.

Samaha, A. M. (2007). What good is the social model of disability? *The University of Chicago Law Review* 74(4), 1251–1308.

Scheyvens, R. (2012). *Tourism and Poverty*. London: Routledge.

Silberberg, T. (1995). Cultural tourism and business opportunities for museums and heritage sites. *Tourism Management* 16(5), 361–365.

Snyman, S. L. (2012). The role of tourism employment in poverty reduction and community perceptions of conservation and tourism in southern Africa. *Journal of Sustainable Tourism* 20(3), 395–416.

Thomson, R. G. (1997). *Extraordinary Bodies: Figuring Physical Disability in American Culture and Literature*. New York: Columbia University Press.

United Nations (2006). *Convention on the Rights of Persons with Disabilities*. Retrieved from www.un.org/development/desa/disabilities/convention-on-the-rights-of-persons-with-disabilities.html on 16 August 2017.

UNWTO (2005). *Technical Cooperation Service Report UNWTO*. Madrid: UNWTO.

World Health Organization [WHO] & the World Bank (2011). *World Report on Disability*. Geneva: WHO.

21

STATE AND STATUS OF WHEELCHAIR BASKETBALL FACILITIES IN ZIMBABWE

Bhekuzulu Khumalo, Johan van Heerden
and Thomas Skalko

Introduction

Environmental design is a determinant of social inclusion and people's participation in life roles and activities. Design that does not cater for a diverse range of ages, abilities and cultures restricts people's access to, and use of, domestic or public premises (Watchorn *et al.*, 2014). This is true for sporting facilities as they should be usable by a range of human ages and abilities. According to Watchorn *et al.* (2014) universal design is an approach that acknowledges diversity of populations and encourages designers to create objects and places that are usable by the greatest number of users. Built environments that are usable by all provide opportunities for engagement in meaningful occupations. Watchorn *et al.*'s (2014, p. 65) study identified four themes toward an all-inclusive environmental design: (1) the difficulties of definition; (2) the push or pull of regulations and policy; (3) the role of formal standards; and, (4) shifting the focus of design thinking. These findings highlighted the complexity of working within policy and regulatory contexts when implementing universal design.

A key aim of equitable access and design in sporting and recreation facilities is that everybody is afforded the same opportunities to participate in all aspects of the facilities, programmes and services and has access to products in an equitable, dignified manner (Office of the Attorney General, 2005). Equitable access to all key elements of sport and recreation facilities must be considered to ensure everyone can participate, and designers must also incorporate other considerations such as economic, engineering, cultural, gender and environmental concerns in their design processes. Universal design is the design and composition of an environment so that it can be accessed, understood and used by all people regardless of their age, size, ability or disability (The Center for Universal Design, 1997). The American Disabilities Act (ADA) Compliance Guide (1991) points out that:

> We are all physically disabled at some time in our lives. A child, a person with a broken leg, a parent with a pram, an elderly person, etc. are all disabled in one way or another. Those who remain healthy and able-bodied all their lives are few. As far as the built-up environment is concerned, it is important that it should be barrier-free and adapted to fulfil the needs of all people equally. As a matter of fact, the needs of disabled people coincide with the needs of the majority, and all people are at ease with them. This implies that, planning for the majority implies planning for people with varying abilities and disabilities.

Physical fitness is important for all human beings irrespective of age or physical ability (Gupta *et al.*, 2007). Staying fit and active enables disabled people to maintain an optimal level of independence and control weight gain which can otherwise have an adverse effect on their independence and quality of life. It is imperative that sports and recreational facilities are barrier-free and adapted to the needs of all people, equally. Often, most facilities are inaccessible, leading to a tendency for disabled people, elderly people and those with physically limiting illnesses to be less active due to reduced mobility. Gupta *et al.* (2007, p. 17) argue that inactivity can lead to:

- a decrease in cardio-respiratory fitness;
- osteoporosis;
- an increase in dependence on others;
- a decrease in social interactions;
- increased depression, tension and anger; and
- secondary complications.

Sports and recreation offer the opportunity to build self-confidence and focus on possibilities instead of dwelling on the impairment. According to Gupta *et al.* (2007) competition improves sports skills; it allows individuals to experience the excitement of competition and the thrill of victory as well as the agony of defeat. These experiences help prepare individuals to face impairment-related adversity and to learn to bounce back in the face of any challenges and changes. Sport instils self-discipline, a competitive spirit and comradeship. Its value in promoting health, physical strength, endurance, social integration and psychological wellbeing is of little doubt (Gupta *et al.*, 2007). It is not difficult to understand why sport is so important for the wellbeing of disabled people. Another important aspect of sport are the opportunities it provides for disabled people to establish social contacts.

Basketball is among the oldest and most established of wheelchair sports (International Wheelchair Basketball Federation [IWBF], 2014). Wheelchair basketball is very vigorous and fast moving and helps develop coordination as the players have to propel the wheelchair and learn to pass, catch and intercept the ball (IWBF, 2014). The sport, which is played on a full-size basketball court, was introduced as a rehabilitation and recreational pursuit for people with spinal cord injuries (Gupta *et al.*, 2007). However, fairly rapidly, it became a much more organised and competitive activity, slowly incorporating among players paraplegics, amputees and people with conditions such as spina bifida, brittle bones, cerebral palsy, multiple sclerosis and persons with sensory impairments such as deafness and blindness. According to the IWBF (2014), wheelchair basketball is played by athletes with lower limb impairments and also by those with 'permanent' injuries that prevent them from running or jumping, limiting the ability of playing the running game of basketball. It is one of the highest profile sports at the Paralympics. Twelve men's teams and eight women's teams qualify through regional qualification games.

Gupta *et al.* (2007, p. 52) cite benefits offered by basketball for disabled people:

- It helps in building a team spirit and builds skill and strategy.
- It can be played as a mixed sport with disabled and non-disabled persons in the team, which enhances inclusion.
- It can be played as a competitive activity with opportunities to participate in International sporting events.
- It helps in maintaining muscle tone and general good health.
- It is an activity with low maintenance costs.
- Basketball can be played both in an indoor court and an outdoor court. The courts built are the same as the courts built for non-disabled basketball.

After numerous years of involvement in paralympic sports at various levels, we observed the various obstacles that persons with mobility impairments faced in their quest to participate in the sport of wheelchair basketball. This prompted the study informing this book chapter, which focused on exposing the discrepancy or the lack of adaptation of the basketball facilities for use by persons with mobility impairments.

The universal access concept

The Convention of the Rights of Persons with Disabilities (CRPD) presents Article 9 (United Nations, 2006), which talks about accessibility:

> Making infrastructure accessible requires implementing and respecting standards and guidelines for accessible buildings and facilities, incorporating inclusive design at planning stages, constructing in compliance with standards, training and raising awareness of stakeholders.

In ergonomics, the science of refining the design of products to optimise them for human use, human characteristics such as height, weight and proportions are considered, as well as information on human hearing, sight and temperature preferences. The International Ergonomics Association (2018) describes ergonomics (or human factors) as the scientific discipline concerned with the understanding of the interactions among humans and other elements of a system, and the profession that applies theoretical principles, data and methods to design in order to optimise human well-being and overall system performance. Defined by Ryan (2013), ergonomics is sometimes known as human factors engineering, and it becomes the backbone of universal design. On the other hand, anthropometrics is the study of the human body and its movement, often involving research into measurements relating to people. It also involves collecting statistics or measurements relevant to the human body, called anthropometric data, and further provides a range of 'building blocks' of specific dimensions detailed for people with various needs.

The cost of not incorporating universal design can be significant to individuals and their communities, as stipulated by the Australian Disability Discrimination Act (Office of Parliamentary Counsel, 1992). For example, people who use a wheelchair can face physical barriers, stigma and discrimination in their local communities. Designing community facilities to be accessible provides an opportunity for people to access education, employment and public life (United Nations, 2006). It also means less reliance on others to be able to participate and it helps reduce stigma. Access to public and private transport is a key factor in breaking down barriers (ibid.). Providing access from home to roads, transport stops and between buildings is critical in ensuring increased access to a wide range of services. Inaccessible environments limit economic, education, health and social opportunities for disabled people and make them more dependent on others. The WHO and World Bank (2011, pp. 42–44) further states that it is important to consider the following three components when working with universal design, with each affecting the economic viability of family units and contributing to a vicious cycle of poverty:

- Direct costs for disabled people, including access to services such as travel;
- Indirect costs to support persons and/or family members of disabled people; and
- Opportunity costs of forgone income for disabled people.

The purpose of the universal design principles is to guide the design of environments, products and communications. The principles can be applied to evaluate existing designs, guide the design process and educate both designers and consumers about the characteristics of more usable products and environments.

As indicated in previous chapters, WHO & World Bank (2011) estimate that over a billion people have some form of impairments, with nearly 3.8% of those 15 years and older having significant difficulties in functioning. Furthermore, the rates of impairments are increasing due to wars, natural disasters, accidents, ageing populations and an increase in chronic health conditions. The United Nations Children's Fund (UNICEF), in a Zimbabwe national survey conducted by Eide *et al.* (2003), pointed out that disabled people are often marginalised and belong to the poorest segments of society. The report revealed that there were approximately a quarter of a million disabled people at that time. The Zimbabwe Population Census of 2002, estimated 7%, approximately 914,287 persons, from a total of 13,061,239, had physical impairments.

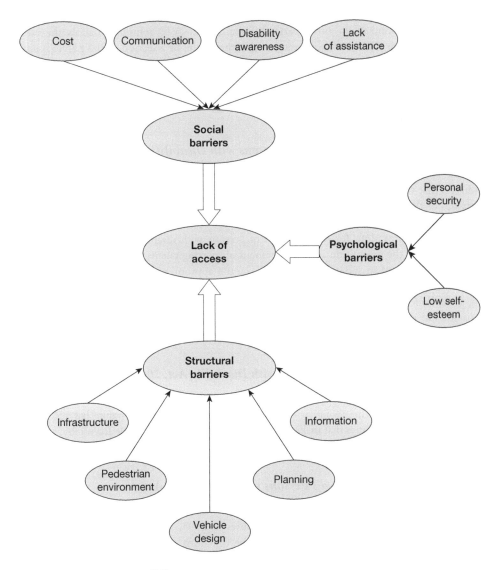

Figure 21.1   Barriers to accessibility

The following examples of country-specific disability legislation were selected on availability from a web search, and we then focused on sections (chapters/divisions) that make specific reference to accessibility to sports, recreation and facilities. It is hoped that the Acts address the barriers to accessibility as illustrated in Figure 21.1.

Australian Disability Discrimination Act

Among the objects of the Australian Disability Discrimination Act are: (a) to eliminate, as far as possible, discrimination against persons on the ground of disability in the areas of: (i) work, accommodation, education, access to premises, clubs and sport; and (ii) the provision of goods, facilities, services and land; and (iii) existing laws; and (iv) the administration of Commonwealth laws and programmes. In division 2 (Section 23) on access to premises it is stated, among other things, that: It is unlawful for a person to discriminate against another person on the ground of the other person's impairment: (a) by refusing to allow the other person access to, or the use of, any premises that the public or a section of the public is entitled or allowed to enter or use (whether for payment or not). Section 28 (sport) states that: (1) It is unlawful for a person to discriminate against another person on the ground of the other person's impairment by excluding that other person from a sporting activity (Office of Parliamentary Counsel, 1992).

India's Rights of Persons with Disabilities Act

Section 30 (Sporting activities) of India's Rights of Persons with Disabilities Act of 2016 indicates that the government shall take measures to ensure effective participation in sporting activities of the persons with disabilities. It also makes it clear that the sports authorities shall accord due recognition to the right of persons with disabilities to participate in sports and shall make due provisions for the inclusion of persons with disabilities in their schemes and programmes for the promotion and development of sporting talents. Without prejudice to the provisions contained in sub-sections (1) and (2), the appropriate government and the sports authorities shall take measures to, (b) redesign and support infrastructure facilities of all sporting activities for persons with disabilities; (c) develop technology to enhance potential, talent, capacity and ability in sporting activities of all persons with disabilities (Ministry of Social Justice & Empowerment, 2016).

Ghana Persons with Disability Act, 2006

Section 6 of the Ghana Persons with Disability Act of 2006 focuses on access to public places. The Act indicates that the owner or occupier of a place to which the public has access shall provide appropriate facilities that make the place accessible to, and available for use by, a person with disability (Government of Ghana, 2006).

Kenya's Persons with Disabilities Act

Kenya enacted an Act of Parliament to provide for the rights and rehabilitation of persons with disabilities to achieve equalisation of opportunities in 2003. Section 7 (1)(b) of the Persons with Disabilities Act of 2003 points out that the functions of the Council shall be, among other things: to formulate and develop measures and policies designed to: (i) achieve equal opportunities for persons with disabilities by ensuring to the maximum extent possible that they obtain education and employment, and participate fully in sporting, recreational and cultural activities and are afforded full access to community and social services. Section 21 (Accessibility and mobility) states that persons with disabilities are entitled to a barrier-free and disability-friendly environment to enable them to have access to buildings, roads and other social amenities, and assistive devices and other equipment to promote their mobility (National Council for Law Reporting, 2003).

Zambia's Persons with Disabilities Act, 1996

Section 6 of Zambia's Persons with Disabilities Act of 1996 mentions one of the functions of the disability agency, which is to: (g) co-operate with ministries and other organisations in the provision of preventive, educational, training, employment and rehabilitation and other welfare services for persons with disabilities. In section 26, the Act refers to the point that, any plans for any premises or amenities approved, after the commencement of the Act, under the Town and Country Planning Act, shall provide facilities that are accessible to persons with disabilities (Republic of Zambia, 1996).

Zimbabwe's Disabled Persons Act

Section 7 of Zimbabwe's Disabled Persons Act (Parliament of Zimbabwe, 1992) indicates that: (1)(a) premises to which members of the public are ordinarily admitted, whether on payment of a fee or otherwise; and services or amenities ordinarily provided to members of the public: including premises owned or services or amenities provided by any statutory corporation or local authority (1(b)) to be accessible. (2) stipulates that where the Board considers that any premises, services or amenities referred to in subsection (1) are inaccessible to disabled persons by reason of any structural, physical, administrative or other impediment to such access, the Board may, subject to this section, serve upon the owner of the premises or the provider of the service or amenity concerned an adjustment order. 1(c) stipulates the period within which the action referred to in paragraph (b) shall be commenced and completed. The challenge however, is non-implementation of such an Act.

Manuals for a barrier-free environment

There are a number of guidelines and standards on accessibility of the built environment and access to information. This section highlights the standards of environmental adaptations as recommended in *Accessibility for the Disabled: A Design Manual for a Barrier Free Environment* produced by the United Nations which recommends universal design standards and is a design guidebook made for the purpose of providing architects and designers with the basic information and data necessary for a barrier-free environment (United Nations Economic and Social Commission for Western Asia [UNSCWA], 2003). The manual is expected to be a stimulus that will lead, in the long run, to the establishment of national building and planning legislation covering access for disabled people. The manual does not cover all the requirements of disabled people in detail, it is simply a straightforward guide expected to be the first in a series of publications having the same theme (UNSCWA, 2003). Practical advice from legal, professional and academic institutions as well as individuals with disabilities is also of the utmost importance in shaping the final form of an accessibility code which can be applied at a national level, as an integral part of the building laws. The manual deals with the technical considerations and design provisions or measures to be taken into account in the planning of the built-up environment. This includes issues related to the design of several complementary domains: open spaces and recreational areas, local roads and pathways, the immediate vicinity of buildings, building entrances and the interiors of buildings (ibid.).

The United Nations manual is meant to provide a basis upon which nations and communities develop accessibility design documents to suit their situation and specific environments and several such documents have been developed around the world, but it is hard to find one such document specific for Africa and/or the developing world. Some countries have gone on to produce documents specific to sports facility designs and access by disabled people. The Americans with Disabilities Act (ADA; United States Department of Labor, 1991), is one such document and it requires new stadiums to be accessible to disabled people so they, their families, and friends can enjoy equal access to entertainment, recreation and leisure.

Aim and significance

The study informing this chapter investigated the levels of adaptation of facilities toward standards for use by people with physical impairments, participating in wheelchair basketball, in selected Zimbabwean cities. Several studies confirm the question of access to the natural and built environment as contemporary the world over (Rimmer *et al.*, 2004; Verschuren *et al.*, 2007; Gray *et al.*, 2008, Buffart *et al.*, 2009, 2010; Chuen & Hui, 2009; Australian Sports Commission, 2010; Hammerschmidt *et al.*, 2011; Roberton *et al.*, 2011; Stanley, Boshoff & Dollman, 2012; Tulloch *et al.*, 2013). However, studies within Africa; particularly Zimbabwe are virtually non-existent. Hence, the need for an audit of wheelchair basketball facilities in Zimbabwe, with the view of informing gatekeepers, planners and users on the state and status of the wheelchair basketball facilities in Zimbabwe.

Methodology

We used a naturalistic approach that sought to understand the phenomena in context-specific settings, where we did not attempt to manipulate the phenomenon of interest. Thus, we inspected the existing indoor wheelchair basketball facilities without any modifications or manipulations. The study targeted those facilities that were in use by wheelchair basketball clubs registered with the Zimbabwe Paralympic Committee (ZPC) by the year 2015. There were 16 such clubs that were drawn from around the country. Five were from Harare, three from Bulawayo and one club each from Victoria Falls, Zvishavane, Gweru, Mutare, Hwange, Masvingo and Beitbridge.

It turned out that only 11 facilities met the inclusion criterion in the visited cities. A Facility Inspection Tool utilised was derived from the *United Nations Accessibility for the Disabled: A Design Manual for a Barrier Free Environment*. The document by the United Nations High Commission for Human Rights is designed to guide and set standards for built environment accessibility by persons with disabling conditions. The manual looks at universal design standards at two levels: (a) urban design considerations (obstructions, signage, street furniture, pathways, curb ramps, pedestrian crossings and parking) and (b) architectural design considerations (ramps, elevators, lifts, stairs, railing and handrails, entrances, vestibules, doors, corridors and rest rooms). The tool was piloted at one high school basketball court within the city of Bulawayo and it reinforced the use of the tool as an effective means to collect information on the accessibility of a given facility.

Recently graduated sports science students, from The National University of Science and Technology (NUST) in Bulawayo, Zimbabwe, were recruited as research assistants. These were trained in the use of the data collection tool. Physical measurements or those derived from construction plans were used to check if the facilities met the recommended basic, standard specifications. The scores used are (+) meets standards, (–) does not meet standards and (o) not available. The data collection period was three months from October to December, 2015. The data were captured using EpiData 3.1, and then posted to SPSS version 16, which was used for analysis. Categorical data are represented using frequency tables.

Participation in this research was by informed consent by the facility owners/managers who had the freedom to choose to participate and withdraw at any stage of the research. All data sheets were coded and presentation is based on the results of statistical analysis so as to conceal participant identity. Ethical approval was granted from the University of KwaZulu-Natal (UKZN) ethics committee.

Results

The results show that all the inspected facilities were single storey and did not have pedestrian crossings, elevators and platform lifts; hence the sections investigating these were excluded in the analysis. Public rest rooms were the best adapted (77.7%), while obstructions, signage, residential rest rooms, pipes and flooring are 51–75% compliant to the universal standards. The other features that are 50% or more adapted toward meeting the recommended standards are non-obstructions, signage, rest rooms, pipes and public rest rooms. Street furniture, public telephones, mail boxes, water fountains, stairs, railings and handrails were the least compliant (0–25%). Features such as street furniture, public phones, mail boxes, water fountains, ramps, stairs, vestibules, corridors, fixtures, faucets, accessories and controls exist in 50% of the facilities and only meet the standards in less than 25% of the inspected wheelchair basketball facilities. Pathways scored 44.39% compliance to standards in terms of being clear of obstructions. Considering being free of steps or stairs, easy to detect, meeting the recommended width of 0.90 metre and having a level surface which is non-slip they meet standards at 81.8%. It was also observed that none of the facilities had automatic doors and only one had an accessible door. There are no accessible indoor parking spaces, as results reflected a 100% non-availability. The results also indicated that there is no enforcement procedure to ensure that accessible parking spaces are not misused or used by non-disabled persons (63.6%). Tables 21.1 and 21.2 provide detailed results.

Table 21.1 summarises the results derived from the facility inspection and the colour coding is explained in Table 21.2.

Discussion, conclusions and recommendations

There is a need to understand the difference between universal design and accessible design, aspects that are likely to lead to misunderstandings by builders and developers and policy makers. Watchorn *et al.* (2014, p. 76) found out that a significant barrier to the implementation of universal design identified by participants was economic pressure, both real and perceived. Many commented that measures aimed at promoting universal design are seen to be more costly, leading to resistance from some quarters. Participants identified a range of socio-cultural trends and changes which have the potential to facilitate the application of universal design. If results of this wheelchair basketball study are used toward improving participation of disabled people in the planning process, then both the concept of universal design and accessible design could be exploited when marketing the need for universal design. A growing awareness of the consequences of exclusion, and its reframing as a human rights issue was also identified as a socio-cultural shift highlighting how essential universal design is to all (Watchorn *et al.*, 2014, p. 76).

Table 21.1 Mean findings and percentage scores for the inspected facilities (N = 11)

Variables	Meets standards		Does not meet standards		Not available	
	$\bar{x}$	%	$\bar{x}$	%	$\bar{x}$	%
1 Obstructions	6.33	57.4	1.33	12.13	3.33	30.33
2 Signage	6	54.55	2.12	19.33	2.87	26.16
3 Street furniture	2.67	24.23	1.5	13.65	6.83	62.12
4 Public telephones	1.8	16.38	2.2	20.02	7	63.6
5 Mailboxes	2	18.2	1	9.1	8	72.7
6 Water fountains	1.5	13.65	2.5	22.75	7	63.6
7 Pathways	5.41	49.21	4	36.38	1.59	14.45
8 Curb ramps	4.56	41.41	1.33	12.13	5.11	46.48
9 Pedestrian crossings	0	0	0	0	11	100
10 Parking	3.47	31.51	2.28	19.39	5.4	49.11
11 Ramps	3.78	34.38	0.78	7.08	6.44	58.54
12 Elevators	0	0	0	0	11	100
13 Platform lifts	0	0	0	0	11	100
14 Stairs	2.14	19.5	1.71	15.6	7.14	64.91
15 Railings and handrails	1.75	15.93	0.25	2.275	9	81.8
16 Entrances	4.75	43.17	1.88	17.06	4.38	39.8
17 Vestibules	4	36.4	0	0	7	63.6
18 Doors	3.64	33.11	2.86	14.29	5.79	52.6
19 Corridors	5	45.33	1.75	15.93	4.25	38.63
20 Public rest rooms	8.5	77.25	0	0	2.5	22.75
21 Residential rest rooms	6	54.55	2	18.2	3	27.3
22 Fixtures	3.33	30.33	1.75	15.93	6	54.53
23 Faucets	4	36.4	0	0	7	63.6
24 Pipes	6	54.5	0	0	5	45.5
25 Accessories and controls	5	45.45	1	9.1	5	45.45
26 Flooring	7.33	66.63	1.33	12.13	2.33	21.23
27 Doors	4.67	42.43	2	18.2	4.33	39.4

Table 21.2 Ranking of compliance to United Nations manual for accessibility of the disabled to a barrier-free environment

Colour code	Percentile range	Meets standards	Does not meet standards	Not available at all
Black	0–25%	9/27	26/27	3/27
Grey	26–50%	12/27	1/27	10/27
Green	51–75%	5/27	0/27	10/27
Yellow	76–100%	1/27	0/27	4/27

Findings from a study by Bringolf (2008) support the view that an association between universal design and the disability paradigm might hinder progress of the application of universal design. A familiar and understandable language was acknowledged to be important to policy development, public perception and academic debate. However, it was also noted to be potentially hazardous to the design of environments that are truly designed for all users and not simply responses to prescriptive accessibility standards (Bringolf, 2011). The variation in terminology is recognised by Steinfeld and Maisel (2012), who argue that while the term is not commonly understood, there is an increasing uptake of design processes which, although not labelled as universal design, better recognise the diversity of abilities within populations and, accordingly, the design of built environments.

There has also been discussion about the value of terms such as universal design and whether industry, educational and other groups should focus more on design that is usable by all or simply talk about good design in general (Moore, 2014). Petrén (2014) prefers to focus on the importance of the implications of universal design on the design process rather than focusing on the preferred terminology. A strong, and potentially negative, connection between the language used when talking about disability and universal design was acknowledged by Bringolf (2008). By acknowledging that an environment should be 'usable by all people, to the greatest possible extent, without the need for adaptation and specialised design' (The Center for Universal Design, 1997, p. 1), specific design elements or features that could be assistive to an individual or specific groups might be discounted (Imrie, 2012). In acknowledgement of this interpretation, Article 2 of the CRPD specifically states that '"universal design" shall not exclude assistive devices for particular groups of persons with disabilities where this is needed' (United Nations, 2006). This was also acknowledged by Bringolf (2008), who identified universal design as a low priority for designers and design schools. Content on universal design may be included as a specific type of design relating to disability and accessibility and not a 'fundamental part of design thinking' Bringolf (2008, p. 47).

Sports England (2010) points out that in facilities such as sports centres and tennis centres, where sports chairs are a key piece of sports equipment for some people and some sports, it is essential that the design of the building and the external works ensures that the sports chairs have unhindered access to all sports activities/facilities. This type of research was driven by the need to provide objective information about the state and status of wheelchair basketball facilities in Zimbabwean cities, toward informing policy on the need for adaptation for use by people with physical impairment. When considering how disabled people will use any part of the facility, it is important to ask the following questions (Sports England, 2010, p. 9):

- How will they find it?
- How will they reach it?
- How will they use it?
- How will they leave the facility?

Contrary to the assumption that attention to the needs of diverse people limits good design, the results of imaginative designers around the world reveal a wide range of applications that delight the senses and lift the human spirit when 'universal design is integral' (Ostroff, 2001). Wheelchair basketball facility inspection revealed that a lot of work needs to be done in the adapting of facilities toward meeting universal design standards, during planning and construction of sporting facilities. Watchorn *et al.* (2014, p. 75) pointed out that many people claim to cater for disabled people and yet there is a need to be more careful because there are various types of impairment-specific needs that should be taken into account. Even with the same type of impairment, it is important to realise that there might be unique individual needs.

Going forward, one would encourage central and local governments to adopt a universal design approach, by ensuring that construction plans clearly show how people with a range of disabilities are to be accommodated in their use of the facility. Colleges and universities offering architectural studies need to include universal design studies in their courses.

Reflective questions

1   How important is the concept of universal design in the provision of sporting facilities for persons with disabilities?
2   Using the United Nations manual for a barrier-free environment, how can your country ensure that it addresses the recreational needs of persons with disabilities?
3   How can the association between universal design and the disability paradigm hinder progress of the application of universal design?

References

Australian Sports Commission (2010). *Participation in Exercise, Recreation and Sport Annual Report*. Retrieved from www.ausport.gov.au/__data/assets/pdf_file/0018/436122/ERASS_Report_2010.PDF on 12 April 2018.
Bringolf, J. (2008). Universal design: is it accessible? *Multi: The RIT Journal of Plurality and Diversity in Design* 1(2), 45–52.
Bringolf, J. (2011). *Barriers to universal design in housing*. Urban Research Centre, College of Health and Science. Retrieved from http://handle.uws.edu.au:8081/1959.7/506910 on 20 July 2017.
Buffart, L. M., Westendorp, T., van den Berg-Emons, R. J. G., Stam, H. J. & Roebroeck, M. E. (2009). Perceived barriers to and facilitators of physical activity in young adults with childhood-onset physical disabilities. *Journal of Rehabilitation Medicine* 41(11), 881–885.
Buffart, L. M., van den Berg-Emons, R. J. G., van Mechelen, W., van Meeteren, J., van der Slot, W., Stam, H. J. & Roebroeck, M. E. (2010). Promoting physical activity in an adolescent and a young adult with physical disabilities. *Disability and Health Journal* 3, 86–92.
Central Statistics Office (2004). *Profile of Persons with Disabilities 2002*. Harare: Central Statistics Office.
Chuen, L. & Hui, S. S. C. (2009). Participation in and adherence to physical activity in people with physical disabilities. *Hong Kong Physiotherapy Journal* 27(1), 30–38.
Eide, A. H. (2013). *Living Conditions among Persons with Disabilities Survey 2013: Key Findings Report*. UNICEF.
Eide, A. H., Nhiwathiwa, S., Muderedzi, J. & Loeb, M. E. (2003). *Living conditions among people with activity limitations in Zimbabwe: a representative regional survey*. Enterprise No. NO 948 007 029 MVA.
Government of Ghana (2006). *Persons with Disability Act 2006, Act 715*. Retrieved from www.gfdgh.org/GHANA%20DISABILITY%20ACT.pdf on 16 March 2016.
Gray, D. B., Hollingsworth, H. H., Stark, S. L. & Morgan, K. A. (2008). A subjective measure of environmental facilitators and barriers to participation for people with mobility limitations. *Disability and Rehabilitation* 30(6), 434–457.
Gupta, S., Sharma, V. & Verma, S. (2007). *A Guidebook on Creating Sporting and Recreational Activities for Persons with Disabilities*. New Delhi: Office of the Chief Commissioner for Persons with Disabilities.
Hammerschmidt, P., Tackett, W., Golzynski, M. & Golzynski, D. (2011). Barriers to and facilitators of healthful eating and physical activity in low-income schools. *Journal of Nutrition Education and Behavior* 43(1), 63–68.
Imrie, R. (2012). Universalism, universal design and equitable access to the built environment. *Disability and Rehabilitation* 34, 873–882.
International Ergonomics Association (2018). *Definition and Domains of Ergonomics*. Retrieved from www.iea.cc/whats/index.html on 16 April 2018.
International Wheelchair Basketball Federation (2014). *Executive Council*. Incheon, Korea: IWBF.
Ministry of Social Justice & Empowerment (2016). *Rights of Persons with Disabilities Act*. Government of India. Retrieved from www.disabilityaffairs.gov.in/upload/uploadfiles/files/RPWD%20ACT%202016.pdf on 16 March 2016.
Moore, P. (2014). A history of UD: today's exemplars and tomorrow's opportunities. *Assistive Technology Research Series* 35, 5–6.
National Council for Law Reporting (2003). *Laws of Kenya: Persons with Disabilities Act*. Retrieved from www.ilo.org/dyn/natlex/docs/ELECTRONIC/69444/115499/F923058%20154/KEN69444%202012.pdf on 16 March 2016.
Office of the Attorney General (2005). *Synopsis of the Irish Disability Act*. Retrieved from www.irishstatutebook.ie/eli/2005/act/14/enacted/en/print on 19 September 2016.

Office of Parliamentary Counsel (1992). *Australian Disability Discrimination Act*. Retrieved from www. legislation.gov.au/Details/C2014C00013 on 23 March 2017.

Ostroff, E. (2001). Universal design: the new paradigm. In Wolfgang F. E. Preiser & Elaine Ostroff (eds) *Universal Design Handbook* (1st edn; pp. 1–12). New York: McGraw-Hill.

Parliament of Zimbabwe (1992). *Disabled Persons Act, Chapter 17:01, Acts 5/1992, 6/2000, 22/2001*. Retrieved from www.parlzim.gov.zw/acts-list/disabled-persons-act-17-01 on 17 September 2016.

Petrén, F. (2014). Turning societal challenges into creative opportunities. *Assistive Technology Research Series* **35**, 11–12.

Republic of Zambia (1996). *Persons with Disabilities Act*. Retrieved from www.parliament.gov.zm/sites/default/files/documents/acts/Persons%20With%20Disabilities%20Act.pdf on 16 March 2016.

Rimmer, J. H., Riley, B., Wang, E., Rauworth, A. & Jurkowski, J. (2004). Physical activity participation among persons with disabilities: barriers and facilitators. *American Journal of Preventive Medicine* **26**(5), 419–425.

Roberton, T., Bucks, R. S., Skinner, T. C., Allison, G. T. & Dunlop, S. A. (2011). Barriers to physical activity in individuals with spinal cord injury: a Western Australian study. *Australian Journal of Rehabilitation Counselling* **17**(2), 74–88.

Ryan, J., Hensey, O., McLoughlin, B., Lyons, A. & Gormley, J. (2013). Reduced moderate-to-vigorous physical activity and increased sedentary behavior are associated with elevated blood pressure values in children with cerebral palsy. *Physical Therapy* **94**(8), 1144–1153.

Sports England (2010). *Accessible Sports Facilities*. Retrieved from www.sportengland.org/media/4508/accessible-sports-facilities-2010.pdf on 15 August 2016.

Stanley, R. M., Boshoff, K. & Dollman, J. (2012). Voices in the playground: a qualitative exploration of the barriers and facilitators of lunchtime play. *Journal of Science and Medicine in Sport* **15**, 44–51.

Steinfeld, E. & Maisel, J. L. (2012). *Universal Design: Creating Inclusive Environments*. New Jersey: John Wiley & Sons Inc.

The Center for Universal Design (1997). *The Principles of Universal Design (Version 2.0)*. NC State University, Author. Retrieved from https://projects.ncsu.edu/ncsu/design/cud/pubs_p/docs/udffile/chap_3.pdf on 10 September 2017.

Tulloch, H., Sweet, S. N., Fortier, M., Capstick, G., Kenny, P. & Sigal, R. J. (2013). Exercise facilitators and barriers from adoption to maintenance in the diabetes aerobic and resistance exercise trial. *Canadian Journal of Diabetes* **37**, 367–374.

United Nations (2006). *Convention on the Rights of Persons with Disabilities*. Retrieved from www.un.org/development/desa/disabilities/convention-on-the-rights-of-persons-with-disabilities.html on 20 January 2014.

United Nations Economic and Social Commission for Western Asia (2003). *Accessibility for the Disabled: A Design Manual for a Barrier Free Environment*. Retrieved from http://static.un.org/esa/socdev/enable/designm/index.html on 12 January 2016.

United States Department of Labor (1991). *The Americans with Disabilities Act (ADA) Compliance Guide*. Retrieved from www.dol.gov/general/topic/disability/ada on 15 June 2012.

Verschuren, O., Ketelaar, M., Gorter, J. W., Helders, P. J., Uiterwaal, C. S. & Takken, T. (2007). Exercise training program in children and adolescents with cerebral palsy: a randomized controlled trial. *Archives of Physical Medicine and Rehabilitation* **161**, 1075–1081.

Watchorn, V., Larkin, H., Hitch, D. & Ang, S. (2014). Promoting participation through the universal design of built environments: making it happen. *Journal of Social Inclusion* **5**(2), 65–88.

World Health Organization & World Bank (2011). *World Report on Disability*. Geneva: WHO.

22

MOBILE OUTREACH SEATING CLINICS

Improving access to wheelchair and support services

Margaret Linegar, Megan Giljam, Shona McDonald and Ronique Walters

Introduction

This chapter shares lessons learned during Shonaquip's 25 years of service to improve the lives of children with mobility impairments in South Africa. Shonaquip was established in 1992 to provide well-fitted, environmentally appropriate wheelchairs for children with mobility impairments, specifically children with complex posture-support needs. This reflection by Shonaquip, illustrates the application of our outreach model in three different contexts. Shonaquip's model has evolved through feedback given by people with disabilities, service providers, community members and partners in the disability sector. Unfortunately, a focus on these perspectives of Shonaquip outreach, while valued, is beyond the scope of this chapter. With potential to be delivered flexibly, we believe lessons shared from Shonaquip's model of outreach services can guide service provision in less-resourced areas.

Shonaquip concurs with the World Health Organization (WHO & UNICEF, 2015) that when children with disabilities are given the same opportunities to flourish as any other children, they too have the potential to lead fulfilling lives. Thus, they can contribute to the social, cultural and economic community activities. Shonaquip addresses medical barriers to access and its main role is to ensure that children with mobility impairments have access to a range of appropriate mobility assistive technology, clinical and technical support services. These can prevent secondary health complications, improve physical function and equip children to benefit from inclusion in everyday activities at home and in broader society. Shonaquip has always prioritised the equalisation of opportunities and the social inclusion of people with disabilities. Through participation in networks of service providers across the different sectors, Shonaquip promotes the reduction of systems barriers and cost effective access to services. Shonaquip adheres to the seating practice of the Guidelines for the Provision of Manual Wheelchairs in less-resourced settings, which sets international standards for wheelchair service provision (WHO, 2008). Such steps typically include referral and appointment, assessment, prescription, funding and ordering, product preparation, fitting, user training and follow-up, maintenance and repairs (ibid.). Shonaquip forms a hybrid social enterprise with Uhambo, which was established in 2010. Uhambo's aim is to raise awareness of the need for early intervention for children with mobility impairments and to fund Shonaquip's community-based work. More specifically, it addresses community barriers to access and ensures that children with mobility impairments, their parents, families, caregivers and communities are empowered and receive the quality information, resources and holistic support needed for their social inclusion. Thus, Uhambo delivers programmes to support individuals, parents, caregivers, early childhood development (ECD) and Day Care Centres, schools and partner organisations.

These reflections focus on Shonaquip's mobile outreach seating service, which provides devices and services to children affected by mobility impairment. Assistive technology (an umbrella term that includes both assistive devices and related services) is recognised as a vital tool to enable rights, dignity and equal opportunities for children with disabilities (WHO & UNICEF, 2015). Assistive technology includes devices for mobility and posture support. Experienced seating practitioners agree that appropriate postural support across the lifespan is key to reducing the burden of care and improving a person's mobility, function and participation. Access to both assistive technology and a range of clinical, technical and support services, is needed for children with mobility impairment to thrive. Together, these promote health, development and participation and open up the world of education, play and socialisation, affording children the opportunity to become valued, contributing individuals (WHO, 2008).

Challenges of access to wheelchair services

The inequalities in client access to health services, including wheelchair services, especially in rural areas across South Africa have been increasingly explored in literature in recent years (Booyens et al., 2015; Schoevers & Jenkins, 2015; Sherry, 2015; Visagie, Scheffler & Schneider, 2013; Mji et al., 2017; Bateman, 2012; Grut et al., 2012). Access to service is constrained by many complex, interrelated variables, not least of which is poverty, which remains rampant in South Africa, denying universal equitable access to healthcare for many (Grut et al., 2012). Rural areas account for almost half of South Africa's population, yet remain the most underserved and marginalised areas in the country. South Africa's Framework and Strategy on Disability and Rehabilitation 2015–2020 highlights the vulnerable position of the poor in rural areas in terms of access to health services. Sherry (2015) established that where poverty and disability intersect, people with disabilities are more prone to multiple health-related risks. Vergunst, MacLachlan and Mannan (2015) noted that there is 'triple vulnerability' resulting from the intersecting of rurality, poverty and disability. Hannas-Hancock and Deghage (2016) reported that families raising children with severe impairments in South Africa are especially vulnerable to poverty, with household income typically only 77% that of comparable families. The cost of purchasing, maintaining and replacing assistive technology, the need for 'round the clock' supervision and care, special transport, the experience of exclusionary community attitudes and practice, increase both out-of-pocket costs and vulnerability of affected households. Bad health outcomes and increasing disability from limited access to health services may incur additional costs to the family should personal assistance or specialised transport become necessary. Barriers to access in urban areas for wheelchair users typically include uneven terrain, transport unaffordability, unreliability and inaccessibility and reluctance of taxi drivers to transport people in wheelchairs. Wheelchair users are especially vulnerable to violence, and during inclement weather or in emergency situations. Rural barriers include hilly terrain, rivers, forests, poor road infrastructure, free running animals and grass-thatched rondavels scattered sporadically across rural areas (Mji et al., 2017). Long waiting times for services, poor drug supply and lack of appropriate referral sometimes result in wasted and repeat visits, illustrating further healthcare process barriers (Sherry, 2015). Long distances to services might lead to dependency on employers for transport or require the need to stay overnight to access services.

The Standardization of Provision of Assistive Devices regulates service provision including that of wheelchair services in South Africa (National Department of Health, 2003). Although access to basic wheelchair services has improved in the past two decades, there are still lengthy delays in accessing the right technologies. The distances travelled to access services cause inevitable delays in the supply of wheelchairs (Visagie *et al.*, 2013). Children with complex needs living in remote areas might have limited access to the necessary level of seating service expertise and are at high risk of developing secondary consequences such as skeletal deformity, pressure sores and lung disorders. Findings from a Northern Cape study revealed the gap between policy and service delivery in rural wheelchair service delivery and in management systems (Visagie *et al.*, 2013). Nearly all WHO-recommended steps of service delivery were reported to be incomplete in implementation. Trained and experienced staff were scarce, distances of local service sites from procurement and maintenance services were vast (as far as 800 kilometres away). In addition, user training, product preparation, fitting and regular reviews/maintenance were found to be superficially executed, compromising safety and well-being of wheelchair users.

Reducing structural and healthcare process barriers is fundamental to improving access. The Framework and Strategy on Disability and Rehabilitation (FSDR) 2015–2020 promotes coordinated action from role players across health, education and social development to disrupt the cycle of poverty and disability to support people with disabilities living productive lives. It also proposes measures to enable services at different levels, preferably at the closest point to where people live (National Department of Health, 2016). More disability awareness workshops, mobile health centres and better collaboration between government, health providers and communities are proposed if we are to move forward (Vergunst, 2016). In a study from the Amathole municipality in the Eastern Cape, Grut *et al.* (2012) urges health strategists to include skilled health professionals in outreach and home-based services to bring health services to people with disabilities and at the same time build capacity of the local healthcare workers. The shortage of skilled staff in remote areas for assistive technology services is one reason WHO promotes this same dual strategy (WHO, 2011).

Outreach services

Outreach services mobilise health workers to provide services to the population or to other health workers, away from the location where they usually work and live. These can be organised through hospitals, private companies, NGOs, local or national authorities. However, they are under-reported in the literature, even in countries where they have been implemented as part of regular activities. Many activities are supported by charitable organisations responding to the demand for access to care from underserved populations (De Roodenbeke *et al.*, 2011).

According to Sherry (2015), the provision of outreach services close to home could go a long way toward secondary prevention of impairments and, in particular, reducing transport costs of healthcare access. This right is entrenched in the United Nations Convention on the Rights of Persons with Disabilities (CRPD), which South Africa has ratified and is making efforts to domesticate through enabling legislation. Sherry (2015) urges the health system in South Africa to respond to the needs of all by including the integration of skilled and appropriate rehabilitation at primary healthcare level.

Shonaquip outreach begins

Shonaquip was founded as a result of the personal experience of the founder, Shona, whose daughter, Shelly, was born with cerebral palsy, a life-long condition requiring high levels of care. Shona soon became aware that Shelly required special equipment to sit upright and move around. Shona drew on her background as a sculptor, and together with the Biomedical Engineering Department of the University of Cape Town, created Shelly's first postural support device. Before long, she became mobile using a customised motorised wheelchair. Although this 'gave Shelly wings', Shona envisaged more for Shelly, wanting her to become part of a much wider community. In seeking this, the family experienced first-hand the systemic barriers faced by people with mobility impairments. Shelly's positive experience at her first inclusive pre-school cemented the family's commitment to inclusion. As Shona walked alongside many families on a similar journey, the benefits of standing together motivated them to start awareness-raising to uphold their children's rights. They began talking to service providers and helping to shape policy affecting the lives of their children.

Parents started to bring their children to Shona's home garage, one of Shelly's carers and a technician (a wheelchair user) and Shona helped design customised devices. Shona began to share her growing expertise with service providers in healthcare institutions. It became clear that for many children, the basic folding frame wheelchair was inappropriate. Hence, fundraising for specialised equipment and services for these children became a priority. Shonaquip staff recall how the lounge became transformed into a rudimentary seating clinic, with children lining the pavement outside as they waited to be seen. Small busloads arrived from special needs schools and care centres, some from as far away as Elim (south of Cape Town), a three-hour drive away. Children, accompanied by their carers and devices were loaded onto the bus and returned home in the evening.

During these years, provision of appropriate wheelchairs was still in its infancy although the Disability Rights Movement was gaining momentum in this area. There were few accepted standards of service provision and no tenders offering the range of options available in South Africa today. Standard folding frame wheelchairs were typically prescribed through state departments following a few key assessments and measurements. Reviews were costly for families, resulting in irregular follow-ups. Poor awareness of the specialised posture-support needs of children often resulted in children acquiring secondary impairments. The possibility of a life beyond the home was lost for those with severe impairments who had no access to special schools. Instead, many were largely immobile in cots and on floors, often excluded from social contact and stimulation. Some were purposefully hidden from the public eye, and locked away in back rooms to avoid attracting the stigmatising attitudes of their community.

Centre staff sometimes used wheelchairs interchangeably between children as they struggled to supply enough of them. Some children were left slumped in their wheelchairs, propped up with blankets, belts or with pillows, battling to keep their heads upright or feet securely in place on footplates. Others faced risks of having secondary impairments from using donor wheelchairs, which although well intended, were sometimes oversized, poorly maintained or unsuited to their complex posture-support needs.

Formalising of Shonaquip outreach services

With growing experience in seating, Shonaquip began to assist therapists to seat children with more complex posture-support needs, as well as trialling emerging rural and off-road devices. These experiences informed early device designs such as the *Madiba*, a robust, easily adaptable buggy geared for children who cannot sit upright without extra support and are unable to propel independently. As demand for the buggies grew, they were sent further afield. Building the capacity of people to use them effectively became a growing priority. During this time, many carers from centres continued bringing children to Shona's home for services, which left too few carers to manage the load of those staying behind. This motivated Shonaquip's earliest mobile outreach clinics. Shonaquip staff had to load spares and devices into the van, as they ventured out on these pioneering trips. This small team did assessments, measurements, fittings, technical adjustments and carer training in how best to use devices.

Working long days, they started to see the difference this made in the lives of these children and their carers. So Shona began approaching donors to fund both devices and outreach programmes, which up until then had had little dedicated funding. Consequently, many children continued using the same devices over many years, despite them being ill-fitting or unsafe. One team member recounts being on her knees in tears seeing children with severe impairments without devices lying on the floor, their bodies crooked and fixed in one position, alone and deprived of change in daily routine. Even children fortunate enough to have their own devices, sometimes spent long hours in them, rendering the child at risk of increasing deformities and discomfort. The inclusion of the *Madiba* buggy on the national tender gave Shonaquip the opportunity needed to influence the state in order to expand the outreach.

Shonaquip currently provides outreach services across many southern African countries. Sites for outreach services are selected dependent on needs identified through Uhambo or our extensive network of government and private service providers, clients and funding partners.

Three case studies are shared to demonstrate how Shonaquip has integrated access to seating into each of these different contexts:

- a public–private partnership of regular outreach mobile seating clinics;
- a short-term seating intervention embedded in a disability training programme in the community;
- a phased centre-based outreach supported by external funding.

Experience in different contexts has informed the development of the current holistic model of service delivery, which guides the planning of Shonaquip outreach services. Each context may require the model to be used in a flexible way to the benefit of the specific beneficiaries.

Shonaquip's current outreach service in the Overberg, Western Cape has developed over 20 years. The earliest visits done in the Overberg had been confined to the Caledon hospital and Elim home. Having seen the benefits of the very early outreach activity, Shonaquip entered into a public–private partnership for a number of years to expand state-funded mobile outreach clinics for the Western Cape Department of Health at district level hospitals, schools and day care centres across South-West Cape. Clinic sites were identified based on needs, funding and compliance and included sites in the Overberg. The outreach team included two seating practitioners and a technician who worked with the specialised Rehabilitation Centre and a key 'host' coordinator with responsibilities split in terms of a Service Level Agreement. Client and device reviews formed the major focus of clinics. Partnership with Sister Meyer enabled services to expand in this region. As a trained orthopedic aftercare sister responsible for mobility services in the Overberg, Sister Meyer had witnessed many barriers facing wheelchair users living in villages and on farms, far removed from specialist services. As such, she has become a key ally supporting mobile outreach clinics. All input from outreach aimed to support the local service providers to manage complex postural issues where standard folding frame wheelchairs fail to meet the child's needs. Trained Shonaquip seating practitioners have comprehensive knowledge of our devices and advocate for the most appropriate devices within the constraints of available budgets or tenders. Over years, the team has seen increased awareness of seating in the community, reduced waiting times for devices and improved continuity of care at grassroots level, which served as motivation to expand services in the Overberg district when the state-funded mobile clinics came to an end due to restructuring in the Department of Health. Sister Meyer, as Western Cape Government Clinical Programme Coordinator for Rehabilitation Services, continued to lobby for a special budget to address her growing long-distance travel concerns of clients for services. Shonaquip responded with a proposal for the development of central seating hubs to provide devices supported by clinical, technical and administrative skills and services to support local staff in their seating, and referral of clients to other services and partners in the outlying communities.

After a successful tender process in 2014, clearly defined responsibilities were allocated between Shonaquip and local 'hosts' for the Overberg clinics. Sister Meyer oversees the outreach programme with clinic sites located as close as possible to where clients live in more densely populated areas, linked to local state hospitals or community clinics. Shonaquip's responsibilities include 'hands-on' clinical mentoring and skills transfer for therapists and technical staff. Services include client assessment, prescription, modification, fitting, client reviews, device maintenance and repair of all assistive devices used for high-risk client groups.

Outreach sites are all approximately a few hours' drive from Cape Town and include Theewaterskloof (Grabouw/Villiersdorp and Caledon); the Overstrand (Hermanus); Swellendam and Cape Agulhas at the southernmost tip of Africa (Bredasdorp/Elim). Clinic venues include children's homes, primary healthcare facilities and rehabilitation outpatient departments linked to state hospitals. Healthnet transport ('Whiskies') carry two or three clients at a time (with carers and devices) to the clinic. The two allocated VW caddies can each accommodate a wheelchair locked in position. One specific driver, with aptitude for handling people with mobility impairments is responsible for most of the clinic transport. His greatest asset is his local knowledge and in-depth understanding of addressing the needs of children and carers he transports. Clinics take place at three-monthly intervals, each accommodating 15 booked clients for the seven-hour clinic. Clients are identified by the district rehabilitation team and Shonaquip helps to track down those needing review, as well as those unconnected to state services or falling between the cracks due to medical aid shortfalls. Each host clinic includes at least two local therapists and one handyman, who take administrative, financial and clinical responsibility for the clinic. They arrange transport, provide the venue, tools for handyman, equipment and spares. Children now seldom have to wait more than four to six months to receive their devices. Team decisions are made on allocation of the most appropriate device from available stock or budget. The local therapist orders devices or parts and keeps records of needs beyond the allocated annual budget and the district looks for funding to address this. This accurate electronic recordkeeping ensures that these needs can be addressed through top-up funding. Additionally, the Shonaquip team issues a summary report following each clinic. Less experienced therapists in remote areas respond well to 'hands-on' mentoring, which helps to build both competences and confidence in seating. Case study 22.1 presents a story of a typical client who has been followed up in this district for almost 20 years.

Case study 22.1   Pieter's story

Pieter* first came to one of the Overberg clinics at around five years old, carried by his mother and a helper from the farm where his family lived. Born with cerebral palsy, Pieter was unable to stand or keep his head and body in an upright position while sitting, neither could he use his hands meaningfully, but from very early he showed he could talk a lot. Mary-Ann, one of the Shonaquip team,

(continued)

(continued)

remembers training Pieter's mother during outreach and now sees his sister who has taken over his care on the farm. Although he battles ongoing stiffness, with one leg shorter than the other, he has always been able to sit and move comfortably, first in a *Madiba* buggy, then in a series of manual wheelchairs, using a customised cushion and footrest supported by special back support and a pelvic strap. Although he has never attended formal schooling, he enjoys an active life in his community and manages his social grant independently. In the past Pieter often used to pay friends to push him out with them, they even once became lost in the mountains and had to stay out overnight! His devices have needed attention by our technician and replacement every few months during his growing years, testimony to his changing needs and active lifestyle. Transported by local Healthnet vehicles, he never misses his review, which is important to prevent further physical deterioration. Pieter was recently prescribed his first motorised Shonaquip Vic wheelchair, giving him greater independence, saving him paying out grant money to friends, and opening up a world of social opportunity. Known for his energetic spirit and sense of fun, he is able to express and share his love of life with all around him, including our team who have become like old friends or family to him. We plan to continue to oversee his seating and accommodate his changing needs to ensure he maintains his active lifestyle. How differently his life may have unfolded without access to regular wheelchair services and the support extended to him consistently over the years.

*not his real name

Role of repair services to the Overberg outreach

The ability to screen devices, do basic device repairs, and understand when a specialised service provider should be consulted are important in any outreach programme. There is currently a trained handyman at Caledon and three wheelchair users there who have been upskilled and who attend their local seating clinic to build their repair skills. They are taught how to change wheelchair tyres or bearings, adjust brakes, lap belts and brackets or replace upholstery, foam, Velcro or rubber. Some have also received further training at a specialist repair workshop at Western Cape Rehabilitation Centre in Cape Town. Case study 22.2 shows how outreach repair services can impact a typical wheelchair user in the Overberg.

Case study 22.2   Oom Japie's story

A request from 'Oom' (Uncle) Japie about his faulty wheelchair used to mean a long drive from the Caledon base (nearly two hours away) to fetch his device, and another drive to Brewelskloof workshop in Worcester (one hour away) a month later when next visiting clients in the area. It would take six to eight weeks for the wheelchair to be repaired and sent back to Caledon and then sent to its owner in Barrydale, who all the time had been struggling to manage without a replacement wheelchair. When Sister Meyer was next in Barrydale some two months later, Oom Japie would finally get his wheelchair back. This fell far short in upholding the rights of wheelchair users to dependable mobility. It is a different story now; the resident therapist responsible for Barrydale, fetches the wheelchair, has it repaired at the local workshop and has it back with its owner within a week.

Embedding seating outreach in community-based programmes

This case study describes how services have begun to be integrated within Uhambo's ECD programmes in children's centres. While some assume that the quality of life improves once a child is seated in an appropriate device, the reality observed is that many children with high posture-support needs remain excluded from learning opportunities. The important effect of appropriate positioning of children with disabilities to enable them to participate more meaningfully, however, cannot be underestimated. Witnessing first-hand how children benefit from different positioning options during activities while, at the same time, relieving caregiver burden, bears testimony to this. Outreach to Eden district (Western Cape) demonstrates how merging even a single intervention of positioning/seating into an externally funded capacity-building programme (in this case, a Uhambo programme) can build awareness of how this can optimise children's participation.

Uhambo's first 2015 visit to the Eden District, introduced carers to the *Ndinogona* (I am capable) kit and structured stimulation programme, which trains carers to promote the development and learning of children with disabilities within an inclusive setting. Utilising children's abilities is key, as is appropriate positioning and simple accommodations to enable participation. Uhambo recognised that a more dedicated focus on positioning options was needed; hence it expanded the team for the five-day follow-up in 2016 to include a seating therapist and a technician. During the visit, Shonaquip checked the set-up of each child's device, identified any repair or modification needs, and also connected with local seating therapists where necessary.

George, Oudtshoorn and Beaufort West (approximately six hours' drive east from Cape Town) were included in this outreach as well as Murraysburg, a smaller, more remote town. In Oudtshoorn, Uhambo began by facilitating their 'Let's Talk Disability' dialogue in which members of the community, parents and peer supporters engaged with social service providers to talk about disability-appropriate interaction and inclusion. Each participant is encouraged to take steps to tackle local barriers in their communities. The team also visited Sonskyn Day Centre, an independent pre-primary school for ECD, which has access to appropriate wheelchairs and positioning devices. While the Uhambo team focused on care, play development and learning for carers, the Shonaquip team targeted positioning routines and devices (such as standing frames, side positioners and vehicle transporters), handling techniques and mobility devices. Seating reviews with local therapists were done at the hospital, assisting them with complex prescription options, and ordering from the tender. *Ndinogona* parents, foster mothers and carers enjoyed supervised practice on how best to position the children to participate during the programme. Following this intervention, a local caregiver has considered the option of qualifying as a teacher for children with disabilities. Partnerships with community-based or child-focused organisations like Association for Persons with Disabilities (APD), Autism Western Cape and Inclusive Education offer potential to embed a greater awareness of seating and positioning into all programmes involving children with mobility impairments.

Centre-based phased outreach in rural Peddie

This case study describes a more comprehensive, holistic, phased intervention using funds derived from different sources. In this case, one funder provided devices, while another supported the capacity building of local stakeholders over four outreach visits. Shonaquip and Uhambo provided outreach services to Nomzamo Centre in Peddie between 2014 and 2016. Peddie is in the Amathole District Municipality (Eastern Cape, South Africa), a two-hour drive east of Port Elizabeth. Nomzamo is very remotely sited, more than 50 kilometres from both

Grahamstown and King William's Town, the nearest large cities. Gravel roads or narrow foot-paths link clusters of small huts dotted across hilly farmlands. Unfortunately, there are no other facilities or schools close to the centre, a harsh reality given that perhaps as many as a quarter of the children could potentially benefit from inclusive schooling.

The Cerebral Palsy Association (CPA) in Port Elizabeth introduced Shonaquip to the centre, which was founded in 1994 as a residential centre for children with disabilities. There are currently over 100 children, ranging from toddlers to young adults with intellectual impairment. Some residents go home during holidays but many live permanently at Nomzamo, having been found neglected, abused or abandoned. As a community-based non-profit institution, Nomzamo aims to cater for children with disabilities from farms in this remote region. Centre Manager, Lizzie, knows each child's circumstances and strives to ensure that each member of staff (irrespective of their role in the centre) is equipped to work with children with disabilities. Demand for a place at the centre has grown over recent years, since its impact has become more visible in the community. Some children receive general therapy at the neighbouring Nompumelelo hospital, but this does not extend to dedicated wheelchair services.

During the first two-day visit in November 2014, the team (including three staff from CPA) arrived to find well cared for children in a clean, spacious, wheelchair-accessible centre. Staff remember feeling shock at the numbers of children lying criss-crossed on the beds, which had been pushed together to form giant cots. A few children were unable to sit in a wheelchair at all due to the severity of their deformities and those who were more mobile could be seen crawling among the others. Children of similar age/ability were placed together in dorms, with older boys and girls in separate dorms. A separate room was allocated for those with severe cerebral palsy. Staff noticed a few oversized wheelchairs being used to transport children to and from a classroom (huts). This presents a real challenge on wet days in muddy conditions. Staff tried hard to stimulate children's learning with the few resources available to them. However, the more severely disabled children remained in a lying position, ill-equipped to draw real benefit from meaningful participation and stimulation. Two seating practitioners accompanied by the CPA therapists screened 50 children with mobility impairments. Only eight children were using a mobility device, of which only two were 'appropriate' for the child's needs. Lizzie and the therapist from the neighbouring state hospital did assessments, hand stimulation and measurements with the assistance of all centre staff. Often, when budgets are stretched, basic folding frame wheelchairs seem the best way to provide for large numbers of children. However, this can be risky to children with complex posture-support needs. Shonaquip problem-solved with local staff to make the most appropriate prescription based on each child's needs. Some positioning devices were ordered for more general use at the care centre. CPA therapists also helped staff group children according to abilities to optimise the benefit from the *Ndinogona* stimulation programme that was introduced to the 18 carers.

During the second five-day visit (six months later), seating practitioners were joined by a technician to fit the new devices. Fitting can be time-consuming when needs are complex and, for some children, seating had seemed impossible. As each child emerged in a new device, he/she was cheered on by the enthusiastic carers, their faces glowing as they greeted those now able to sit upright in their new device for the first time. Carers enjoyed the ease with which they could now transport children around the centre and grounds.

During the third visit three months later, each child and the device were reviewed. It is recommended practice that growing children be reviewed regularly because they might need more frequent adjustments to the device (Schoevers & Jenkins, 2015). The gardener, displaying a natural aptitude for 'fixing', stayed after hours to learn the repairing skills from our technician. Carer training was integrated throughout the programme, with staff working alongside

Shonaquip, practising safe techniques to lift, transfer and position children, cut pre-ischial shelves into foam cushions, adjust devices, screen them for faults and do basic repairs. Learning about the purpose and use of positioning devices facilitated the development of a 24-hour positioning routine at Nomzamo. The centre manager led her staff by example, participating fully at each visit. Uhambo staff mentored carers in how to use the *Ndinogona* kit optimally with the children at the centre, selecting one as a 'key' facilitator to implement the programme. Two areas have since been set up to provide stimulation as part of daily routines. Each child rotates through one of the stimulation rooms where they enjoy learning opportunities in a small group with two trained carers. Following the outreach, children are reported to be more responsive to their environment. For example, one blind 15-year-old, also with athetosis, used to be confined to bed and was unable to engage with others. However, now he is able to sit upright in a buggy while, at the same time, responding to auditory stimuli.

In March 2016, Shonaquip attended the 'handover' event at Nomzamo where funders were handing over devices. All the children, mobile in their new devices, reviewed and correctly positioned, were present for the event. This gave funders the opportunity to engage directly with the children, and to witness the impact of their new devices. Local residents, their families, community members, social department representatives, CPA, as well as the local mayor and tribal leader were also invited to attend. It was also a form of awareness-raising event where all stakeholders were encouraged to support the centre as locals. It was disappointing that parents, most of whom live far from the centre, were unable to participate in training. Likewise, more staff from the neighbouring hospital could have been invited to join the 'Let's Talk Disability' training to promote inclusive attitudes in the community. CPA, on a visit to the centre a few weeks after assessment, reported back positively about the progress the centre had continued making following the outreach. They continue to assist the centre with follow-ups. Case study 22.3 illustrates the impact of the phased intervention on one resident, Andile.

Case study 22.3   Andile's story

Andile★ is a 6-year-old boy with dystonic cerebral palsy at Nomzamo. Andile is a friendly, interactive and fun-loving little boy. Although not able to speak, he understands well and can follow basic instructions. Before age 4, he had never owned a wheelchair and shuffled along the ground with his legs in a 'frog-like' manner. Six months later Andile became the proud owner of a Sully wheelchair. With the correct posture support to sit upright, he could use his arms to push himself. Able to move around outdoors for the first time, his world opened up. Thrilled by his independence, he was reluctant to get out of his wheelchair at bedtime. Staff were also trained to position Andile in the centre's standing frame each day and shown how to facilitate activities in a standing position. Three months later Andile had learned to pull himself up on furniture into standing. He had learned to push himself independently to the stimulation centre and staff reported that he had also started assisting them with dressing and washing. He was also able to feed himself independently and no longer needed nappies. Prior to our next visit, we received an excited phone call from the centre manager. Andile had started walking with the assistance of a walking frame. It was apparent that strengthening Andile's physical abilities, sense of control and independence had also improved his participation in daily routines. Sadly there is no local school for Andile to attend in this isolated area but we are satisfied that he is well able to participate in any of the stimulation activities.

★not his real name

Box 22.1 provides key lessons learned from Shonaquip outreach service, including stories presented in this chapter.

Box 22.1 Key lessons learned from Shonaquip outreach service

- Mobile outreach clinics connect service providers to users and carers 'on the ground' which helps uncover emerging needs which inform the design of products and services.
- A dedicated 'host'/local coordinator is key; someone to lead through example. Challenges of outreach include high staff turnover, which requires a dedicated ally to recruit new staff to the programme and ensure relevant upskilling. This should not stand in the way of the full involvement of all staff in programme implementation.
- Sub-districts involved in outreach should ideally assume administrative, clinical, technical and financial accountability for services. This builds local sustainability and empowers local staff to map action when a child needs more specialised equipment.
- Children deprived of early intervention are at risk of developing deformities which makes seating more complex for practitioners, especially when there is no technical backup.
- Some users assessed to require intermediate seating devices can make use of more basic devices if more complex modifications and adjustments are carried out efficiently at district level. This is enabled through mentoring.
- Outreach provides opportunities for mentoring of therapists, and enables advocacy around budgets, waitlists, ordering of spare parts, maintenance and refurbishment of devices. Following outreach, Shonaquip prioritises ongoing communication with local staff and regular contact with the outreach team is supported telephonically, via email or through SKYPE.
- CPD (continuing professional development) points increase therapists' motivation to participate in outreach clinics.
- Liaison with transport drivers, carers or assistants, local handyman, educators and therapists is pivotal, enabling integrated networking and service across sectors to solve local challenges.
- Involving local hospital staff and therapists 'hands-on' during all stages of intervention deepens local awareness of seating and disability issues, increasing sustainability of outreach.
- Informal networks between users, carers and families are a positive spin-off from outreach and boost local peer support. Wherever possible parents should be urged to participate in training offered to carers. This provides opportunities for parent champions to be identified who can drive local parent advocacy and support for children.
- The sequence of inputs in outreach is important. Foundational activities like 'Let's Talk Disability' (disability dialogue), child handling and positioning techniques prepare participants to derive benefit from the *Ndinogona* stimulation programme. Involving community partners builds local external support for changed practice.
- Positioning awareness and skills embedded into community-run programmes enable children with mobility disabilities to benefit from inclusion. Collaboration with local partners can streamline services for families and improve sustainability of outreach.
- To fully realise their rights, children benefit not only from devices but from wheelchair services and support from their empowered carers and inclusive, disability-friendly communities.

- There is undoubtedly much to do in rural areas such as the Northern Cape where remote communities know little about disability, rights for people with mobility impairments, the role of positioning or the capacity of ordinary people to influence change.
- Scaling community-based outreach services depends on innovative funding mechanisms within a nationally driven service plan aligned to rights entrenched in the CRPD.

Concluding comments

The current model of service delivery expands Shonaquip's original mobile outreach seating clinic model, which focuses on comprehensive wheelchair services, including follow-up to ensure positioning and mobility devices met users' needs across their lifespan. Mindful that vast numbers of children are beyond reach of specialist wheelchair services, during outreach trips Shonaquip locates children with posture-support and mobility needs through key workers in communities, at local clinics or hospitals, social services, schools, ECD centres, individual households or residential facilities.

Wheelchair services and mentoring of local seating practitioners and technicians is now ideally embedded within broader capacity-building interventions to sensitise parents, carers, service providers and community members to disability. This helps to build awareness of how positioning can equip children for participation and inclusion. Wherever possible, local parent and advocacy groups are promoted during outreach to support and link families affected by disability to existing community resources (Visagie, Duffield & Unger, 2015). Together, in upholding the rights of children with disabilities, they can help shift the community closer to the goal of being more inclusive and barrier free.

Reflective questions

1   What barriers prevent people with mobility impairments from accessing wheelchair services in your region and what action can be taken to reduce these barriers?
2   To what extent do local service providers in your region have the seating and technical capacity and necessary support to provide the full spectrum of quality wheelchair devices and services recommended by WHO for low-resource settings? What steps can be taken to improve the quality of service provision?
3   How can service providers work together in your region to ensure posture support and mobility are embedded in existing programmes to equip children with severe mobility impairments to participate more fully and benefit from inclusive opportunities?

References

Bateman, C. (2012). 'One size fits all' health policies crippling rural rehab therapists. *South African Medical Journal* **102**(4), 200–208.

Booyens, M., Van Pletzen, E. & Lorenzo, T. (2015). The complexity of rural contexts experienced by community disability workers in three southern African countries. *African Journal of Disability* **4**(1), Art. #167.

De Roodenbeke, E., Lucas, S., Rousaut, A. & Bana, F. (2011). *Strategies to increase access to health workers in remote and rural areas.* Geneva: World Health Organization. Retrieved from http://apps.who.int/iris/bitstream/10665/44589/1/9789241501514_eng.pdf on 20 March 2017.

Grut, L., Mji, G., Braathen, S. & Ingstad, B. (2012). Accessing community health services: challenges faced by poor people with disabilities in rural communities in South Africa. *African Journal of Disability* **1**(1) Art# 19. Retrieved from http://dx.doi.org/10.4102/ajod.v1i1.19 on 23 March 2017.

Hannas-Hancock, J. & Deghage, N. (2016). Elements of the financial and economic costs of disability to households in South Africa: a pilot study. In *Best of UNICEF Research*. Florence: UNICEF Office of Research Innocenti. Retrieved from www.unicef-irc.org/publications/pdf/Best%20of%20 UNICEF%202016_web.pdf on 22 March 2017.

Mji, G., Braathen, S., Vergunst, R., Scheffler, E., Kritzinger, J., Mannan, H. *et al.* (2017). Exploring the interaction of activity limitations with context, systems, community and personal factors in accessing public health care services: a presentation of South African case studies. *African Journal of Primary Health Care & Family Medicine* **9**(11) a1166. Retrieved from www.phcfm.org/index.php/phcfm/article/view File/1166/pdf_1 on 20 March 2017.

National Department of Health (2003). *Standardization of Provision of Assistive Devices in South Africa*. Pretoria: Department of Health, South Africa.

National Department of Health (2016). *Framework and Strategy for Disability and Rehabilitation Services 2015–2020*. Pretoria: Department of Health, South Africa.

Schoevers, J. & Jenkins, L. (2015). Factors influencing specialist outreach and support services to rural populations in the Eden and Central Karoo districts of the Western Cape. *African Journal of Primary Health Care & Family Medicine* **7**(1), 1–9. Retrieved from www.phcfm.org/index.php/phcfm/article/view/750 on 22 March 2017.

Sherry, K. (2015). Disability and rehabilitation: essential considerations for equitable, accessible and poverty reducing health care in South Africa. SAHR 2014/15, 89–100. Retrieved from www.rhap. org.za/wp-content/uploads/2015/10/Disability-and-rehabilitation-Essential-considerations-for-equitableaccessible-and-poverty-reducing-health-care-in-South-Africa.pdf on 22 March 2017.

Vergunst, R. (2016). *Access to health care for persons with disabilities in rural Madwaleni, Eastern Cape, South Africa*. PhD Thesis, Dept. of Psychology, University of Stellenbosch. Retrieved from http://scholar. sun.ac.za/handle/10019.1/98408 on 22 March 2017.

Vergunst, R., MacLachlan, L. & Mannan, H. (2015). 'You must carry your wheelchair': barriers to accessing health in a South African rural area. *Global Health Action* **8**. Retrieved from www.ncbi.nlm.nih. gov/pmc/articles/PMC4592846/ on 20 March 2017.

Visagie, S., Duffield, S. & Unger, M. (2015). Exploring the impact of wheelchair design on user function in a rural South African setting. *African Journal of Disability* **4**(1), 8 pages [online]. Retrieved from www. ajod.org/index.php/ajod/article/view/171 on 20 March 2017.

Visagie, S., Scheffler, E. & Schneider, M. (2013). Policy implementation in wheelchair service delivery in a rural South African setting. *African Journal of Disability* **2**(1), Art. #63.

World Health Organization (2008). *Guidelines on the provision of manual wheelchairs in less resourced settings* [online]. Retrieved from www.who.int/disabilities/publications/technology/wheelchairguidelines/ en/ on 20 March 2017.

World Health Organization & UNICEF (2015). *Assistive technology for children with disabilities: creating opportunities for education, inclusion and participation. A discussion paper*. Geneva: World Health Organization. Retrieved from www.unicef.org/disabilities/files/Assistive-Tech-Web.pdf on 20 March 2017.

PART VII

Narratives from disability activists

In Part VII, disability activists share their vivid personal stories on how they face and deal with exclusionary practices in their everyday lives and the coping mechanisms they use to overcome such practices.

PART VII

Narratives from disability
activists

23

A CITIZEN OF TWO WORLDS

Irene Sithole

Introduction

'Irene, have you seen the paper? Did you read what they are saying about you?' That was my elder sister calling me from the lounge. 'Yes, I did,' I calmly answered because I knew what she was referring to. This was about an interview that my colleague and I had with a journalist from one of the local daily newspapers. The journalist had described my colleague as being blind, which she is; and me as being partially blind. The 'partially blind' description ascribed to me is the one that had shocked my sister because the term has never been used in my family to describe my condition.

Before this incident, I had co-facilitated a workshop for blind women and one of the things the women wanted to know about me was whether I was sighted or not. So I told them that I can see but in partiality. These two incidents got me on the path of writing this book chapter. I realised that throughout my life, I have always been dealing with, and even in the future I will always deal with, the question of my sight. Do I see or not with my physical eyes? The journalist from the daily newspaper was right to say that I am partially blind. If I close my right eye, everything becomes dim and hazy. If I try to walk, I will most probably crash into something. My left eye cannot see anything distinctly. I am blind in that eye. At the same time, I was right to tell those workshop participants that I am sighted. My sister had every reason to be shocked by the way I was described in that newspaper article because I have been raised as a sighted person. My right eye is the one that I use to do all my seeing though it also has limited sight.

I then started thinking about all my experiences, particularly the challenges that I have gone through because I am both blind and sighted. I can see and at the same time I cannot see. I thought I should share these experiences on what it is to belong to the world of sighted people and that of blind people – to be a citizen of both worlds. The purpose of this book chapter is not to elicit pity or sympathy, but having personal insight into both worlds to some extent qualifies me to assist both sides to understand each other. It is hoped that when sighted people read this book chapter, they will appreciate, support and treat blind people with dignity. Similarly, it is hoped that when blind people read this chapter, they will understand some of the attitudes of sighted people; they will cooperate with them on how they can best support each other.

First encounters with adversity

I believe that one of the unique things about me is that I remember the day I was weaned. A baby gets weaned at two years or younger and how many people can remember what happened when they were two years old? That makes me unique. I do remember very clearly all of us sitting on the veranda of our house, my mother, brothers, sisters and myself. There was such a palpable air of expectancy around. I am not sure how, but somehow I knew that the thing that was about to happen had something to do with me. That is when my mother took me on her lap and started breastfeeding me. The moment the milk got into my mouth I started yelling because my mother had smeared some chilli on her breasts, a very effective way used in those days to dissuade babies from breastfeeding. From that day, I never came to my mother for breast milk because I believed that her milk was full of chilli and too hot for my taste buds.

Despite remembering the day I was weaned, I do not have a similar vivid memory regarding my sight. While doctors later told me when I was 12 years old that I had congenital cataracts, a condition that existed at my birth, I am unable to place a timeframe to when I became conscious of the fact that I could only see partially. All I recall are snippets from incidents that occurred when I was five years or younger, which proved to me that there was something wrong with my sight. I remember walking with two of my sisters through an area where bricks were being moulded. I then stepped on some wet bricks without seeing them. Needless to say, the owners of the bricks were really mad at me and called me names in spite of the fact that my sisters apologised profusely on my behalf. I had just experienced my first baptism of insults and name calling.

Another thing that I remember from those early years is that failure to see caused me to be very accident-prone. It was common for me to be seen walking with a limp after stumbling upon a rock or tree root. After all, I was staying in the rural areas where rocks, tree stumps and roots are a common occurrence. I also bled easily each time I got injured and I would be really scared when I saw my blood. At that tender age, I believed that bleeding meant that I was seriously injured and I would cry a lot each time I looked at the bleeding wounds. As a precaution to the stumbling accidents, my mother made sure that my travelling or any walking outdoors after dark were minimised. I suppose wearing shoes might also have provided some protection during such accidents, but which 'kids' like wearing those things? At that age, walking barefoot is such fun and I did have some fun, bleeding toes and all.

Going to school was another experience to be remembered as it holds both painful and joyful memories. Growing up in the village, we did not have crèches and our home was also isolated from the other homesteads in the village. This means that my preschool years were more or less sheltered and I played and interacted mostly with my siblings. I did not get opportunities to be around other kids. School was a different story. The moment I got there, everybody noticed that I squinted. So began the question that has since become an everyday part of my life: 'What happened to your eyes?' they all wanted to know.

On the bright side of things, my class teacher did not ask about what happened to my eyes. Probably my mother had briefed him on my condition. Because of my short sightedness, he made sure that I got to sit in front of the class near the blackboard where he wrote most of the stuff that we were supposed to learn. Where textbooks were not enough to go around and pupils had to share, I got to read the teacher's copy so that I could put the book as close to my face as I needed to enable me to read. Tests or examinations were written on the blackboard that covered most of the front wall of the classroom. Even the blackboard was too wide for me to read its contents while sitting on one end of the classroom. So when writing tests, I got to sit on the teacher's chair, which I would move from one end to the other whenever the need arose.

This worked very well for my first school year, which was grade one. I managed to pass all my tests and to have first position in my class throughout that year. The problem arose when I got to second grade and changed teachers. My parents got the shock of their lives when I told them at the end of the first school term that I was number 33. They could not understand how this could have happened. My new teacher had not been briefed of my impairment-specific needs and I did not think it was my duty to enlighten him. So, come test time, I only answered the questions on the part of the blackboard that was close to me. The teacher did not know that I needed to move around and, hence, I did not move. There were about 50 pupils in grade two that year and looking back, I always marvel that I even managed to score more in the tests than some 17 pupils who could see the whole blackboard.

While the teachers understood, it was a different story among my classmates. I guess it is because 'kids' will always be 'kids' and they do cruel things maybe without understanding that they are being cruel. It could also see that the teachers did not explain to the other kids that I had such impairment and this was not something to be made fun of. We used to do some group work and, particularly during the early grades, I was a very shy and a reserved person. These are not the qualities that teachers look for when selecting group leaders. This meant that I was never selected to lead groups during group work. However, I was also highly intelligent and smart, which meant I got most of the answers correct. This did not go down well with my group leaders who felt outsmarted. I remember one group leader who used to call me a *n'anga* (witch doctor). He said this was because he could not understand how I could get all answers correct when I could not see. According to him, I had some super powers that showed me the answers. Most of the time, I would not volunteer the answers and he even avoided me, but when the group was stuck, he would say '*n'anga tiudze*' (witchdoctor, give us the answer). The other group members would laugh and no one ever bothered to defend me.

Those were 'kids' but that does not mean that the adults have been angels. I have already mentioned those who called me names for stepping on their bricks and outside school. There was also the rather annoying challenge of being talked about as if I am not there. Often times, as I moved around the community, after enquiring about what happened to my eyes, people would start talking about my performance at school which was known to be very good. Then, they would go on to commiserate and say, '*Mwari haanyimi zvese chokwadi*', meaning that though God had not given me sight, he had given me intelligence, and such a discussion would go on and on without asking for any input from me.

One thing that has always puzzled me is the way people assume to know the solution to my impairment. While the question about what happened to my eyes has become an integral part of my life, some people do not even bother to ask. They will just order me to wear spectacles in order to correct my eyesight. I remember one incident while I was on a bus and, as my habit is when travelling, I was reading a book. The man who was sitting on a seat across from me then started telling me to wear spectacles. He even offered to buy them for me and he was a total stranger. To avoid saying something rude, I ignored him completely and continued with my reading. When we were getting off the bus, the man could not wait to tell my sister with whom I was travelling of my rudeness in not responding to his spectacles conversation. It is incidents like these that leave me really baffled. My sister went on to question me about why I had not answered the man. She supported the notion that I had been rude. I kept asking myself, in the first place, is it not rude for people to just assume that I need spectacles without seeking to understand whether my condition can be rectified by spectacles or not? Is it not rude to just make assumptions about a person's sight when you are strangers and you do not know anything about that person? How come I am the one labelled as rude if I keep quiet?

In all honesty, I have to concede that there are times when I have been rude in answering questions about my sight and I am not proud about those times. Sometimes, when you have gone through a lot of insults and stigmatisation, you develop a tendency to hit out at society in general and that is something that most disabled people have to work on, myself included. I believe I am getting better and, with God's grace, there will be a day when someone will walk up to me and say, 'Hey you, why don't you wear spectacles?' and I will answer them nicely with a wide smile.

The nightmare of travelling

The challenge in being counted among sighted people is that the expectation of the sighted is that a person should have perfect sight. This is why people will push me to wear spectacles because they believe every eyesight problem can be rectified. I remember, from a very early age, one of my brothers would try to stop me from squinting simply by asking me to watch the way he opened his eyes and imitate him. I would try my best but, once he stopped, I would go back to squinting because that is the way I am able to focus on objects and people and see them better.

My way of seeing has also resulted in people being impatient with me. For instance, when I drop something on the ground, particularly something small and I have to pick it up, I tend to do it in slow motion and not instantly. First of all, I have to figure out the general area where the object has fallen. Then I have to try to locate the object in that area and, with my poor sight, it normally takes a bit of time. Sometimes, I might even use my hands to assist me in locating the object. In the meantime, if there is a sighted person watching me nearby, that is when they get impatient with me because they will be seeing the object perfectly. More often than not, the person will shout at me and say, 'There it is', and, 'Can't you see it?' This makes me more flustered and distracted resulting in it becoming more difficult for me to see. Of course, by then my instinct would be to shout back and say, 'No, I can't see it!' But usually I just hold back and concentrate on the business of finding the fallen object.

As a sighted person, I have to walk on my own, read on my own and generally attend to all the affairs of my life without assistance. In this regard, I have faced some challenges, particularly in travelling. Long ago before the era of commuter omnibuses with touts who shout the destinations, we used to travel using buses. This was the time I was attending a boarding school. I had to stand at a bus stop to wait for the bus. I had to read the destination board at the front of the bus to avoid getting on the wrong bus. At such times, especially when schools were opening, there would be many people travelling and some pressure would have to be applied in order to get on the bus. This means you had to read the bus destination while it was still some distance away so that you could rush to the door as it stopped. I was then at a disadvantage because I could only see the destination board when the bus had stopped. Even then, I had to literally go to the front of the bus, look at the destination board, then rush to join the queue if it was the right bus. Now with commuter omnibuses, life is easier because the touts shout the destination while it is still some distance away from the bus stop.

Travelling by public transport is now easier, but walking on foot in the central business district of Harare is now a nightmare. There is so much traffic on the roads and crossing these busy roads is difficult. The only traffic lights that I can see clearly are the big ones, particularly the solar ones along Sam Nujoma street (a street passing through Harare city centre). With most of the roads, I have to watch the traffic or simply follow others, trusting that whoever will be crossing the road at that time knows what they are doing. In a world where both motorists and pedestrians seem to have developed a habit of flouting traffic rules, there have been several near misses from being struck by cars while crossing roads.

Travelling by air also presents its challenges. When I first travelled by plane, someone announced the arrival and departure of the various planes via an intercom at the airports. You just had to listen to the voice and you would know when and where to board your plane. These days, all the information and flight timetables are displayed on boards which passengers have to read for themselves. The boards are usually too far up and the print is too small for my short sight, which means it is now very difficult for me to travel alone. I will have to ask strangers for assistance and this is both a risk and a challenge.

At one time, I had to travel to Rome, Italy and the travel agent alerted me to this challenge since it was my first time travelling to Europe. She booked me on a special assistance ticket. The first leg of my journey would take me to Johannesburg, South Africa then Germany and finally Rome. Since I had travelled to Johannesburg before, on arrival I just got off the plane with others and I did not wait for special assistance. I was amazed by the reaction of the person at the check-in counter where I went to collect my boarding pass for the next leg of the journey. When she realised that I was booked for special assistance, she was shocked to see me standing in front of her without assistance. She then phoned for someone to come and assist me and she was practically screaming saying, 'I don't know how she got here on her own'. My assistant came but this time it was my turn to be shocked. The lady had a wheelchair and she expected me to get on it. It took time for me to explain and for her to understand that it was my eyes and not my legs that had a problem. Next, it was her turn to be shocked when I further told her that she did not even have to hold my hand, she could just lead the way and I would follow. I guess it baffled her as to why I needed special assistance if I could see on my own. I could not make her understand that my challenge was not seeing where to place my feet but reading the signs and directions on where to go.

However, despite the initial shocks and hiccups, the trip was really great. I did not go through all the hassles and queues associated with air travel. The airline staff assisting me whisked me through on a golf cart when we got to Germany and when we got to my final destination in Rome I was helped through customs and immigration. All things considered, I had a smooth trip because of the special assistance. It made me realise that with the right kind of support it is not so dark out there for blind people.

Reading price tags in shops has also been a challenge. The world of technology has resulted in a pricing system where prices of goods are put on shelves and not on the product itself. The problem is that some shelves are too high for me to see the prices. I would have to climb on a chair to look at the price. Some shelves are too low. I would need to kneel on the floor in order to see the prices. My predicament has been exacerbated by the economic challenges the nation is facing, which have caused most businesses to cut down on employees, including shop assistants. Most of the time, I find myself in a supermarket standing by the shelves trying to read the price of a product with no assistant in the vicinity to help me. I have to take the product to the till to get assistance from the cashier. The irony is that before computerisation, when stickers would be placed directly on the products, I used to ward off unnecessary help from the shop assistants. A shop assistant would see me holding something, it could be a soap tablet or some tooth gel, while contemplating whether I wanted to buy it or not. He/she could mistakenly assume that I could not see the price and would approach me and say, 'That's going for $10' or whatever the price was. I would then hasten to let them know that I had seen the price. Now I need help because I cannot see the prices but help is not available anymore. At the till, the cashier adds up the purchases and looks at me expectantly waiting for the money. I have to read the total on my own from his/her computer screen but, being short sighted, the computer is beyond my vision. So unless it is one item, I always have to ask verbally for the total price of any goods purchased so that I know how much money to hand over.

The reading dilemma transcends the issue of prices of goods as I face the same challenges with most public documents. I have been to offices where all visitors are required to sign in and the book where you are required to fill in your personal information will have some headings in small print. To make matters worse, the reception area will be dimly lit. The same applies for forms one is required to fill in when applying for documents such as passports and visas. As a sighted person, I am expected to fill in these forms by myself. However, because of the size of the print, most of the time I have to ask someone to assist me. I find this embarrassing since I am highly literate and, with the right print size, I could easily do this by myself. If only someone in the administrative ladder could be sensitive enough to have forms in large print, it would make life easier for people like me. However, this is not just a story of woes. My experiences, both negative and positive have led me to reflect on my two worlds, that is, the world of sightedness and the world of blindness. Belonging to both worlds, I have realised that I might be able to contribute in clearing up some of the misunderstandings between the two worlds. I came to a point where I asked myself the question, what is it that the two worlds want or expect from each other?

What do the two worlds want?

Being partially sighted means that I have to think both as a sighted person and a blind person. I have also interacted with both sides. My advantage is that citizens of both worlds talk to me freely because they consider me as one of their own. The main view held by sighted people is that generally blind people are bitter people. Sometime back, one of my sighted friends was complaining about a blind lady in our community. Her complaint was that the said lady is always bitter and suspicious of people around her. This notion is often dramatised in a common joke about a blind person who was always complaining to his family about the quantity of meat served to him. When he got three pieces, for instance, he would assume that the others had more. He was convinced that he was getting less meat because he could not see what the others had on their plates. So the other family members decided to give him more meat. When he saw the increase in his portion, he then exclaimed, 'If I got so much meat today, it means the others are having a whole goat per person'. It is true that the bitterness might be there, but the important thing is that its existence within a particular blind person must be evident and not assumed to be there just because the person is blind. In other words, it is wrong to assume that every disabled person or every blind person is bitter toward society. This is one of the stereotypes that fuel stigma and discrimination against blind people. There are other factors that shape and influence a person's character besides their impairment. This is the reason why there are also bitter people among sighted people. So not all disabled people are bitter and those who are bitter might have become so because of other disadvantages and negative experiences that have nothing to do with their impairments.

It is also crucial to understand how blindness can result in bitterness. Even in this modern world, there are still ways of thinking in our society where blindness is viewed as a curse. From an early age, a child with visual impairment is exposed to the thinking that his/her condition is a punishment by some supernatural power that is angry at his/her family. Since this will be considered as a spiritual problem, the visually impaired child will be dragged to all sorts of healers and is made to go through a lot of rituals to reverse the curse. Such ordeals can breed bitterness.

The constant insults and negative words from people also cause bitterness. I have already narrated my experiences of being insulted and being labelled a witch doctor by one of my peers at school. There are various other incidents where insults have been thrown at me because of my visual impairment and this phenomenon is not unique to me but it happens to every visually impaired person. The insults are also evident in the names and descriptions given to disabled people in general and blind people in particular. In Zimbabwe and in the Shona language, a blind person is called '*bofu*'. This term is derogatory and insulting because it is used with the pronoun 'it'; thus making a blind person an object, not a person.

Another cause of bitterness is the discrimination experienced by blind people. I have already alluded to verbal insults; but sometimes the non-verbal communication is even worse. Imagine people treating you as if you are not there, treating you as if you do not matter in any way. You are not consulted in any decisions made about your life and people even talk about you as if you are not there. Sometimes when I am walking with my blind friend and her assistant, I have seen people addressing questions about her blindness to the assistant. They are somehow reluctant to talk to her directly. These are the day-to-day experiences of blind people. Their opinions are rarely asked for because people assume that they are not able to make any meaningful contributions and, in any case, society knows their needs so there is no need to bother consulting them. The test to find out if any action or practice is discriminatory is simple. Before carrying out the action or performing the practice, a person must ask himself or herself the question, 'If this deed was performed against me, how would I feel?' For instance, 'If I were the one being talked about as if I am not there or if decisions are made about my life without consulting me, how would I feel?' If you feel outraged about that, then it gives you an insight into the behaviour of blind people whom you condemn for being bitter and grumpy.

These are just a few examples of how the negative attitudes and perceptions of society have contributed to the bitterness found in blind people. I will never forget a statement made by one prominent politician in my country when talking about how his experiences shaped his current life. This was at a function held in his honour and it was common knowledge that he was a person who rarely smiled. Someone mentioned this fact jokingly and when it was time for his speech, the politician saw fit to explain why he did not smile. Apparently, he had gone through solitary detention for many years during the national liberation struggle. He described how horrible it was and then said, 'When you have gone through such things, you don't smile.'

At one meeting that I participated in, one blind acquaintance narrated her humiliating ordeal at another meeting she had attended. She narrated how someone had messed up the toilet seat with menstrual blood and everybody assumed that she was the culprit because she was blind; and she was the only blind lady at that meeting. She tried to convince the group that she was not the one responsible and that it was not even that time of the month for her. No one believed her and the leader of the group took her to the bathroom for a physical examination to prove her innocence. It should be noted that the other group members did not undergo this physical examination. This is just an illustration of how people thoughtlessly invade the privacy and violate the dignity of blind people simply because they are blind.

In essence, disabled people have gone through a lot of pain, hurt and disappointments in their lives. By the time you meet them, if they lash out at you, sometimes it is not about you as an individual, but a response to a deep rooted bitterness festering over time. So when you wonder why they are not always cheerful and smiling, remember it is because of their experiences. When you have been insulted, discriminated against and stigmatised all your life, you do not smile.

The positive thing is that this bitterness does not have to be a permanent feature in a person's life. This is my message to my fellow colleagues with disabilities: we can work through this and overcome the hurt and bitterness. Personally, I have realised that I need to treat individuals who ask questions about my impairment separately and desist from treating any questions and issues about my impairment as the voice of society. For instance, I do not have to be angry when people ask me about the condition of my sight because the person who asks me today is not the same person who asked me yesterday. I also must restrain myself from assuming that any person wanting to know about my sight has a bad motive or that the person is doing it out of malice. In other words, not everyone out there is out to harm us or look down upon us. Some people have a genuine desire to understand our conditions so that they can support us if need be.

As I am writing this, I am reflecting on that incident that I earlier narrated of the man I ignored on the bus when he asked me why I did not wear spectacles. Maybe if I had answered him, he could have suggested other viable solutions to rectify my eyesight that I have not heard of before. The man could even have been an eye specialist; but I will never know now. The fact is that I let my emotions take over and I did not give him a chance to explain himself. Even those who hurt us might do so without realising it. Hence, there is a need to respond to their issues. People of good character will apologise if they hurt another person unintention-ally. Rules of etiquette also apply in how sighted and blind people interact with each other. Generally, it is a well-established principle that you do not ask personal questions to strangers. Imagine just walking into a hospital and asking patients what they are suffering from or just approaching a fellow shopper in a supermarket and asking them what they are buying. It is not normal, it is strange and awkward and that is how it is when you ask a disabled person whom you have just met personal questions about their impairment. The important thing is that both sighted and those with no sight or limited sight, need to work on their attitude toward the other group. Visually impaired people need not look at sighted people as the enemy. Neither should sighted people view the visually impaired as bitter and resentful people.

Another point of contention between the two worlds relates to the support to be provided to the visually impaired and other disabled people. A family member came home one day relating an incident that occurred at her workplace, which had really puzzled her. A colleague of hers who was very short had shouted at a woman who had tried to assist him in opening a door. The door was a staff entrance that members of the public were not allowed to use. He had rebuked the woman for daring to open such a door although she was doing it for him. What puzzled my relative was why the colleague would refuse assistance since he was very short and could not reach the door handle on his own. This man had been at this workplace for many years and used that door every day. The question is therefore; 'How did he open it every day?' He probably had developed his way of doing it, which is why he resented the woman's assistance.

I have highlighted this story to answer the question of when should a disabled person, or in this context a blind person, be assisted. The best way is to get guidance from the person on what kind of support they need. That was the mistake made by the woman trying to assist the man in the incident narrated above. She was standing by the door, she looked at the man's height and concluded that he could not reach the door handle and therefore he needed help. It would have been better to ask the man if he needed help or, better still, to wait and see how he was going to handle this seemingly impossible situation before even offering to help. As I have already stated, the man had worked at the place for a long time and is most likely to have developed his own coping mechanisms.

Assuming that a person needs help and defining the help needed is one of the mistakes made by the sighted. It is like what happened to me at Johannesburg airport when that lady assumed that I needed a wheelchair and later that she needed to hold my hand to guide me to the board-ing gate. She could have asked me first what assistance I needed. I will dare to say that all visually impaired people do not like to be dependants. In this regard they have developed their ways of dealing with their disability depending also on the level of disability. Even among those with total blindness, there are those who walk with their white canes and they do not need someone to physically hold their hands to guide them. I have already alluded to my challenges in crossing the busy streets of Harare, but this does not mean that I need someone to hold my hand in order to cross the roads. A verbal communication that the traffic light is green and the road is clear will do it for me. However, if I am walking in a dark place with ditches and rocks at night, I might need someone to physically guide me. So it is up to me as a visually impaired person to state the kind of support which I require in any particular situation.

This is part of the consultation process which I earlier said could cause bitterness if it does not take place. The sighted can also become bitter if they feel that their support is being rejected while the visually impaired will feel bitter that they are being offered support which does not meet their needs. A case study used in the development arena to emphasise the need for consultation is also relevant here. It is said that a development partner decided to provide a borehole for a certain community. They consulted the community leaders, who were men, concerning the site for the borehole. In Zimbabwean society, the role of fetching water is generally carried out by women. The men decided that a central location in the middle of the village would be best. After the borehole was sunk, the women who were mainly responsible for fetching water ignored it and continued to walk long distances to fetch water which baffled everyone concerned. When they were finally consulted, it came out that they felt that they could not communicate freely, particularly on marital matters, at the borehole which was at the village centre where they could be overheard by the men.

Lack of consultation always results in irrelevance and frustration for everyone concerned. Instead of being appreciated, the unsolicited support might actually end up hurting the feelings of the recipient. One visually impaired friend who is a professional and gainfully employed once shared about an incident where she was in a supermarket and someone offered her a 50-cent coin. She tried to refuse but the person insisted and she ended up accepting the money. The person went away happy, probably considering it his good deed of day while my friend felt somehow offended and humiliated. She was not given an opportunity to decide and someone just assumed that because she is blind she needed a cash donation. The lack of consultation at individual level is also reflected at group level where visually impaired people are excluded in development programmes and processes.

The lack of consultation is even displayed in churches. When preachers see a blind person, they will just say to the blind person's neighbour, 'Bring that person here for prayer.' I once had an uncomfortable experience when I visited a country in East Africa. We went to see a group of women who had been affected by violence and one of their leaders suddenly laid hands on my eyes and started praying in her language. Our local escort is the one who told me that the woman had been praying for me. I do not even know what she prayed about or whether she shares the same faith with me. From a Christian perspective, it is not prudent to let anyone lay hands on you. It would have been nice and proper for her to ask me first before laying hands on me. I believe it is every visually impaired person's lifetime dream to receive sight but all the healing processes, spiritual or medical, should be done through a consultative process.

When it comes to financial support, blind people are the ones who confuse sighted people through the practice of begging. The act of begging for money, food and the basics is a declaration by blind people that they are not capable of looking after themselves. It sends confused messages to the sighted world because, in one breath, blind people are saying they are equal with sighted people, implying that they have the same rights and obligations. In the next breath, the same blind people then beg for financial support from sighted people. The language used is not a reflection of that equality. You hear the blind person saying words like '*ndinokumbirawo rubatsiro, kurarama kwangu ndimiwo hama dzangu*' (May you help me please, I depend on you for my livelihood) and many such similar words. How then are sighted people expected to treat blind people with dignity when they themselves are the ones saying we are not equal to you?

I acknowledge the root of the problem that generally blind people are discriminated and disadvantaged when it comes to access to resources and economic opportunities. However, begging compounds the problem instead of solving it because it makes blind people more dependent upon sighted people. Maybe begging can be a temporary measure when things are really hard, but it should not be viewed as a lifetime occupation. Blind people should demand equal access to resources and economic opportunities and not beg for handouts. Visually impaired people are not helpless dependants and that is the message that must be communicated clearly. They have talents, skills and abilities that can be developed and used to their own benefit and that of their families, communities and nations.

Conclusion

In conclusion, it is important to note that just like any other grouping in society; disabled people are not homogeneous. To begin with, there are different types of impairments that require different responses and support. In addition, there are different levels of impairments. For instance, among visually impaired people, there are those who cannot see at all, some have sight in one eye and some have limited sight in both eyes. Families also respond differently to impairment. Some families do not know how to impart life skills to the disabled person and such a person will require rehabilitation. On that premise, the specific needs of each group and each individual will vary. It is for this reason that this book chapter has zeroed in on key principles without going down to specifics. When our society is guided by the principles of non-discrimination and respect of the human rights and dignity of all people, including disabled people, it will not go wrong. Furthermore, the relationships between the sighted and those without sight will be more cordial and less confrontational. It is through understanding each other that the two worlds become one world, where respect and tolerance become the unifying factors and not points of departure.

24

DISABILITY ADVOCACY THROUGH MEDIA

Action Power

*Lovemore Chidemo, Agness Chindimba
and Lincoln Matongo*

Introduction

The inaccessibility of information to deaf people is synonymous with genocide, as lack of it makes deaf people feel like they are being caged and choked to death. This is because information empowers and opens the mind to new thinking. As Helen Keller puts it, 'Deafness means the loss of the most vital stimulus – the sound of the voice that brings language, sets thoughts astir and keeps us in the intellectual company of man'. With the advent of technology, information was brought within the reach of many, albeit in formats not accessible to the majority of deaf people. Mass media brought about opportunities that could be exploited through transmission of Sign Language programmes. This chapter explores the challenges faced by disabled people, in particular deaf people, in accessing information, and chronicles the birth of *Action Power*, a disability-focused television programme that is broadcast in Zimbabwe. Before focusing on our personal experiences, we provide some background information on the right to access to information; challenges with access to information for disabled people; deaf people and access to information; raising disability awareness; disability and media advocacy television for deaf people in Zimbabwe.

Right of access to information

On the issue of access to information, Article 21 of the United Nations Convention on the Rights of Persons with Disabilities (CRPD) states that:

> State parties shall take all appropriate measures to ensure that persons with disabilities can exercise the right to freedom of expression and opinion, including the freedom to seek, receive and impart information and ideas on an equal basis with others and through all forms of communication of their choice, as defined in Article 2 of the present Convention.
>
> *(United Nations, 2006)*

Deaf people miss out on information that is often gained through hearsay due to lack of Sign Language in the mass media. Hearing people assume that every deaf person knows what they term general knowledge (Chiswanda, 2001). Experience has taught us that hearing people assume that all deaf people can lip-read and that they can speak vernacular language such as Shona, Ndebele among others. Many people also assume that all deaf people can read written language in English, Shona and Ndebele.

Apparently, deaf people have divergent ways of accessing information as some can lip-read, write and read vernacular languages, while others cannot. Sign Language, despite the differences in origination, is one language that brings deaf people together. With Sign Language, deaf people are equal as they can make informed decisions on their own. Sign Language promotes deaf people's right to collective space within society; to pass on their language and culture to future generations (Lentz, 1995). Being involved in the Deaf community and culturally identifying as deaf has been shown to significantly contribute to positive self-esteem in deaf individuals (Jambor & Elliot, 2005). Sign Language forms the backbone of all communication among deaf people and those who can hear. The right of access to information is also enshrined in the Bill of Rights in the Zimbabwe Constitution of 2013 which states that information is a right to everyone; this includes disabled people. Without access to information it is impossible for disabled people to enjoy other rights (Miti, 2008).

Challenges with access to information for disabled people

Lack of access to information is one of the major reasons why disabled people remain marginalised. One of the major challenges with lack of access to information stems from attitudes toward disability by service providers. Deaf people require information in Sign Language and those with blindness require information to be made available in Braille. The HIV/AIDS pandemic demonstrates clearly how lack of access to information impacts on persons with disabilities. Many of my colleagues are dying of diseases such as cancer, HIV/AIDS, Ebola and cholera because information has not been made readily available in Sign Language, Braille or other accessible formats. During major disease outbreaks, information on prevention measures does not reach many persons with disabilities as many cannot access it on television, books and newspapers. The government and other service providers usually make excuses such as the costs of making information accessible to all, cost of hiring interpreters or Braille transcription services. As a result of lack of access to information, disabled people are unable to participate fully in their communities. They are not able to access opportunities for work or other economic or social activities. As a result, disabled people continue to live as second-class citizens in their communities with very little knowledge of what is happening around them; let alone around the world.

Deaf people and access to information

The term 'deaf' has different meanings ascribed to it. When used in the uncapitalised form 'deaf' refers to the condition of being unable to hear, while in the capitalised form (referred to as Big 'D') it refers to the cultural identity of deaf people. The condition of being unable to hear sounds has different degrees of severity ranging from moderate hearing loss to profound hearing loss. The most striking effect of profound hearing loss is the lack of development of spoken language, with its impact on daily communication; this, in turn, restricts learning and literacy (Marschark & Wauters, 2008). Thus, profoundly deaf people rely solely on Sign Language as their mode of communication. They find it difficult to communicate through written language as most of them graduate from high school with fourth grade level of English proficiency (ibid.).

It has to be realised that while hearing people have the ability of acquiring more than one language most deaf people have to be content with Sign Language as their mode of communication in their day-to-day endeavours; be it home or business environment. It has to be commended that Zimbabwe as a country has acknowledged the existence of Sign Language as a language on its own for deaf people, by the inclusion of Sign Language as one of the 16 official languages (Government of Zimbabwe, 2013). Thus, the inclusion of Sign Language is a clear indication of the government's recognition of its importance.

Sign Language is a language that chiefly uses manual modality to convey meaning as opposed to acoustically conveyed sound patterns. Sign Language is visual and television is one mode of transmission that is visual, which can be used to transmit messages to both deaf and hearing people. However, television in Zimbabwe lacks Sign Language on its programmes and they lack captioning as well, save for the main news bulletin. Yet, captioning allows deaf people to read the dialogue on screen, albeit not all can understand it; still, half a loaf is better than nothing.

Raising disability awareness

Raising awareness is an important part of disability advocacy and Article 8 of the CRPD specifically targets that aspect (United Nations, 2006). The challenges that many disabled people face stem from societal attitudes toward disability, which include long-held myths about disability. Raising awareness is therefore important to address these myths and attitudes. Disabled people have previously been perceived as requiring medical help or handouts. The new thinking in disability advocacy looks at disability as a social construct and disabled people as rights holders (United Nations, 2006). Shifts from the long-held positions require a lot of advocacy and awareness-raising effort. Article 8 of the CRPD requires State Parties to invest in awareness-raising programmes. However, budget cuts and lack of commitment by most governments result in them abdicating their responsibilities to civil society, particularly on issues to do with disability. Hence, it is left to Disabled Persons' Organisations (DPOs) and disability advocates to step in and fill the gap. Funding for awareness-raising programmes is scarce because, in most cases, donors want to see immediate and quantifiable results. However, raising awareness is a long-term issue that does not yield immediate results as attitudes take time to be dismantled.

Media and disability advocacy

Media play a very important role in disability awareness. Unfortunately, disability issues continue to be under reported in mainstream media due to a number of reasons. Such reasons include lack of awareness on disability among media practitioners. While, for example, the Rio 2016 Olympics were given considerable coverage with special channels introduced dedicated to the sport extravaganza, the subsequent Paralympics passed with very little coverage in the media. In addition, there are very few disabled media practitioners who can champion the case of disabled people. In Zimbabwe for instance, we have Soneni Gwizi and Langton Mugova who present on radio. However, the challenge is that radio programmes are not visual, making it difficult for deaf people to follow her programmes. Much needs to be done to include more disabled people in the mainstream media, and specifically, visual media.

Lack of awareness on disability issues among media practitioners manifest in continued use of disempowering terms in the media. Such terms as *Chirema and zvirema* in Shona are disempowering. *Chi* is used to signify objects and the use of such words in society and in the media continues to reinforce the perception of disabled people as sub-humans. Media practitioners also continue to use terms like 'deaf and dumb' or 'deaf-mute' when referring to deaf people. Such terms suggest that deaf people are stupid (dumb) or that they do not have a language (mute).

While the media have continued to have negative effect on how disability is perceived in society, it also presents a big opportunity in terms of disability advocacy if it is correctly harnessed. Media campaigns can be used to raise awareness about disability; that is in both print and electronic media. An advert by a detergent manufacturing company in Sign Language during the Rio Paralympics raised a lot of interest among viewers, at the same time drawing attention to accessibility issues for deaf people and Sign Language. Social media and new media technologies also present new opportunities for disability advocacy. Social media is cheap and pervasive even in the rural areas. Disabled people and DPOs can use social media to run effective disability-awareness campaigns at minimum cost.

Television for deaf people in Zimbabwe

Access to television in Zimbabwe has always lagged, with very few programmes having been made specifically for the deaf audience. Television lends itself well to Sign Language broadcasts due to its visual nature. Most of the content on television, however, has no subtitles and there is very little Sign Language interpretation, which is limited to two or three news broadcasts per day. Lack of subtitles on television is exacerbated by delays in implementing the digitilisation process in Zimbabwe, which makes subtitles readily available. While news and information are widely available through the print media, this is inaccessible to deaf people due to low levels of literacy in the spoken languages. A combination of these factors work to ensure that deaf people are largely ignorant of what happens around them, and much less to what is happening in the world. This situation can be explained by lack of funding from the national broadcaster, a very common and overused excuse, and lack of capacity to produce Sign Language programmes. It is against this background that Zimbabwe Deaf Media Trust began broadcasting Sign Language programmes in 2012.

The birth of Zimbabwe Deaf Media
Trust and *Action Power*

Zimbabwe Deaf Media Trust (ZDMT) was formally registered as a disability advocacy trust in April 2010. The major objectives of ZDMT are, among others, to disseminate information about deafness and to provide information to the deaf community in a language that they understand through the promotion of the use of Zimbabwe Sign Language. The primary target is deaf people, although we aimed to raise awareness about disability in general. Funding challenges hampered immediate implementation of the project. The funding environment in Zimbabwe has been challenging for organisations working in various sectors. In 2011, we obtained some funding from the Open Society Initiative for Southern Africa (OSISA), which allowed us to commence our project. In January 2012, we visited South Africa on a learning tour to The New Production Company that has been producing the popular DTV (Deaf Television) programme for deaf people on the SABC 3 television channel. This visit allowed the ZDMT team to learn about producing television programmes for deaf people. On 13 February 2012, we held a stakeholders' meeting in Harare, which brought deaf people from across the country to discuss the birth of *Action Power*. The name was derived from a similar programme that had, however, suffered stillbirth in 2008, falling victim to the demise of the declining Zimbabwean dollar. On 23 April 2012, *Action Power* was broadcast for the first time during Prime Time on Zimbabwe Television (ZTV). The very first episode of *Action Power* discussed the causes of deafness and feedback from viewers was overwhelming.

Action Power synopsis

Action Power is a weekly, 30-minute magazine programme, which is done in Sign Language, covering a variety of topics that are of interest to deaf people in the country. Although the programme is mainly in Sign Language, it also caters for the hearing and blind people through subtitles and voice over; which is a model for accessibility as the programme is accessible to all. The programme is produced by a predominantly deaf crew and is mainly run with an advocacy theme aimed at raising awareness on deaf people and issues that they grapple with on a daily basis. *Action Power* also addresses issues affecting other impairment-specific groups. It has now evolved into an entertainment, lifestyle and informational programme for deaf people in the country. Episodes include interviews (studio and out of studio interviews with deaf people and hearing people) and Sign Language lessons. The programme also profiles deaf and hearing people or institutions of note. Hearing guests are provided with interpreters.

Achievements and challenges

From the day *Action Power* was broadcast for the first time in April 2012, the programme has continuously been on the screens. We started *Action Power* without much technical knowledge of television production. So we focused on producing the programme while external consultants worked on the technical aspects. With our first grant, our focus was on capacity building; hence we bought camera equipment and laptops. We also sent three of our deaf crew to college to learn filming and editing in preparation for production by a deaf crew. From January 2013, we began producing *Action Power* with the help of an external consultant who helped with sound editing, while training our deaf crew. *Action Power* has continued to thrive and now our studio is almost complete.

Action Power soon began to focus on all impairments, in line with the theme of being inclusive. One of the major focuses of *Action Power* was the promotion of Sign Language and lobbying for its official recognition. As a result of our efforts, and many others working with deaf people, Sign Language was officially recognised in the Zimbabwe new Constitution adopted in 2013, taking its place among 15 other languages. We also lobbied for the signing and ratification of the CRPD, which yielded results when Zimbabwe ratified the Convention on 23 September 2013. To promote awareness about the CRPD by disabled people and policy makers, in 2015 we started a new series entitled *ENABLED* to raise awareness on the Convention. Disabled people have remained ignorant about the CRPD and what it means for their rights. Thus, *ENABLED* was an attempt to take the CRPD to the people and to lobby for its domestication and alignment with countries' laws.

Action Power has played a part in raising awareness about issues that affect deaf people and also promoting the status of Sign Language in Zimbabwe. As a result there has been an increase in interest in Sign Language as seen by enquiries that we, and other deaf organisations, receive for training in Sign Language. For example, ZDMT partnered with the University of Zimbabwe's School of Social Work students to introduce training in Sign Language. In addition, we have trained healthcare and childcare workers. Such trainings ensure that deaf people can access social services.

ZDMT has also been willing to harness the power of art to promote disability awareness. In 2015, ZDMT introduced the Deaf Arts Festival, which brought together deaf learners from across the country for performances in Harare. Media houses were invited to report on the festival. Deaf learners explored topics such as disability rights, inclusion, language rights and disability awareness. While the festival provides a platform for deaf learners to express their artistic talents, it also challenges perception of society about what disabled people can do.

Issues covered on *Action Power*

Action Power has engaged with many issues. For example, we managed to visit various rural areas in Zimbabwe, which include Juru, Mutare rural district, Zvishavane rural areas, Dotito and Chiundura among others, and highlighted the challenges that disabled people in rural areas face. They are often ignored as service providers often concentrate on urban areas. The narratives of disabled people in rural areas often remain untold. One of the issues that we discussed and addressed at length in our programmes is that of deaf education where deaf learners are usually disadvantaged due to lack of Sign Language in schools. As a result of our advocacy efforts, and that of other organisations working with deaf people, the Ministry of Primary and Secondary Education invited us and the deaf community to present on how Sign Language can be included in the school curriculum under the curriculum review that was initiated in 2014. This is an important development as the educational outcomes of deaf learners hinge on the use of Sign Language.

Action Power provides a forum where experts, deaf people and other disabled people can engage with each other on how best to implement inclusive programmes, for example inclusive education. The signing and ratification of the CRPD has been a welcome development for the disability sector in Zimbabwe. Unfortunately, most disabled people, who are the rights holders, remain ignorant about the Convention and what it means for them. To take the Convention beyond conference and academic halls, we embarked on raising awareness on the Convention through a television series that was aired over two seasons on national television. We sought to use the media to explain what the Convention entails and to challenge authorities on its implementation.

Challenges facing *Action Power*

The biggest challenge that we have faced is that of funding; a phenomenon that is not peculiar to our organisation only. However, raising awareness about disability is an important task, which we continue to fulfil through creative ways of funding to ensure that our programmes remain on television screens. Other challenges include negative attitudes to disability within societies, which affects our programmes. For example, authorities at times are reluctant to engage us. While the national television station has availed us airtime, sometimes we have to fight them on issues of scheduling when the programme is being pushed to time slots not favourable for our intended audiences. However, we have managed to stand our ground as the programme has constantly been aired during prime time, although more slots would help to ensure that disability issues are understood by our society.

The road ahead

The signing and ratification of the CRPD presents exciting opportunities for advocacy and advancement of the rights of persons with disabilities. While our initial focus has been on deaf people, we also continue to include other types of impairments in our programming as deaf advocacy is centred on broader disability advocacy. New technologies continue to emerge within the media sector and, as an institution, ZDMT will take advantage of the cheaper technologies to create disability awareness within Zimbabwe and beyond its borders. Social media channels such as Facebook and Twitter can be used effectively in disability advocacy, especially when raising awareness about disability in communities. We are already embracing new technologies through the creation of a Facebook group, WhatsApp group and YouTube channel to disseminate our programmes on disability advocacy. In addition, we are also collaborating with mainstream media to ensure that it plays a role in raising disability awareness in communities. It is our hope to raise disability awareness in Zimbabwe so that disabled people in general and deaf people in particular, access social services and contribute to national development. This can only be possible if our disability-awareness efforts continue to change the attitudes of the general public toward disabled people so that they see them as fellow rights holders in Zimbabwe and beyond. Our ultimate vision is to ensure that disability is viewed as a cross-cutting issue at every level, hence promoting sustainable inclusive development.

Conclusion

DPOs and individuals can take advantage of the media to raise awareness about disability and to run advocacy programmes. The way media portrays disabled people is important to how society perceives them. Media have the power to influence perceptions. DPOs should not wait upon the governments to initiate awareness programmes. However, they seek to establish partnerships with media houses to implement disability-awareness programmes, while lobbying and advocating for disability inclusion in mainstream television programmes, hence promoting inclusive development in Zimbabwe and beyond.

References

Chiswanda, M. V. (2001). Education for the deaf and hard of hearing in Zimbabwe. In R. Chimedza & S. Peters (eds) *Disability and Special Needs Education in an African Context* (pp. 62–73). Harare: College Press.

Government of Zimbabwe (2013). *The Constitution of Zimbabwe*. Government of Zimbabwe, Harare.

Jambor, E. & Elliot, M. (2005). Self-esteem and coping strategies among deaf students. *The Journal of Deaf Studies and Deaf Education* **10**(1) 3–81.

Lentz, E. (1995). *The Treasure: ASL poems DVD*. San Diego, CA: In Motion Press and Dawn Sign Press.

Marschark, M. & Wauters, L. (2008). Language comprehension and learning by deaf students. In M. Marschark & P. C. Hauser (eds) *Deaf Cognition: Foundations and Outcomes* (pp. 309–350). New York: Oxford University Press.

Miti, L. (2008). Language rights as human rights and development issues in southern Africa. *Open Space* **2**(3), 39–48.

United Nations (2006). *Convention on the Rights of People with Disabilities and Its Optional Protocol*. Geneva: United Nations.

25

DISABILITY ADVOCACY IN ACTION

Why I built an accessible house in Zimbabwe

Edmore Masendeke

According to Maslow (1943), shelter is one of the basic needs. However, many disabled people rarely realise this need despite it being clearly articulated in Article 19 of the 2006 United Nations Convention of the Rights of Persons with Disabilities. Article 19 states that disabled people have the right to live independently and be included in the community. Thus, as disabled people, we should have the opportunity to choose our place of residence and where and with whom we should live on an equal basis with others. However, due to the scarcity of disability-friendly or accessible houses in Zimbabwe, securing appropriate accommodation is a major challenge for disabled people and their families. They face many barriers in the housing sector, including lack of physical accessibility; ongoing discrimination and stigmatisation; institutional hurdles; lack of access to the labour market; low income; and lack of social housing or community support. Having encountered some of these barriers myself, I developed a passion to ensure that the housing needs of disabled people are met. This chapter explains the steps that I took toward the attainment of Article 19.

When I began to explore the possibilities of living on my own as a disabled person in 2006, I faced a lot of obstacles, including being turned down by landlords who did not want me as a tenant and being ridiculed by those around me who undermined my ability to cook or look after myself. This, however, did not deter me from pursuing my dream; instead, it strengthened my resolve to stay on my own as I saw it as one of the ways that I could begin to challenge some of the misconceptions that people hold concerning disabled people. It took me four years to find the right accommodation and at that time I left home and started living on my own – cooking and caring for myself – and have continued to do so ever since.

The challenges that I faced during my search for accommodation made me realise that not much was being done to promote independent living among disabled people in Zimbabwe. Hence, I decided to also address some of the challenges that reduce disabled people's chances of being independent in adulthood, namely lack of education, unemployment and social segregation.

Thus, in 2010, the same year that I started living on my own as a tenant, I decided to start an organisation called 'Endless Possibilities' that would address some of these challenges and also empower disabled people to determine their own fate in life. Since then, I have had to move to a new place twice. I was more comfortable in my first home than in the latter two. What made them less comfortable was their inaccessibility.

My second and third accommodations were on the first and second floors, so climbing the flight of steps was a challenge; more so at night because there were no lights in the staircases. My second accommodation had an inaccessible kitchen. It was small and did not have counters for me to work on. The only place that was available to work on was the kitchen sink. I could not fit an extra table in the room and I found it too much of a hassle for me to have to work in the other room and then return to the kitchen to do the cooking. Hence, I was no longer able to do most of my cooking – it was done by my helper and visiting family members and friends. In addition to having issues with the stairs and the kitchen, there was poor drainage at that place. Whenever it rained, there were puddles stretching from the main gate to the entrance hall. Some of the residents created a staggered path to walk on using bricks and big stones. However, I am not good at balancing, so I often ended up walking in the puddles.

In 2013, I came across an advert in which a local housing development company was offering to build people garden flats upon payment of a deposit on the property value and the balance over a ten-year period. I asked the housing development company to make alterations on its designs to make them more suitable for me and wheelchair users in general. Some of the alterations that I asked the housing development company to make to the flat's design included installing ramps at the main entrance and exit to the garden; installing non-standard (wide) doors throughout the unit; lowering door handles, light switches and the electricity box to wheelchair height; installing easy-to-turn taps in both the kitchen and bathroom; combining the toilet and bathroom; installing grab bars around the toilet seat and bathtub; and installing a bathroom door that opens outwards.

Since I chose the finish-to-taste option, I was responsible for the flat's floors, cupboards and walls. I chose to put ceramic tiles with a wooden finish throughout the flat. I specifically chose this type of tiles because they are not slippery and do not need to be waxed after they have been swept and mopped. Oh, and they look good too. When it came to designing the kitchen, I asked the carpenter to install two sinks at different levels – one at the standard height, which one can use while standing, and another one that is about a metre high, with an open space underneath. The latter can be used by someone who is seated on a chair or wheelchair. The hob is also about a metre high and has an open space underneath. The open spaces that are underneath the kitchen sink and hob enable a person that is seated on a chair or wheelchair to move close to the hob or kitchen sink without bumping their legs into anything. I also installed an oven with a side-opening door. I also have a moveable storage cabinet in my kitchen. In the bedrooms, I installed pull-down closet rods.

In addition to the above architectural changes and installations, I equipped my house with several items of assistive technology. These assistive technologies include a vegetable slap chopper, an automatic can opener, cool drink and milk bottle holders, a food guard, a pot holder, an assistive chopping board, a side-opening oven; and a talking microwave. I do not need or use all these assistive technologies, but I bought them so that I can show them to others who might need them.

In September 2015, I made a video of my house which went viral on social media. One of the people that watched, shared the video and commented:

> To my friends in the UK [United Kingdom] and the rest of the developed world, this may not be a big deal. But the fact that this has been done in Africa, by an African completely blows me away. This is what I came back for. To see PWDs [people with disabilities] from my own continent get the same opportunities and services as those from richer parts of the world. It won't happen overnight, but we will get there in the end. We have to!!!

The above statement is on point. The reason why I built an accessible house in Zimbabwe is because I also want to see disabled people from my own continent getting the same opportunities and services as those from richer parts of the world. I also agree that it will not happen overnight, but we will get there in the end. We have to! Thus, my house is a clear demonstration that it is possible to build houses that are responsive to the needs of everyone, including disabled people. Therefore, the government and society as a whole has no excuse for failing to ensure that disabled people have access to houses in which they can live independently with dignity and respect. However, this is not going to happen until we change our attitudes toward disabled people and put in place laws that protect their rights in general and their right to adequate housing in particular. This is what I am fighting for in building an accessible house and filming it for the world to see. That is why I built an accessible house in Zimbabwe. To watch the video on YouTube, readers can visit: https://www.youtube.com/watch?v=L2MuQCQ1d3M. I hope that you will watch, listen and learn. Also, share this link as part of an advocacy tool. Yes, we can embrace diversity in Africa. Yes, we can accommodate all our citizens in accessible houses. What is needed is to change our mind sets.

References

Maslow, A. H. (1943). A theory of human motivation. *Psychological Review* **50**(4), 370–396.

United Nations (2006). *Convention on the Rights of Persons with Disabilities.* Retrieved from www.un.org/development/desa/disabilities/convention-on-the-rights-of-persons-with-disabilities.html on 14 April 2018.

26

THE SECURITY GUARD WHO TURNED THE LAWYER INTO A DISABILITY ACTIVIST

Abraham Mateta

Introduction

I do not even for a single moment believe that there is anyone born an activist. Life gives us various challenges and how we respond to those challenges often creates what kind of people we end up becoming. As a person who became blind before the age of two, I know that I have always lived a life of struggling in order to fit within the system. During most of my early years, my fight was characterised by the desire to ensure that I could be as acceptable as possible. Little did I ever imagine that I was pandering to the whims and caprices of the ablest society. In this chapter, I shall share a little story that was my turning point as a Zimbabwean blind person. I will share a story that then defined the kind of activism I have undertaken for the past ten years and, after the story, I will briefly share some of the work that I am currently doing as an activist.

Life after graduation

About nine years ago, I completed my studies and graduated with an LLBS (honours) degree from the University of Zimbabwe. In much simpler terms, I graduated with a Bachelor of Law honours degree. Oh! What a wonderful feeling it was! Since grade six, I had harboured and nurtured the desire to be a lawyer. I had withstood the pressure of the harsh academic atmosphere, which was characterised by serious shortages of Braille material since primary school to the university. Hence, I had energetically developed myself into a formidable presenter. My graduation was, therefore, supposed to be a source of pride. Wasn't I supposed to be singing a melodious song of victory? Unfortunately, my joy was short-lived. I soon realised that my degree transcript and certificate were like initiation certificates into long and gruelling fights, which still form part of my life even now.

When I got my degree, I was thinking like a young law graduate of my time. I intended to work for the government and gain a little experience and then join private practice in which I envisioned myself as a brilliant legal mind who would be trusted with all kinds of litigation. I therefore applied to the government and in a few days I was called for an interview and subsequently advised that I had got a job as a law officer in the Ministry of Justice. Oh, how good it felt. 'So easy', I thought to my sweet innocent self. I happily went to the Human Resources (HR) department in the ministry, hoping to be deployed like all the others. It was at that point that I was reminded that since I was blind, I was supposed to have an assistant. I was, therefore, advised to bring someone who had five Ordinary level passes including English to work as my aide. 'Welcome to the real world of dependence', I said to myself. However, this was not very difficult for me to understand because, throughout my education, I had worked in many cases with sighted assistants owing to the unavailability of literature in accessible formats. While at college, I had made sure to teach myself the computer and by the time I graduated, I had enough computer skills to make myself both independent and marketable. However, in government where I got my first job, most of the things were done manually, which implied that my job would require me to interact with a lot of printed literature on paper.

My work experience

I did not face any trouble finding someone meeting the minimum requirements set for my assistant and, with such a person, I went back to the HR department from where I expected a deployment letter. At that point, I was then exposed to serious discrimination camouflaged as bureaucratic requirement. I was advised that my deployment depended on a meeting, which was supposed to be held at the then Public Service Commission (PSC) by the commissioners. The meeting would produce the authorisation necessary for what was then termed 'the treasury concurrence' which would allow the government to pay that extra person called the aide. You see, dear reader, when discrimination takes place it wears very sophisticated smart tags so that, if the one being discriminated against is not careful, he or she might even begin to consider discrimination as a tolerable thing. However for me, that situation meant that I could not assume duty with my colleagues who got jobs at the same time as me, presumably because of the absence of the treasury concurrence. This had the effect of rendering me unemployed on grounds of my impairment.

After one month of frequent visits to the HR department in which I continued to receive the same sad news, I lost my calm and started grilling the officer who had been assigned to do my case by drawing her attention to the anti-disability discrimination provisions in the country's Labour Act and the Disabled Persons Act; and how the government's conduct was incompatible with the said Acts. I also made use of our old Constitution (defective as it was), making it clear that it also prohibits discrimination. Since the right to be protected from discrimination is a political right, which should not be subjected to progressive realisation, I felt that the Ministry of Justice had no excuse in being part of the perpetuation of this unlawful conduct. The argument was so forceful that she took me to her director with whom I engaged in a similar discussion. The director tried to lecture me on bureaucratic practice, blending her talk with those lessons on patience that one would get during a Holy Sabbath or Sunday service. However, on that day, I would have none of that. I insisted that the government cannot be seen to be failing to enforce its own laws. We finally agreed that I should physically go to the PSC and possibly meet one or two commissioners to urge them to consider my case more quickly.

Becoming an activist

I went to the PSC the next day looking forward to a productive engagement. There, I was directed to a floor where some secretaries listened to my case. Treating me to another lesson on how busy the commissioners could be, the number of issues commissioners had to look at and how weighty such issues were in comparison to mine, they also pleaded with me to be patient. Again, the lawyer in me was reactivated. 'What is heavier than a government department which by its rules or Acts of omission perpetually breaks the law of the land?' I asked. I reasoned therefore that for the sake of the integrity of the Commission, the inviolability of my right and the respect for the law, the Commission should quickly deal with my case. The secretaries gave in at that point and directed me to the tenth floor where I was advised that I would meet at least one of the commissioners.

On the tenth floor, I was welcomed by two guards who enquired what I wanted. I indicated that I wanted to see a commissioner. Suddenly, one of the guards ranted like a rabid jackal. 'Do you know how important the commissioners are? Blind as you are, how do you want to see the commissioner?' When I had last been reminded of my blindness at the Ministry of Justice, it had not been so infuriating. This time, I felt like someone was piercing a fiery arrow into the heart of my heart. One of my lecturers for Clinical and Practical Skills had taught me that a good lawyer must in all circumstances remain composed. I therefore held my own. The other security guard who sounded sober-minded asked me to explain my case. I narrated the case in the simplest possible way. I did not want to confuse my simple listeners with the law because of their background. As I finished, the rowdy security guard was at it again.

'What is your problem, you blind people are difficult to help. You are saying they have offered you a job? So you can't just wait? After all it was their sympathy to employ you. Can't you understand?'

I felt the argument had taken an ugly twist. Reasoning was no longer a useful tool. I thought for a moment that if I had an iron bar, I would have inflicted maximum damage to him. Even with such boiling emotions, I still managed to calmly say to him, 'But do you realise that I am educated and qualified to do the job?' 'It doesn't matter', he shouted. 'You are blind. That is the point. You must be grateful.' He said that, closing the door to the entrance. I had two thoughts. One of the thoughts was to just start making a noise and chanting revolutionary songs. However, the lawyer in me prevailed. I would make myself prone to be viewed as unfit for the legal profession by such conduct, I thought. I therefore went home.

At home, I entered my room, closed the door and locked it. I sat down and started thinking. Why was that security guard so rough to me? I even thought of suing him. As I was developing my thought, a more powerful thought came to mind. I benefited nothing from thinking of this security guard as an individual. The guard was a representative of a wicked and discriminatory system – a system where one is either sighted or blind. For me, that was a system in which if you are blind, it does not matter whether you are educated, you can still receive treatment worse than that of a beggar or vagabond. So like the biblical Moses, I found myself saying, 'So who am I to fight a system?' When I had gone to school, toiling and sweating, I had imagined myself as a bright smart lawyer. Yet the system still expected me to be a grateful beggar. Had I gone to school in vain? I cried real tears and failed to eat that day.

I admit that sometimes I struggle to make it clear to other people that the major challenge for disabled people like myself is that the system does not respect abilities, but rather looks at our impairments and further creates our disabilities through attitudinal, structural and physical barriers after which it wants us to be grateful. Even if this might sound too abstract to some, at least it is one thing that transformed me into a full-blown activist and gave me a new direction to go. In the last part of this story, I will be sharing the new direction that I then decided to take.

The new direction

After three months from the date of getting the confirmation that I had got a job, I was finally called, the treasury concurrence having been secured, to work as a law officer in the office of the Public Protector. In that office, we were responsible for handling complaints of members of the public against government and other public officers. We facilitated for the resolution of matters and helped the government to avoid being sued. I decided during that period to join organisations for and of persons with disabilities, and after about two years it dawned on me that the government was one of the chief violators of the rights of persons with disabilities and it would be very difficult to work in government while at the same time offering adequate constructive criticism befitting an activist that I was. I therefore resigned from my job and joined the civic society.

In 2009, I started working for an organisation known as the Zimbabwe National League of the Blind as a disability rights and advocacy officer. While part of my job was to help the organisation craft policy and legislative positions, the bulk of my work revolved around getting into the community and designing as well as implementing disability-awareness training. This job was a departure from the model lawyer that I had envisioned myself as when I was young. The job brought me face to face with real stories, successes and challenges of disabled people. It gave me access to various government departments with which I interacted either in an advisory capacity or as part of the lobbying and advocacy strategies of the organisation. One such institution was the Zimbabwe Youth Council in which I served as a board member between 2009 and 2014. One of the tangible results was that I pushed for the inclusion of disabled youths in the processes of coming up with the National Youth Policy. Hence, the current youth policy is very disability inclusive.

The second area with which I was heavily involved during the same period was the electoral reform process. First, I was one of the applicants in the celebrated case of Simon Mvindi and others versus the President of Zimbabwe and others in which we challenged the way in which blind voters were supposed to vote. We argued that the way in which we were required to vote did not respect our right to the secrecy of the ballot. The Supreme Court eventually ruled in our favour. I have worked in the Zimbabwe Electoral Commission Technical Team, which developed the *Voter Education Manual* (Zimbabwe Electoral Commission, 2013) that was used for the 2013 elections. One of the features of that manual was that it included issues of disability. I also had the opportunity to move with the Commission's staff, testing the suitability and readability of the *Voter Education Manual*. We also took the opportunity to encourage many persons with disabilities to participate in the voting process.

The third area in which, as an activist, I was able to participate was the Zimbabwean Constitution-making process. This process started when I was still working for the government and I played a role of mobilising disabled people to ensure that disability would be thought of as a thematic area. Toward the conclusion of the Constitution-making process in 2012, I was tasked to present the position of disabled people on the whole Constitution. Although I must point out that the Constitution gave us far less than we had bargained for and still falls short of the standards set out in the United Nations Convention on the Rights of Persons with Disabilities (CRPD), there are certain provisions that can be used progressively. In fact, at present, part of my activist's work is to conscientise the society on 'how it can make lemonade out of the lemon called the Constitution'.

In 2014, I got a scholarship and went to study at the University of Leeds for my Masters in International and European Human Rights Law with a special emphasis on disability. There I was exposed to disability rights experts. I did a dissertation analysing the participation of persons with disabilities in Zimbabwe in keeping with Articles 4 (3) and 33 of the CRPD. In the United Kingdom, I gained valuable experience in disability issues and that knowledge has continued to be very useful in my work.

Joining a law firm

After completing my Master's degree, I came back home and decided to retrace my steps back to the profession. I therefore decided to do something which I had failed to do out of anger with the system, and that is registering as a legal practitioner. I joined a law firm and got a practising certificate and I am currently in private practice. As I do so, I now have a new vision of myself. While I am currently involved with general litigation, disability rights remains in my heart. As a result, I have come together with other like-minded individuals to form the Lawyers with Disabilities Association Zimbabwe (LDAZ), in which I am currently the secretary. In that organisation, our aim is first and foremost, to promote the rights of disabled lawyers to participate at an equal level with their non-disabled counterparts. Second, we aim to ensure access to justice for all persons with disabilities in general and we hope to develop the jurisprudence on disability by taking up cases in which disability is an issue and effectively litigating them.

I also believe firmly that social media can be a powerful attitude transformation platform. Through platforms such as Twitter and Facebook, I often post thought-provoking posts on disability. Some of my posts are based on true personal experiences such as 'my blind life in a sighted world', which I usually post on Facebook. I also run another blog called *Disability Rights with Abraham* in which I also deal with issues of disability from a rights-based approach. What is rewarding is to learn that there are quite a lot of people who are being touched by the discussions that I start in my blogs or on social media platforms.

Conclusion

I have no illusions about the fact that the practice of law is indeed something that I naturally like. However, it was the security guard's conduct that served as an initiation for me to a higher calling and that calling is to be a disability rights activist. I therefore view myself as a legal practitioner by training and a disability rights activist by calling. I am very sure I am yet to reach greater heights but those two things are what make my world go round.

Reference

Zimbabwe Electoral Commission (2013). *Your Vote Is Your Voice*. Harare: Zimbabwe Electoral Commission.

27

'FOR I KNOW THE PLANS THAT I HAVE FOR YOU'

The story of my life

Rachel K. Kachaje

My background

My story starts with a Scripture from the Book of Jeremiah 29 verse 11, '*For I know the plans I have for you,*' declares the LORD, '*plans to prosper you and not to harm you, plans to give you hope and a future*'; because that is my personal journey, my destiny.

My father is Boston Kamchacha and my mother is Esther Chimseu Kamchacha. They are both from Malawi. Initially, we were nine children; five boys and four girls. The first born was a boy who died at a tender crawling age. The second and third children were boys. My mother started lamenting for a baby girl. When the time came, she became pregnant and her wish was granted, hence I was born. Later in my life, I overheard her telling her friends that the pregnancy that was to result in me was different from the other three pregnancies, but I did not fully understand what that meant.

When the time was due for the baby to be born, she gave birth to a girl. The joy and desire of her heart of having a baby girl was manifested on 5 May 1958. It was a special day indeed for her. As she shared her experiences with her friends, she indicated the baby was beautiful; her hair was like that of a newly born goat, pure black and shiny. The baby was indeed gorgeous, energetic and looked clever. She was really a source of joy to a mother who was so desperate for a baby girl. I belong to a matrilineal Chewa tribe where giving birth to a girl child is an assurance of the continuity of lineage.

As I was growing and walking up and down, many people admired me because of my beauty as my mother told me. As a result of my beauty, my mother said she experienced ridicule from the community, making one wonder if it is wrong to bear a beautiful baby. When I started walking at the age of 11 months, I was told that she used to go for traditional dances with her aunts. They would carry me on their back. This was in a village called Linga under Chief Mwase. At the age of three years, tragedy struck my family, as my mother recounted. There was an outbreak of polio and, sadly, I was also affected. All my body parts were rendered useless. My body parts were lifeless and my neck was falling backwards. The only part that was alive was my heart, which was still beating. It was a shock to the family, especially to my mother as I was a source of her happiness. Her only hope and source of inspiration was my heartbeat, which encouraged and gave hope to my mother. The following months were hell on earth for my mother. She received all sorts of insults. Friends, neighbours and even some of my relatives were urging her to throw me away or bury me as I was a useless being. She was a laughing stock for clinging to what, to them, was a 'dead thing'. My mother would carry me on her back and cycle five kilometres to the hospital every fortnight for physiotherapy.

My education and aspirations

Most children do not really know why they go to school. One day I asked my niece, Tisungane, why she goes to school and she said she did not know. However, she was certain that she was sent to school and did not go willingly as she did not see the purpose or importance of going to school. Her response made me think that parents have a great role in discussing issues with their children and helping them in shaping their destiny. In my case, I knew I needed education at an early age because, as a disabled girl, I felt that I would not be able to go to the farm, to the well to draw water and to fetch firewood as part of the daily chores around the home. These are expectations of any girl in Malawi. No matter the challenges I went through because of my physical impairment, interacting with the environment (e.g. lack of mobility aids, inaccessible buildings and roads), I did not lose focus of what I wanted. One thing I knew then was that I needed education to expand my mind and achieve my dream. I always dreamed of becoming a soldier. Every time I saw our Malawi Defence Force, it motivated me to become one of them. However, there were two challenges to this dream. At that time, the laws in Malawi did not allow female soldiers. As a result, I thought of having a second dream of becoming a doctor. I was always inspired when my mother took me to Queen Elizabeth Hospital for physiotherapy. From the loud speakers, I could hear a call for Dr Boxten. And the uniform, wow! I said I will become a doctor so that I will also have to be called 'Dr Rachel Kamchacha'. Just the thought of being called 'Dr Rachel Kamchacha' made me value education dearly. Regrettably, my two dreams (soldier and medical doctor) could not be accomplished because of my impairment. God's time was the best. His plan was not my plan.

I started primary school education at the age of eight at Kanjedza Primary School in Blantyre, a government school that was two to three kilometres from our house. I was in the same class with my young sister who came after me. She used to carry me on her back to and from school. After writing and passing my standard eight examinations, I was then selected for form one at Henry Henderson Institute Secondary School in Blantyre, which is a mission secondary school. It was a challenge, as the school was very far (about 10 kilometres) from where I was staying. The school was not accessible as it was a double storey structure, which meant that I could not access any of the facilities in that building without being carried. Now when I look back, I cannot even imagine myself being carried. This is like being dehumanised simply because society does not take into account the diverse needs of every individual. Regrettably, even up to now, the situation has not changed much as most public places are inaccessible to disabled people.

Let me get back to my story. My father arranged for me to transfer to Chichiri Secondary School, which was a bit closer to my home. The major challenge that I faced was that I had to cross the Naperi River. During that time, there were no bridges. Rather, there were poles that served as crossing points, a kind of a makeshift bridge. The school also was not accessible. However, I managed as it was much better than Henderson Institute Secondary School.

Come rain season, it was tough for me. It was not easy to walk on the muddy road to school. I remember this other day, it rained heavily while I was at school. When we knocked off to go back home, the river was overflowing and one of the poles was half way in the river. I had to figure out how to cross, as walking on the remaining two poles was not possible for me. I took my school bag and threw it on the other side and tried to cross. Unfortunately, I missed and went down into the river. I was drowning and, by the Grace of God, I held on to the grass and struggled to get out. That experience did not deter me from going back to school the following day. One thing that kept on coming to my mind was that I should be educated so that someday I would be independent and become somebody in life. To be honest, I still wanted to be that soldier or doctor, the professions I was always admiring. Education was my only passport, thanks to my precious mother who always encouraged me to take education seriously despite living in a disabling environment. She used to tell me not to engage in any relationship with boys, because if I became pregnant that would have been the end of my dream. She always reminded me that I would have to go back to the village and that life would be tough for me as I would be expected to draw water from the well or river, fetch firewood and till the land. So I made up my mind to concentrate on education so that I should be somebody someday and, maybe, escape these social rites.

My employment experiences

After my secondary education at Chichiri Secondary School, I stayed home for one year. In 1978, I registered with the Malawi Council for the Handicapped, which was established by an Act of Parliament, the Handicapped Persons Act, in order to enable disabled men and women to be recognised as equals within Malawi society. The Council was registering disabled people with the aim of training them in different skills. Through that process, five of us – two females and three males – were given employment by one of the financial institutions in the country as telephone operators. One day, I received a call. As usual, as a polite and well-trained telephone operator, I answered the call. The man on the phone said, 'My God, your voice is so sweet, can I come and see you please? And who should I say I need to see?' I told him how he could find me. One hour later, he was there at the counter; he called for me. When I stood up to go and see him, I introduced myself and he was kind of shocked to see the woman with a beautiful voice but disabled. I saw the disappointment on his face. He did not stay long and went back to his office and called me again and said, 'Is it really you that I saw when I came at the bank?' Obviously, this man is not alone. Societal attitudes toward disabled people are still negative up to this day, although they are gradually changing.

Four years down the line, I was not satisfied with the work of answering phones. I enrolled for evening classes with the Malawi Polytechnic to train as a secretary. I qualified a year later and I wrote a letter to my employers asking them to upgrade me from the telephone operator to a secretary position. It took seven years for my employers to consider me for that position. They looked at the physical impairment and not my ability. Later on, the company was going through a restructuring process and it decided to retrench me. Jeremiah 29 vs 11 as indicated earlier declares: 'For I know the plans I have for you,' declares the LORD, 'plans to prosper you and not to harm you, plans to give you *hope* and a *future*' (my emphasis). God had a totally different plan for my life. My life was in that bank! In my mind, I could not see the other door that God had opened when the door of the bank closed in my face. It was just a matter of me getting out of the bank's door and entering the other door that God had opened. I never thought that there was life after the bank. So, at times, we need to be moved out of our comfort zone in order to see the greener side of our lives, and this is what happened to me.

Soon after walking out of the bank's premises, the Ministry of Persons with Disabilities was in the process of developing a disability policy document and reviewing the Malawi Council for the Handicapped Act of 1971. I was in the taskforce of drafting that policy. This process kept me busy as it required the Committee to travel across the three regions of Malawi to consult on the policy and the Act. I was also kept busy with the work at Southern Africa Federation of the Disabled (SAFOD). SAFOD is an umbrella organisation in the SADC region, it advocates for the rights of persons with disabilities, as well as nurturing and strengthening its affiliates and other stakeholders in the region. This is to ensure the promotion of inclusive development and human rights of persons with disabilities in the SADC region. I was the first SAFOD female chairperson, from 2002–2007; thus breaking the 16-year circle of male dominance within the organisation. I was also re-elected in 2015 as chairperson.

My relationship

When you are a disabled person, it is not easy to have a relationship, let alone raise a family. Society has a strong belief that marrying a disabled person is a taboo. Thus, most people in Malawi, and I guess in other parts of Africa and beyond, believe that children born to this type of marriage will also become disabled. By the way, I am a happily married woman with my own children. I know people would want to know more about how I met my husband and I am glad to share that with the readers.

We met at Scripture Union Retreat. Prior to that, we did not know each other. He told me that as we were in the conference, he heard the voice telling him that I am the one to replace his late wife; but he said he refused to listen to this voice. However, the voice became stronger and stronger up until he felt like his heart wanted to burst. He left for his room and prayed a prayer of acceptance and he felt relieved. From there, he came back and at tea break, he came to me and asked me jokingly if I know how to make tea. So I thought he wanted me to make tea for him. That is how it all started and the rest is history.

I remember very well that after my husband proposed to me, whenever he came to see me at the office people would be calling each other to come and see the man who had proposed to a disabled woman. Some were asking me directly how and where I met him and whether there were no other women there who were not disabled women he could propose to. Even his relatives were not happy. I remember it took my father-in-law three years to come to my house. One day he came and he welcomed me as his daughter-in-law. This shows how attitudes can change for the better as long as people begin to understand and appreciate disability issues and the capabilities [and limitations] of disabled people. My marriage has been a blessed one and we are a happy couple together, if I can blow my own trumpet!

My source of inspiration

One key to becoming successful is to admire people who have been successful. Some of the people I admire and who have been a source of encouragement to me include Joni Erickson Tada, an American. I have read her book where she talks about her life, the way she became disabled, and what she went through and how God has raised her up to achieve a lot in life despite her impairment. She was involved in a diving accident in 1967, which left her without the use of all her four limbs (quadriplegia) and a wheelchair user. She is an internationally known mouth artist, a talented vocalist, a radio host, the author of 17 books and an advocate of disabled people worldwide. The way she struggled to accept God's design in her paralysis inspired me. Proverbs 27 verse 19 says: 'A mirror reflects a man's face, but what he really is, is shown by the kind of friends he chooses.' Therefore, it comes as no surprise that she is my source of inspiration, as she is a wheelchair user.

Many times I ask myself, who am I to be brilliant, gorgeous, talented and fabulous? Actually, I should be asking myself, 'Who am I not to be?' I am a child of God who knew my destiny as per God's plan (Proverbs 29 v11); hence playing small does not serve the world. I have no doubt that I was born for a purpose, just like each one of us. The important step is for every one of us to identify our purpose of being on earth. As I let my own light shine, I unconsciously give other people permission to do the same. As I am liberated from my own fears, my presence automatically liberates others; hence, everyone needs to do the same.

There came a time when I felt that things were not going well in the disability sector and I became disappointed and made up my mind to quit. I thank God because my husband encouraged and advised me to keep on. I also pay tribute to a few people who were, and are, a source of encouragement to me. There have been moments when I have wanted to quit because of the pressure, intimidation, insults and slanderous remarks from my fellow disabled people. I felt that enough is enough, I should just quit. I remember Fred Mzoma saying: 'Rachel, do not quit, it is better for you keeping on fighting while you are still inside, because the moment you are outside the movement, your voice will never be heard.'

My husband, Gibson, Fred Mzoma, Mussa Chiwaula and the late Alexander Phiri have been the central pillars of my life and success. Therefore, I told myself that I will focus on my dream. My dream is for disabled people to live in a nation that embraces equality and equity. These people remind me of a story in the Bible about Moses when he was fighting his enemies. When Moses raised his hands up, there was victory on his side, but when he got tired and dropped his hands, his side was defeated. So there were two men who held his hands up when he got tired. In so doing, they conquered the enemy. I have cherished this support and encouragement that these four men have given me, hence the saying: 'He who walks with wise men will be wise, but the companion of fools will suffer harm.'

In November 2006, my sister was admitted to a referral hospital after she fell sick. As I was going to visit her, I met two pastors from our church who were amazed at seeing me in a wheelchair. They greeted me and my husband. They specifically asked me how I was feeling and when I responded that I was fine, they asked why I was in a wheelchair and if I was okay. Even the church has problems with disabled people. When I entered the hospital, the nurse at the hospital enquired which ward was I admitted in. I responded that I was not a patient, but that I was visiting my sister who was admitted. Then she said, 'But you are in the wheelchair'. I said yes, this wheelchair is for my mobility. Again, the assumption that all disabled people are 'sick' and they need medical attention, is still ingrained in most people.

One thing that I have learned in life is that we should never ever undermine each other because you never know another's destiny. I never knew that my country was watching what I had been doing in promoting the rights of disabled people. In 2004, I was given an Award by the Malawi Human Rights Commission for championing the rights of disabled people. In 2008, I was also given a Diversity Leadership Award for my achievements. In 2013, I was appointed as Minister for Disability and Elderly Affairs. One interesting thing is that I was appointed not because I was affiliated to the party, but because of my expertise in disability issues.

As I indicated earlier, I broke the record in 2002 when I was elected the first woman to the position of SAFOD chairperson. I have twice been deputy chairperson of the Disabled People's International (DPI) and in 2015 I became the chairperson. I am also the secretary of the board of the Africa Disability Forum (ADF) as well as the founder and executive director for the Disabled Women in Africa. It is these milestones that keep me energised and I know the sky is the limit. As a disability activist, I have dedicated my life to breaking institutional, physical and societal barriers that prevent disabled people from living their lives like other citizens. My conviction is that every individual has got the right to be treated equally and discrimination resulting from, for example, gender, social status, race, age, illness and impairment, should not be used to exclude people in accessing services or participating in community and national development processes. It is my hope to live in a society where diversity is embraced and every individual is treated with dignity and respect. My favourite Bible verse from the Book of Jeremiah, chapter 29 verse 11 – 'For I know the plans I have for you' keeps the flame in me burning to ensure that I do my part to ensure that this world becomes more inclusive. I am glad that I am living a purpose-driven life.

28

CONCLUDING REMARKS AND FUTURE DIRECTION

Tsitsi Chataika

Introduction

This chapter brings the handbook to a conclusion by drawing lessons, challenges and opportunities proposed by various authors. Key to this conclusive chapter, is the need to reflect on how each chapter feeds into the sustainable development agenda, which is the focus of this handbook, and how the conclusions can inform future directions (i.e. policy and practice), with possible implications for improved livelihoods of disabled people in the southern African region and beyond. Hence, links and connections from each chapter that promote sustainable inclusive development in southern Africa are identified. Also, gaps have been identified in this handbook and suggestions of closing them down have been outlined. Areas for further research have been recommended, which can potentially promote disability inclusion in southern Africa.

Concluding remarks and the way forward

It is argued in this handbook that poverty and disability reinforce each other, contributing to increased vulnerability and exclusion (WHO & World Bank, 2011). The authors are in agreement with existing evidence that exclusion in one area of life can have negative repercussions in other areas (Mitra, Posarac & Vick, 2013; Groce, Kett, Lang & Trani, 2011; WHO & World Bank, 2011). It is also evident that disability manifests itself through the interaction of individuals with impairments with attitudinal, environmental and institutional barriers imposed by society (Bruijn et al., 2012; Wapling & Downie, 2012; WHO & World Bank, 2011). This is unfortunate since nearly one billion disabled people in the world, with the majority of them in the global South, struggle to access education, employment and health services (WHO & World Bank, 2011). Consequently, new ways of thinking about disability have provided a platform to shift spaces and reorient the planning of environments in ways that build a culture of support, raise awareness to overcome stigma, change belief and value systems and generate organisational commitment to disability-inclusive policies and practices. Thus, the debate on disability is likely to be raised to the next level by engaging key people on issues policy and programme implementation.

Interesting in this book is how the seven parts and the individual chapters feed into each other as the book progresses. The next subsections provide conclusions and recommendations drawn from each section.

Part I: Disability inclusion and sustainable development

Part I mapped out key conceptual, theoretical and disciplinary domains or spaces within the disability and development agenda. It focused on issues of disability inclusion with implications for policy and practice and promoting inclusive sustainable development. In Chapter 2, Koistinen reflected upon the experiences and practices based on the work of Disability Partnership Finland (DPF) on disability mainstreaming since 2013, using case studies drawn mainly from Malawi and Mozambique. She argued that disabled people have been largely invisible in poverty-reduction programmes and in the development agenda. Hence, the continued invisibility of disabled people by national governments and international development agencies remains one of the great gaps in poverty-reduction efforts (Groce, 2011).

Focusing on work done in Malawi and Mozambique, Koistinen argued that the development agenda has started embracing disability inclusion in line with the global vision, with the aim of creating a world where no one is left behind. It is this kind of world that would allow disabled people to participate equally and equitably in community, national and interventional development activities. She further argued that disability mainstreaming is still rather new as an approach for many organisations as they are taking their first steps toward disability inclusion. Hence, monitoring and evaluation of this progress is critical. Koistinen emphasises the need for collecting and sharing good practices on disability mainstreaming, an aspect that other authors have also proposed (Coe & Wapling, 2010; Bruijn, 2013; van Veen, 2014). Documenting such success stories might assist development partners in coming up with development programmes and tools that can benefit disabled people and their diverse needs in the global South. Koistinen emphasised that no sustainable development initiative can afford to leave disabled people at the periphery of its agenda, if the SDGs are to be achieved in southern Africa and beyond.

In Chapter 3, Sefuthi and Sekoankoetla reflect on the development of the disability mainstreaming plan in Lesotho. They argued that a successful partnership between disabled people's organisations (DPOs) and policy makers marks a major achievement in any national development initiative. However, they noted that disability activists and DPOs should be capacitated on disability mainstreaming in order to convince the government about the need to develop the national disability mainstreaming plans (Wazakili *et al.*, 2011). Sefuthi and Sekoankoetla emphasised that in the process of disability mainstreaming, all stakeholders should be involved in order to ensure that all citizens, including disabled people, are part of the national development processes. However, they observed that many government officials are not aware of disability issues and perhaps do not have enough time to learn about disability inclusion and mainstreaming. Hence, the development of the disability mainstreaming plans could be delayed and/or hampered due to lack of awareness and lack of capacity to deal with such processes (Wazakili *et al.*, 2011). Hence, DPOs and their allies become crucial in raising disability awareness and also to provide the government with full support toward the development of a national disability mainstreaming plan. Second, it should be indicated from the very beginning that disability mainstreaming does not only require specialist expertise but, rather, political will (Chataika, 2012). Key to the whole process is to understand disability as a human rights and development issue rather than a social welfare issue (WHO & World Bank, 2011). Thus, it requires intensive advocacy, lobbying and time to change the mindset of policy makers for them to view disability as a human right, cross-cutting and development agenda.

In Chapter 4, Chivandikwa analysed the unrecognised (and private) resistive powers or 'hidden transcripts' (Scott, 1985, 1990) of young disabled people and how this power and agency can be nurtured and appropriated for transition into the public domain (resistive public transcript) in Theatre for Development (TfD) discourses. He argued that the 'hidden transcripts' as resistance are necessary for the liberation and self-construction of disabled young people in publicly challenging their oppression and marginalisation.

From his case study, Chivandikwa argued that it is important for facilitators to inspire, motivate and challenge disabled participants intellectually in order to access and engender forms of radical resistance which can give them the skills and confidence to challenge 'grand truths' at the public level. This challenging of 'grand truths' can happen in preliminary and surrounding events such as meetings, workshops and informal research processes.

Chivandikwa noted that it is important to gain the trust and confidence of disabled participants in order to access what goes on 'backstage'. Also, the activities and events that take place before the 'actual' theatre work are valuable sites in which to access and nurture coherent and organised forms of private resistance. Another aspect is that since 'hidden transcripts' are not 'perfect', it is important for the facilitator to expose disabled participants in TfD to radical disability discourses to equip them intellectually and socio-politically for the public confrontation with power-laden dominating discourses and practices that denigrate their embodied lived experiences. To a large extent, this transitional phase, or 'restricted public transcript', equipped disabled students to come up with ideologically, intellectually, aesthetically and socio-politically engaging public theatre productions which defiantly challenged disability oppression.

Chapter 5 presented experiences from South Africa, Mozambique, Zimbabwe and Angola. Here, Irvine focused on the development and implementation of policies aimed at increasing the social inclusion of disabled people during conflict transformation. Thus, she explored the relationship between the inclusion of disabled people and sustainable communities by focusing on the experiences of societies that have undergone conflict transformation in southern Africa. Four key similarities have been identified in the experiences of conflict transformation in southern Africa: the role of the disability rights movement in challenging the status quo; the importance of participatory decision-making; the need to build capacity for not just people with disabilities, but also for their families, organisations, communities, and decision-makers; and that introducing policies is not enough to ensure the realisation of equal rights (African Union, 2018).

Irvine noted that in all of the four countries, the organisation of disability rights activists has a distinct impact on the political recognition of disability within the redevelopment of state and society. She emphasised the need for the participation of disabled people as a key component of building sustainable communities. It is against this background that Irvine argued for the development of the capacity of disabled people in order to enable them to participate in meaningful ways in inclusive development processes (WHO & World Bank, 2011).

From this chapter, there are areas of building sustainable communities in which little evidence on the participation of disabled people has been found. For instance, Irvine noted that environmental concerns are rarely connected to the disability rights movements and there is widespread failure to plan for not just the current needs of citizens with disabilities, but also their future needs. Irvine emphasised the need to do better at building more inclusive post-conflict communities, as none of the experiences demonstrated a clear, sustainable model. Despite the opportunities for change located within policy and legislative reform, there seems to be a failure to capitalise on the opportunities for implementation. Limited financial resources, international pressures, national tensions and competing interests have been identified as the inhibiting factors. Hence, the need to think more creatively about how countries can build sustainable communities that can thrive and, at the same time, acknowledging disabled people as full and equal citizens (African Union, 2018).

In Chapter 6, Manhique and Giannoumis considered accessibility as a precondition for enjoying all other substantive rights as prescribed by the CRPD (United Nations, 2006).

They examined the experiences of persons with disabilities in Mozambique in relation to CRPD the SDGs. They concluded that ICT is an important tool for the social inclusion of disabled people. However, the results also suggest that the design of, and access to, ICT prevents persons with disabilities in Mozambique from using it, with implications for their participation in public life. In addition, the current approach to ICT legislation is yet to address ICT accessibility for disabled people in Mozambique. Hence, Manhique and Giannoumis proposed a holistic approach to examining ICT accessibility, which combines an investigation of both social regulations and redistributive policies if disabled people are to fully participate in national development in Mozambique. This is because accessible ICT is effective in addressing the concerns of individuals facing social exclusion, lowers employment barriers, enhances learning experiences and decreases skill gaps between the average user and those with unique needs (G3ict, 2017). Accordingly, Article 9 of the CRPD requires Member States to ensure that technology design takes into account accessibility and usability features (United Nations, 2006). This is meant to protect and promote the human rights of disabled people in all policies and programmes. It is from this understanding that Manhique and Giannoumis propose a holistic approach to examining ICT accessibility in order to ensure that diverse needs of disabled people are addressed.

Part II: Access to education

In Part II, authors discussed issues of access to education of disabled people from early childhood to secondary education. They have provided evidence suggesting that existing education systems in southern Africa are not accommodative and responsive to the diverse needs of all learners, especially children with disabilities. Hence, disabled people cannot reap the benefits of the expanded services to all citizens due to the inadequacy of support systems. This is because several factors are contributing to the non-inclusion of disabled children and these are embedded in attitudinal, environmental (physical and communication) and institutional (policy and programming) barriers (Chataika, 2012). The British Council Ethiopia director indicated that the British Council believes that the inclusion of children and young people with disabilities in mainstream education systems of their respective countries is an entitlement and a fundamental human right (Brown, 2018). He also emphasised that if the inclusion of such groups is to be successful and sustainable, then it must be predicated on an approach that is achievable, empowering, and based on a thorough and sensitive understanding of the current context of the particular school and education system. The commitment to developing inclusive practice therefore requires a multi-tiered response that addresses policy, practice and culture at all levels within the education system (Brown, 2018).

Peta's Chapter 7 explored the extent to which disabled women accessed early childhood education during their early years. It is deliberate to expand on this chapter as no other chapter has addressed early childhood education. Considering challenges that surround early childhood learning for children with disabilities, Peta noted that it is evident that some families might find themselves stuck, unable to find appropriate early childhood education centres within their communities. Consequently, they live with the guilt of keeping their disabled children at home or delaying such enrolment until the children are of primary school going age or beyond. Yet, children's learning is cumulative and early childhood education determines future learning outcomes (Moore, 2014).

Peta's concern is that the early childhood education sector is likely to be infiltrated by opportunists, who set up sub-standard centres in order to cash in on desperate parents. Hence, she recommended that the Ministry of Primary and Secondary Education should establish machinery that conducts periodic checks on the status of all private and public early education centres. Also, the delivery of the curriculum, staff and well-being of the children should be supervised. Teachers who are capable of catering for children with and without disabilities should be appointed if there are chances of realising positive learning outcomes and child development. It becomes important to ensure the capacity development of teachers to ensure that they competently address the diverse needs of all learners (Howell, McKenzie & Chataika, 2018).

Peta challenged the Ministry of Primary and Secondary Education to re-examine the broader aspects of inclusion in early childhood education and pay more attention to key aspects such as support, access and participation. In line with Moore (2014), educational policy and practice should stretch beyond professional development, to include appropriate implementation of inclusive practices that support disabled children. It becomes necessary to consciously create support platforms, upon which opportunities for collaboration and communication between families and educational staff can take place to ensure high-quality early childhood education. Also, access can be achieved by offering a diversity of environments and activities, which cater for the needs of all children including disabled children. Both physical and attitudinal barriers ought to be dealt with, within contexts that offer different and multiple ways of promoting early childhood learning and development to ensure effective participation. Also, Peta emphasised the need for the creation and sustenance of early childhood programmes that use different mediums of instruction, so as to promote engagement of disabled children with disabilities in inclusive learning and playing environments.

With regard to policy, Peta recommended that all stakeholders need to raise awareness about the value of early childhood education to all children, including disabled children. Such awareness will enable families and communities in both rural and urban areas to realise the need for including children in such programmes. The involvement of families and communities is an acknowledgement that children do not live in isolation; the well-being of the children's families is likely to enhance the success of the children's learning experience, which is evidently linked to the home environment (McKenzie & Chataika, 2018). Families need to realise that having any form of impairment does not mean that a child should start school later than his or her non-disabled peers. It becomes imperative to ensure that the government's two years of early childhood education are more inclusive in order to ensure that disabled children's needs are also addressed (UNESCO, 2006). Such an approach tends to promote holistic development of children and allows them to be ready for formal education.

Children enrolled at early childhood education centres could be assessed at the beginning of the year by a transdisciplinary team of practitioners. This is a step further from Peta's suggestion of a multidisciplinary team. Thus, a transdisciplinary team is one in which members come together from the beginning to jointly communicate, exchange ideas and work together to come up with solutions to problems (Davies, 2007). This is contradictory to the famous multidisciplinary team, in which members use their individual expertise to first develop their own answers to a given problem and then come together, bringing their individually developed ideas to formulate a solution (King *et al.*, 2009). This is because disabled children have complex needs that usually require the expertise and knowledge of different professionals. Unfortunately, the reality of providing services across multiple disciplines sometimes means that the child receives fragmented services. This fragmented service might not translate into functional outcomes for disabled children since goal attainment might not be generalised across people, materials and settings. Hence, the transdisciplinary approach integrates a child's developmental needs across the major developmental domains and involves a greater degree of collaboration than other service delivery models (Davies, 2007).

The primary purpose of this approach is to pool and integrate the expertise of team members so that more efficient and comprehensive assessment and intervention services can be provided. The communication style in this type of team involves continuous give-and-take between all members (especially with the parents) on a regular, planned basis. Professionals from different disciplines teach, learn and work together to accomplish a common set of intervention goals for a child and family (King *et al.*, 2009; Davis, 2007). The role differentiation between disciplines is defined by the needs of the situation rather than by discipline-specific characteristics. Assessment, intervention and evaluation are carried out jointly by designated members of the team. This teamwork usually results in a decrease in the number of professionals who interact with the child on a daily basis.

A detailed assessment report would then be used to determine the child's needs, including their unique educational needs. Considering that UNESCO (2006) recommends a holistic approach that integrates educational activities with additional services such as nutrition, health and social services, the involvement of transdisciplinary teams would go a long way in offering a wholesome early childhood education programme, which eases the transition into primary school. In any case, early development of a child begins from birth to school-entering age. Therefore, a full package with more benefit for early childhood education programmes would yield more results (Davies, 2007).

In resonance with the above assertion, King *et al.* (2009) argue that the multidimensional nature of early childhood learning calls for the removal of barriers among separate domains if the comprehensive nature of child development is to be effectively attended to. The Ministry of Primary and Secondary Education should consider the establishment of a holistic policy, which directs synergy of education, nutrition, health and social welfare so as to provide a wholesome supportive and rich experience for all children, including children with disabilities. However, while there is growing international interest in the early learning of children, the topic of early childhood education of disabled children is minimally researched within the global South. Hence, Peta calls upon interdisciplinary scholars to undertake further research on this valuable topic, particularly within African contexts.

In Chapter 8, Musengi and Nyangairi analysed the inclusion of deaf children in mainstream and special secondary schools in Zimbabwe. They examined the evolution of the concept of the least restrictive environment with particular focus on deaf learners. It is evident from this chapter that inclusive education should not only be about placement, but also participation in the learning process. Also, the practice of inclusive education for deaf children should enable not just their physical access to schools, but also access to the mainstream curriculum regardless of whether this occurs in mainstream or special schools, aspects that are also raised in Chapter 15.

Musengi and Nyangairi established that resource units for deaf pupils that were created in mainstream schools seem not to meet the criteria of 'schools for all' as there is inadequate training of teachers in Sign Language, shortage of Sign Language materials and financial resources. They argue that such inadequacies need to be addressed by government in order to create school environments suitable for the education of deaf children in both mainstream and special schools. It also emerged that deaf school-leavers from both mainstream and special school settings were dissatisfied by their educational experiences. This implies that the educational setting itself does not make education inclusive or discriminatory. What makes education inclusive are practices that make academic content accessible (United Nations, 2006). The authors noted that reverse inclusion in special schools for deaf pupils should be judged to be inclusive only if there is optimal learning by both hearing and deaf pupils.

In Chapter 9, through an analysis of survey and qualitative data of the Zambia disability study conducted in 2015, Azalde *et al.* used the International Classification of Functioning, Disability and Health (ICF) model in changing the discourse of disability to promote inclusive education in Zambia. They argued that by viewing functioning as continuous, and in interaction with its surroundings, the ICF model can help create opportunities and enabling environments in schools to ensure that all children learn to their potential regardless of vulnerability.

In Chapter 10, Gweme and Chataika examined the effectiveness of the special class model in improving the learning outcomes of primary school children with specific learning difficulties in Hwange urban in Zimbabwe. They noted several factors that either facilitate or hinder its effectiveness. Such factors include the understanding of the special class model, eligibility of learners and challenges in implementing the model. These have implications for learning outcomes of children with specific learning difficulties. The authors highlighted the lack of understanding of the special class model among teachers, parents and learners, thus compromising its good intentions. Negative attitudes, lack of understanding and the selection of learners have adversely affected the implementation of the special class model. Hence, the need to raise awareness and capacitate teachers, parents and learners so that such a class is not labelled so that it does not work against improving learning outcomes (Howell *et al.*, 2018). Gweme and Chataika believe that a larger scale study that evaluates the effectiveness of this model, would allow policy makers and implementers to come up with more effective ways of supporting learners with specific learning difficulties.

Part III: Inclusion in higher education

Part III brought out the challenges, opportunities and threats faced by disabled students in accessing higher education in southern Africa. Riddell, Tinklin and Wilson (2005) argue that having a university qualification is a gateway to professional employment, the underrepresentation of disabled people in higher education underlines an immense social injustice still existing in the current education system. Hence, Chapter 11 focused on disability and higher education in southern Africa. Matshedisho noted that southern Africa is trying to recognise disability rights in general; it has an opportunity to learn from challenges of other disability rights movements elsewhere. He suggested the need to attend to these challenges by raising the profile of disability rights and services in southern Africa.

In Chapter 12, Pretorius, Bell and Healey presented the current state of inclusion within South African higher and further education institutions, focusing on access and reasonable accommodation in order to promote equity and inclusion. They allowed disabled students to share their lived experiences in higher education. Although they acknowledged some progress has been made in disability inclusion, they argued that a consolidated framework needs to be implemented in the sector in order to ensure and regulate access, equality and full inclusion of all South African disabled students. They also noted a gap in the transition of disabled students to the labour market after graduation that has not been addressed and recommended it as an interesting area for further research.

Part IV: Disability, employment, entrepreneurship and CBR

Part IV addressed the employment and entrepreneurship issues affecting disabled people and the relevance of community-based rehabilitation (CBR) in promoting sustainable development. In Chapter 13, Ntinda *et al.* drew lessons from several southern African countries to argue for CBR as a preferred development strategy in promoting disability-inclusive social development. They argued for the implementation of socially inclusive CBR development strategies that promote full participation of disabled people. Such disability-inclusive community development strategies are likely to create and sustain structures that optimise the participation of disabled people, rather than expecting them to fit in within pre-defined arrangements (WHO & World Bank, 2011). Also, the authors argued for the collaboration of government and civil society in the design and delivery of community development initiatives where disabled people can actively contribute. Such partnership forms a basis for any successful CBR programme. Ntinda *et al.* also recommended resourcing CBR for sustainable development in the SADC region through inter-organisational, intra-organisational and social organisation for the appropriation of national resources. To them, this kind of resourcing prioritises the interests and well-being of average citizens, including disabled people.

In Chapter 14 Charema explored options of self-employment, entrepreneurship and sustainable development among disabled people, drawing examples from southern African countries. This is because disabled people are marginalised and have limited access to education, transportation, vocational training, employment, decent living and good medical health services (WHO & World Bank, 2011). He examined the roles of the governments, educational institutions, vocational and industrial institutions. Charema established some socio-economic factors that are likely to impact on disabled people's livelihoods, as well as challenges they face that expose them to social and employment discrimination. He argued that with proper planning and government support the process of consumer empowerment and the impact of the entrepreneurship programmes on the lives of disabled people can benefit the country and individuals involved. This is because there is dignity in work, which contributes to an individual's self-worth and self-respect and offers a sense of purpose and accomplishment. Charema recommended the establishment and implementation of entrepreneurship programmes in high schools, institutions of higher learning, vocational centres and training institutions as a way of addressing unemployment among disabled people.

In Chapter 15, Mutswanga, explored the role of guidance and counselling in empowering deaf people to have realistic hopes and aspirations for socio-economic sustainable development. Deaf students' responses reflect a high mismatch between pursued subjects and desired vocational interests. She also revealed that district career guidance days were of less help in informing deaf students to have realistic hopes and aspirations. Mutswanga also established the need for robust and fully funded policies which mandate positions of career guidance counsellors. She further recommended Zimbabwe's Ministry of Education of Primary and Secondary Education to engage skilled counsellors if the produced scholars are to meaningfully contribute to the socio-economic developments of the country. Mutswanga also recommends the use of visual guidance such as Becker's (1988) *Reading-Free Vocational Interest Inventory*, where deaf individuals identify their vocational choices using pictures from an informed background through counselling interventions. Such procedures are likely to empower all people in selecting their career paths and produce a marketable workforce for Africa where everyone is included in sustainable socio-economic development matters.

Part V: Religion, gender and parenthood

In Part V, parenthood, gender and religion were discussed to illustrate how they intersect with disability, resulting in the exclusion of disabled people; hence, the importance of promoting inclusive sustainable development. Chapter 16 explored how the interpretation of Judaeo-Christian and African Traditional religio-cultural traditions can impact on the well-being of disabled people in Zimbabwe. Machingura advocated for a liberative approach to indigenous traditions, biblical traditions, biblical texts, beliefs and practices on disability. He also engaged and interrogated cultural beliefs that fuel the negative beliefs and practices toward disabled people. Machingura's main argument is that all human rights initiatives come to nought if men and women of God or religious practitioners in their 'holy talks, spaces, places, platforms and scriptures', do not interrogate certain cultural, religious beliefs, practices and teachings where disability is taken as a sign of sin, curses, disobedience, evil spirits, demons and witchcraft. He recommended that the broader mainstream society must be conscientised on the beauty and strength that nations have the moment there is an inclusive society that is built on honesty, trust and respect of all members including disabled people. Religions, civic organisations and government should create an inclusive environment that gives hope to the excluded, vulnerable, disfranchised, disabled people and women. Religions, traditions, beliefs, history and culture are always changing because they are dynamic; the changes must also influence the way we look at and understand disability. Thus, culture, tradition and religion should assist in bringing respect, inclusiveness, equality and dignity to all people and avoid any disabling texts that undermine disabled people.

In Chapter 17, Lehtomäki, Okkolin and Matonya examined the global approaches, processes and (policy) frameworks on disability and gender, focusing on similarities and differences over decades and how they intersect. They focused on what can be learned by looking at the intersection, rather than individual dimensions as independent entities in order to improve and implement enabling inclusive development initiatives. Their argument is that by analysing disability and gender together as intersecting issues in education (Chataika, 2013), research can better inform policy and practice about critical factors in development toward equality and equity with the southern African region and probably beyond.

The authors have argued that both gender-inclusive and disability-inclusive developments call for engaged approaches, while the interface of gender and disability seriously challenges education development. They also recommended multiple types of evidence and perspectives of all stakeholders, such as families, persons with disabilities, men and women with disabilities to ensure that quality education is provided for all. There is an emphasis on stakeholders' participation both in service development as well as data collection being essential for ensuring equality of conditions, equality of experience and institutions' commitment to non-discrimination. Thus, through engagement in the development processes and evidence production, stakeholders should use their capabilities and freedoms to grow agency that is needed for sustainability of equality, equity and inclusion in education.

Rugoho and Maphosa discussed the factors that have caused women with disabilities to remain at the periphery of society in Zimbabwe in Chapter 18. They attributed institutionalised discrimination and the weakness of the disability movement as the major factors responsible for the marginalisation of disabled women (Chataika, 2013). The interrogation of legal instruments on gender and disability and their level of implementation (or non-implementation), to some extent, seem to contribute to the perpetuation of the marginalisation of disabled women. They concluded the chapter by proffering some recommendations on how women with disabilities achieve self-representation in development processes. These include the need to clearly spell out the rights of disabled women in the Constitution, policy makers taking a leading role in promoting the rights of disabled women and giving them access to the means of production. The authors also emphasise that decision-making bodies should adopt a quota system so as to guarantee the inclusion of disabled women in all areas of development and access to services.

In Chapter 19, Neille explored the experiences of disabled people in the establishment and maintenance of long-term intimate relationships and their experiences of pregnancy and child-rearing with disabled adults with various impairments in rural South Africa. She established that contextual and stereotypical beliefs regarding sexuality among disabled people, together with a high incidence of violence, negatively impact on identity development. These results highlight the need for contextually relevant information which supports freedom of choice, while at the same time, protecting disabled people from becoming victims of violence. Neille argues for a need to evaluate ways in which human rights policies are put into practice and the extent to which they relate to contextual beliefs pertaining to disability, intimacy and parenthood. She is also concerned that limited research into this field has resulted in narrow understandings of the challenges and experiences of disabled people in establishing resilient identities where they are able to enjoy rights to freedom and equality in all spheres of life. Neille believes that incorporating these issues into research serves to acknowledge and validate the reality of living with impairments in rural areas.

Part VI: Tourism, sports and accessibility

In Part VI, authors have challenged discrimination of disabled people in tourism and sports and suggested ways of increasing accessibility with a view to increasing participation in recreational activities. In Chapter 20, Chikuta and Kabote explored policies related to disability and tourism in four southern African countries (Botswana, Zambia, Zimbabwe and South Africa). The common element within these countries, as in most low-income countries, is lack of implementation and enforcement framework (Wazakili *et al.*, 2011; WHO & World Bank, 2011). Without properly laid down policies and pieces of legislation on disability and tourism, implementation becomes difficult. The authors challenged southern African countries to take disability issues seriously if disabled people's needs are to be addressed. Of concern in this chapter is that in all the tourism policies discussed, there is little or no mention of disability issues. However, legal documents developed in these countries since the 1960s, have helped shape organisational mandates to serve disabled people by offering tailor-made services.

Khumalo, van Heerden and Skalko's Chapter 21 is informed by a survey conducted on wheelchair basketball facilities in selected Zimbabwean cities. They investigated the levels of adaptation of facilities toward standards for use by people with mobility impairments. The authors established that the majority of the expected features fall short of the specifications or are non-existent. They emphasised the need to understand the difference between universal design and accessible design, aspects that are likely to be misunderstood by builders, developers and policy makers (Watchorn *et al.*, 2014). They recommended the need for educating those responsible for designing and constructing buildings and sports facilities, the disabled people's needs and the fundamentals of universal design. They also urged central and local governments to adopt a universal design approach, by ensuring that construction plans clearly show how people with a range of impairments are accommodated in sports facilities. Also colleges and universities offering architectural studies need to include universal design studies in their courses in order to ensure that graduates are more accommodative to the diverse needs of all people engaging in sporting activities. It is evident that if recommendations proffered in this chapter are adopted, then both the concept of universal design and accessible design could be exploited, thus increasing the uptake of sports by disabled people.

In Chapter 22, Linegar, Giljam, McDonald and Walters illustrated how mobile outreach seating clinics, run by trained seating practitioners, can increase the access of children with posture-support needs to assistive equipment and holistic services close to where they live. They shared internal reflections of Shonaquip's holistic model of service delivery that has evolved over 25 years' experience in diverse contexts and communities across South Africa. It is evident that an appropriate wheelchair is widely recognised to be a fundamental right and an important pre-requisite for the participation, health and well-being of a person with mobility impairment (Vergunst, 2016). When accompanied by sustainable seating services, and supported by empowered parents, skilled carers and a disability-aware community, the authors argue that each child is better placed to develop, learn and flourish as a valued member of their community. In upholding the rights of disabled children, the authors believe that it enables communities to be more inclusive and barrier free (Sherry, 2015).

Part VII: Narratives from disability activists

In Part VII, disability activists shared vivid personal stories on how they face and deal with exclusionary practices in their daily lives and the coping mechanisms they use to overcome exclusion. My argument for including this section is based on the notion that narratives give our lives meaning. It is only through narratives that oppressed people resist by identifying themselves as subjects, by defining their reality, shaping their own identity, naming their history and telling their story (Walker, 2004).

In Chapter 23, Sithole walked with us the journey of her life as a disabled person, which has given her both positive and negative experiences in society. Being partially sighted has allowed her to view the world through the lens of sighted and blind people. She has experienced the stigma and discrimination faced by blind people, as well as experiencing the frustration that sighted people face in trying to understand blind people. This story is about her personal experiences in both worlds of sightedness and blindness. It is an expression of her hope and desire that the misunderstandings and lack of trust between the two worlds can be cleared when each group makes a deliberate effort to understand each other. Sithole concludes by challenging the two worlds to work together for the development of humanity.

Chidemo, Chindimba and Matongo's Chapter 24 is based on their journey of starting up a disability advocacy television programme, *Action Power*, in Zimbabwe. They share their successes, lessons learned, challenges and what lies ahead in their quest to ensure that the rights of disabled people in general, and deaf people in particular, are upheld in Zimbabwe.

In Chapter 25, Masendeke explained the steps that he took toward the building of an accessible house that meets his impairment-specific requirements, which is a first of its kind in Zimbabwe. Masendeke unpacked Article 19 of the CRPD (United Nations, 2006), which focuses on disabled people's right to live independently and being included in the community. He argued that disabled people should have the opportunity to choose their own place of residence, including where and with whom they should live on an equal basis with others. However, due to the scarcity of disability-friendly or accessible houses in Zimbabwe, Masendeke argued that securing appropriate accommodation is a major challenge for disabled people and their families. Hence, part of his advocacy work is on promoting the building of accessible houses in Zimbabwe in order to ensure that disabled people's right to accessible shelter is addressed.

In Chapter 26, Mateta believes that no one is born an activist. However, life gives us various challenges and how we respond to those challenges often creates what kind of people we end up becoming. He shared a story that was his turning point as a Zimbabwean blind person and how it defined the kind of activism that he has taken for the past ten years, as well as some of the work that he is currently doing as an activist. In Chapter 27, Kachaje emphasised that addressing attitudes people have toward disabled people should be an ongoing process, which starts in the family and spreads to the community. She takes us on a journey through her personal experiences as a disabled woman in Malawi; her challenges, achievements and how she has managed to live a purpose-driven life. The narratives in this section serve to make us realise that disability issues are best achieved through understanding how life is perceived by those experiencing stigmatisation and exclusion (Chataika, 2005). It then becomes apparent for us to pay more attention to the voices of disabled people and ensure that they are a formidable part of decision-making processes in families, communities and national development processes.

Conclusion

It is my hope that readers find this handbook engaging and challenging. I also hope it opens up spaces for critical thought, research and practice in southern Africa and beyond. This handbook is neither complete nor comprehensive, but I feel that a complex and diverse thematic area such as disability perhaps never can be, particularly in southern Africa. Having said this, I hope that this project is one step toward an ongoing quest of amplifying the traditionally silent voices of upcoming disabled African authors. It is also a step toward challenging exclusion and marginalisation, with a view to promoting inclusive development in southern Africa, where diversity is embraced through critical praxis and transformative decolonising revolution.

As indicated in Chapter 1 and earlier in this chapter, a visible gap in this volume is the limited work on early childhood education, which is crucial in preparing children with disabilities for meaningful adulthood, where they can have more access to inclusive and equitable education and, eventually, employment opportunities. Also, the absence of research on people with intellectual impairment, albinism and dyslexia is of great concern, as these categories are among the most marginalised in southern Africa. Thus, these areas and others that might not have been covered in the handbook are recommended for research in order to create critical connections, close gaps and promote inclusive sustainable development in southern Africa and beyond.

In the process of finalising this handbook, the African Union adopted the *Protocol to the African Charter on Human and Peoples' Rights on the Rights of Persons with Disabilities in Africa* (African Union, 2018) in January 2018. The protocol is intended to complement the *African Charter on Human and Peoples' Rights* and address continued exclusion, harmful practices, and discrimination affecting those with disabilities, especially women, children and the elderly. This protocol is the culmination of the African Union's focus on the rights of persons with disabilities, which began in 1999 with the declaration of the African Decade for Persons with Disabilities and the creation of a working group tasked with drafting this new instrument. The protocol lays out the rights of persons with disabilities, drawing from the CRPD but also addressing additional issues specific to Africa (e.g. increased rates of poverty; systemic discrimination; and risk of violence and abuse, particularly for those with albinism and women and girls with disabilities (Modern Ghana, 2018)). It is therefore important to make reference to this ground-breaking protocol when reading this handbook and see how disability rights can be prioritised in our personal spaces and at policy-making levels in southern Africa and the rest of the continent.

Acknowledgements

I would like to thank Edmore Masendeke for drawing key themes emerging from some of the chapters in this handbook that have informed this concluding chapter.

References

African Union (2018). *The Protocol to the African Charter on Human and Peoples' Rights on the Rights of Persons with Disabilities in Africa*. Addis Ababa: African Union.

Becker, R. L. (1988). *Reading-Free Vocational Interest Inventory, Manual*. Columbus, OH: Elbern Publications.

Brown, P. (2018). Foreword. In *British Council, Connecting Classrooms: Inclusive Education Symposium*. Addis Ababa: British Council, p. 3.

Bruijn, P. (2013). *Inclusion works! Lessons learned on the inclusion of people with disabilities in a food security project for ultra-poor women in Bangladesh.* Retrieved from www.licht-fuer-die-welt.at/sites/default/files/inclusionworks.pdf on 15 September 2016.

Bruijn, P., Regeer, B., Cornielje, H., Wolting, R., van Veen, S. & Maharaj, N. (2012). *Count me in: include people with disabilities in development projects: a practical guide for organisations in North and South.* Veenendaal: Light for the World. Retrieved from www.light-for-the-world.org/sites/lfdw_org/files/download_files/count-me-in-include-people-with-disabilities-in-development-projects.pdf on 15 September 2016.

Chataika, T. (2005). *Narrative Research: What's in a Story?* Paper presented at the Nordic Network Disability Research Conference, 14–16 April, Oslo, Norway.

Chataika, T. (2012). Postcolonialism, disability and development. In D. Goodley & B. Hughes (eds) *Social Theories of Disability: New Developments and Directions* (pp. 252–269). London: Routledge.

Chataika, T. (2013). *Gender and Disability Mainstreaming Training Manual: Prepared for Disabled Women in Africa.* Germany: GMZ and GIZ. Retrieved from www.diwa.ws/index.php?option=com_phoca download on 14 November 2017.

Coe, S. & Wapling, L. (2010). Practical lessons from four projects on disability-inclusive development programming. *Development in Practice* **20**(7). Retrieved from www.jstor.org/stable/20787356?seq=1#page_scan_tab_contents on 15 July 2017.

Davies, S. (ed.) (2007). *Team around the Child: Working Together in Early Childhood Education.* Kurrajong: Early Intervention Service.

G3ict (2017). *2016 CRPD ICT Accessibility Progress Report: A global analysis of the progress made by States Parties to the Convention on the Rights of Persons with Disabilities to implement its dispositions on the accessibility of information and communication technologies and assistive technologies.* New York: UN DESA.

Groce, N. E. (2011). *Disability and the Millennium Development Goals: A Review of the MDG Process and Strategies for Inclusion of Disability Issues in Millennium Development Goal Efforts.* New York: United Nations. Retrieved from www.un.org/disabilities/documents/review_of_disability_and_the_mdgs.pdf on 15 August 2016.

Groce, N., Kett, M., Lang, R. & Trani, J.-F. (2011). Disability and poverty: the need for a more nuanced understanding of implications for development policy and practice. *Third World Quarterly* **32**(8), 1493–1513.

Howell, C., McKenzie, J. & Chataika, T. (2018). Building the capacity of teachers for inclusive education in South Africa and Zimbabwe. In Y. Sayed, C. Howell & A. Badroodien (eds) *Continuous Professional Teacher Development in Sub-Saharan Africa: Improving Teaching and Learning* (pp. 127–150). London: Bloomsbury Academic.

King, G., Tucker, M., Desserud, S. & Shillington, M. (2009). The application of a transdisciplinary model for early intervention services. *Infants & Young Children* **22**(3) 211–223.

McKenzie, J. & Chataika, T. (2018). Supporting families in raising disabled children to enhance African Childhood Development. In K. Runswick-Cole, T. Curran & K. Liddiard (eds) *The Palgrave Handbook of Disabled Children's Childhood Studies* (pp. 315–332). Basingstoke: Palgrave Macmillan.

Mitra, S., Posarac, A. & Vick, B. (2013). Disability and poverty in developing countries: a multidimensional study. *World Development* **41**, 1–18.

Modern Ghana (2018). *African governments urged to ratify Africa Disability Protocol.* Retrieved from www.modernghana.com/news/834251/african-governments-urged-to-ratify-africa-disability-protoc.html on 2 February 2018.

Moore, T. G. (2014). *Understanding the nature and significance of early childhood: new evidence and its implications.* Presentation at Centre for Community Child Health seminar on Investing in Early Childhood, 25 July, The Royal Children's Hospital, Melbourne. Retrieved from www.rch.org.au/uploaded Files/Main/Content/ccch/PCI_Tim-Moore_Understanding-naturesignificance-early-childhood.pdf on 14 April 2018.

Riddell, S., Tinklin, T. & Wilson, A. (2005). *Disabled Students in Higher Education: Perspectives on Widening Access and Changing Policy.* New York: Routledge.

Scott, J. C. (1985). *Weapons of the Weak: Everyday Forms of Peasant Resistance.* New Haven, CT: Yale University Press.

Scott, J. C. (1990). *Domination and the Arts of Resistance: Hidden Transcripts.* New Haven, CT: Yale University Press.

Sherry, K. (2015). *Disability and rehabilitation: essential considerations for equitable, accessible and poverty reducing health care in South Africa.* SAHR 2014/15, 89–100. Retrieved from www.rhap.org.za/wp-content/uploads/2015/10/Disability-and-rehabilitation-Essential-considerations-for-equitableaccessible-and-poverty-reducing-health-care-in-South-Africa.pdf on 22 March 2017.

UNESCO (2006). *Strong Foundations: Early Childhood Care and Education*. Paris: UNESCO.

United Nations (2006). *Convention on the Rights of Persons with Disabilities*. Retrieved from www.un.org/development/desa/disabilities/convention-on-the-rights-of-persons-with-disabilities.html on 18 March 2017.

van Veen, S. C. (2014). *Development for All: Understanding Disability Inclusion in Development Organisations*. Hertogenboscg: BOXPress.

Vergunst, R. (2016). *Access to Health Care for Persons with Disabilities in Rural Madwaleni, Eastern Cape, South Africa*. PhD thesis, Dept. of Psychology, University of Stellenbosch. Retrieved from file:///C:/Users/tsitsi.chataika/Downloads/vergunst_access_2016.pdf on 22 March 2017.

Walker, (2004). Knowledge, narrative work and national reconciliation: storied reflections on the South African Truth and Reconciliation Commission. *Discourse* **25**(2), 279–297.

Wapling, L. & Downie, B. (2012). *Beyond Charity: A Donor's Guide to Inclusion – Disability Funding in the Era of the UN Convention on the Rights of Persons with Disabilities*. Boston, MA: Disability Rights Fund.

Watchorn, V., Larkin, H., Hitch, D. & Ang, S. (2014). Promoting participation through the universal design of built environments: making it happen. *Journal of Social Inclusion* **5**(2), 65–88.

Wazakili, M., Chataika, T., Mji, G., Dube, A. K. & MacLachlan, M. (2011). The social inclusion of persons with disabilities in poverty reduction policies and instruments: initial impressions from Malawi and Uganda. In A. H. Eide & B. Ingstad (eds) *Disability and Poverty: A Global Challenge* (pp. 15–29). Bristol: Policy Press.

World Health Organization [WHO] & the World Bank (2011). *World Report on Disability*. Geneva: WHO.

INDEX